Addiction Medicine

An Evidence-Based Handbook

Addiction Medicine

An Evidence-Based Handbook

Darius A. Rastegar, M.D.
Assistant Professor of Medicine
Center for Chemical Dependence
Johns Hopkins Bayview Medical Center
Baltimore, Maryland

Michael I. Fingerhood, M.D.
Associate Professor of Medicine
Center for Chemical Dependence
Johns Hopkins Bayview Medical Center
Baltimore, Maryland

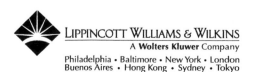

LIPPINCOTT WILLIAMS & WILKINS
A **Wolters Kluwer** Company

Philadelphia • Baltimore • New York • London
Buenos Aires • Hong Kong • Sydney • Tokyo

Acquisitions Editor: Sonya Seigafuse
Developmental Editors: Nancy Winter and Francis Murphy
Marketing Manager: Kathleen Neely
Production Editor: David Murphy
Compositor: Publication Services, Inc.
Printer: R.R. Donnelley

© **2005 by LIPPINCOTT WILLIAMS & WILKINS**
530 Walnut Street
Philadelphia, PA 19106 USA
LWW.com

Printed in the USA

Library of Congress Cataloging-in-Publication Data
Rastegar, Darius A., 1962-
Addiction medicine : an evidence-based handbook / Darius A.
Rastegar, Michael I. Fingerhood.
    p. ; cm.
    Includes bibliographical references and index.
    ISBN-13: 978-0-7817-6154-3 / ISBN-10: 0-7817-6154-9 (alk. paper)
1. Substance abuse—Treatment. 2. Compulsive behavior—Treatment.
3. Evidence-based medicine.
    [DNLM: 1. Substance-Related Disorders. 2. Behavior, Addictive.
3. Evidence-Based Medicine. WM 270 R229a 2005] I. Fingerhood,
Michael I., 1960- II. Title.
RC564.R36 2005
616.86—dc22
                        2005026799

10 9 8 7 6 5 4 3

Preface

Our goal with this handbook is to provide a practical, evidence-based resource for the non–addiction specialist. We also hope that this handbook will be a useful resource for those who are more experienced in caring for individuals with substance use disorders. Addiction is a common medical problem and one of the leading causes of preventable morbidity and mortality world-wide. We hope that this book will help practitioners feel more comfortable with—and be more competent in—evaluating and treating their patients with substance use disorders.

Over the years, a number of our colleagues have encouraged us to develop a handbook that makes addiction more accessible to others. As primary care physicians who are also involved in addiction treatment, we have incorporated addiction treatment into our own primary care practice, and this has provided us with a unique perspective on this problem. We believe that this experience has helped us to present this issue in a manner that "makes sense" for other practitioners. We have found that treating addicts is challenging but, at the same time, gratifying and that these patients are generally appreciative of practitioners who show interest in their problems and treat them with respect. We have also been involved in teaching house staff about addiction and found that trainees' attitudes toward and comfort with treating addicts can improve with experience and positive role modeling.

At the beginning of this project, we decided to make our handbook "evidence-based"; by this we mean that the information we present is based on primary data, whenever possible. We began this project with an extensive review of the literature in each of the topic areas we covered. Furthermore, we have done our best to explicitly present our sources and to critically evaluate them. It is for this reason that we have provided numerous references and have included additional details in the form of annotation for many of them.

We would like to acknowledge the help and support of our colleagues who encouraged us to undertake this project and reviewed earlier drafts of this book. This book would not have been possible without the inspiration of our mentor, Donald R. Jasinski, who introduced us to the field of addiction treatment. Finally, the support of our families was essential, as always.

CONTENTS

1

Introduction

Overview of Addiction   *1*
Addiction is a common medical problem and an important cause of preventable morbidity and mortality.
Legal Issues   *4*
The use of many psychoactive substances is limited and regulated by a variety of laws.
A Note on Terminology   *5*
There is a confusing and overlapping array of terms used to describe substance use disorders. The DSM-IV recognizes two general categories: "substance abuse" and "substance dependence."
References   *5*

OVERVIEW OF ADDICTION

The use and misuse of a variety of psychoactive substances is very common. In fact, if one includes caffeine, it is an almost universal experience. Table 1.1 provides data from the United States' 2003 National Survey of Drug Use and Health (NSDUH) (5). This

Table 1.1.   Substance use and dependence among Americans aged 12 and older: 2003 estimates

Substance	Lifetime Use	Recent Use (past month)	Dependence (past year)
Tobacco	172,843 (72.7)	70,757 (29.8)	35,700 (15.0)
Alcohol	197,533 (83.1)	118,965 (50.1)	7,563 (3.2)
Tranquilizers (1)	20,220 (8.5)	1,830 (0.8)	196 (0.1)
Sedatives (2)	9,510 (4.0)	294 (0.1)	112 (0.0)
Marijuana	96,611 (46.4)	14,638 (8.2)	2,520 (1.1)
Hallucinogens	34,363 (14.5)	1,042 (0.4)	135 (0.1)
Opioids			
Heroin	3,744 (1.6)	119 (0.1)	169 (0.1)
Prescription pain relievers (nonmedical)	31,207 (13.3)	4,693 (2.0)	943 (0.4)
Stimulants			
Cocaine	34,891 (14.7)	2,281 (1.0)	961 (0.4)
Methamphetamine and others (nonmedical)	20,798 (8.8)	1,191 (1.0)	112 (0.1)
Inhalants	22,995 (9.7)	570 (0.2)	37 (0.0)

Numbers are in thousands, percentages in parentheses.
(1) Includes benzodiazepines, muscle relaxants, prescription antihistamines.
(2) Includes barbiturates, temazepam, chloral hydrate.
Source: 2003 National Survey on Drug Use & Health (NSDUH).

Table 1.2.   Selected scheduled drugs*

Schedule	Opioids	Sedatives	Stimulants	Hallucinogens & Others
Schedule I (High potential for abuse, no currently accepted therapeutic use)	Diacetylmorphine (heroin)	Gamma hydroxybutyric acid (GHB), methaqualone	Cathinone (Khat), methcathinone (Cat)	MDMA (Ecstasy), lysergic acid diethylamide (LSD), marijuana, mescaline, psilocin
Schedule II (High potential for abuse, but does have accepted therapeutic use)	Codeine, fentanyl, hydromorphone, meperidine, methadone, morphine, oxycodone	Pentobarbital (Nembutal), secobarbital (Seconal)	Amphetamines (Dexedrine, methamphetamine), cocaine	Phencyclidine (PCP)
Schedule III (Moderate abuse potential)	Buprenorphine, codeine and hydrocodone combination products (Tylenol with codeine, Vicodin, Lortab)	Butalbital (Fiorinal, Fioricet)		Anabolic steroids, dronabinol, ketamine

Schedule IV (Low abuse potential)	Butorphenol (Stadol), propoxyphene (Darvon)	Phenobarbital, benzodiazepines, chloral hydrate, dichloralphenazone, eszopiclone, zaleplon, zolpidem	Modafinil (Provigil), phentermine
Schedule V (Lowest potential for abuse)	Codeine preparations—100 mg/100 ml (cough syrups), diphenoxylate (Lomotil), Opium preparations—100 mg/100 ml		

*Not all substances are listed; selected brand or street names appear in parentheses.
Source: U.S. Drug Enforcement Administration (www.usdoj.gov/dea).

is a survey of households, so it does not include homeless or institutionalized adults and likely underestimates the true prevalence of these problems. A brief review of the data shows that—by far—tobacco dependence is the most common problem. After tobacco, alcohol is the most common substance of dependence in the United States. Illicit drugs, including marijuana, opioids, stimulants, and a variety of other agents, are less common but important nonetheless. Substance misuse is also responsible for a tremendous amount of preventable morbidity and mortality; smoking alone is believed to be responsible for millions of premature deaths worldwide each year.

While addiction treatment has traditionally been viewed as the province of specialists (generally psychiatrists), primary care providers and other practitioners are on the front line of dealing with this problem. It is clear that many practitioners do not feel comfortable in addressing this issue (1) and that this problem goes unrecognized for many patients (2). This is largely due to lack of education, experience, and role models during training (3). This is exacerbated by the fact that addicts are an ostracized group and addiction treatment is often looked down upon by health care professionals. One reason for this is that addiction is often seen as a "behavioral" problem, one that would go away if addicts simply changed their behavior. However, it is more accurate to look at addiction as a chronic illness that has an important behavioral component, as well as genetic and environmental factors (4). The same can be said for many illnesses that are in the mainstream of medicine. For example, type 2 diabetes mellitus is a common illness that is largely a consequence of an individual's behavior and choices (diet, exercise, etc.), as well as genetic and environmental factors. Addiction, like type 2 diabetes, cannot be "cured," but there are effective treatments.

LEGAL ISSUES

Addiction intersects with the law in a number of ways. The most obvious is that the use of many substances is illegal. In the United States, the Harrison Narcotics Tax Act of 1914 was the first federal law that regulated psychoactive substances (opium and coca); it allowed a physician to prescribe narcotics "in the course of his professional practice only." What constituted proper "professional practice" was, of course, subject to interpretation. The use of alcohol was banned during Prohibition in the United States from 1920 to 1933. In 1970, the Controlled Substances Act consolidated a number of laws regulating the manufacture and distribution of a variety of legal and illegal psychoactive substances; the Drug Enforcement Agency (DEA) was created in 1973 to enforce this law.

The Controlled Substances Act divides psychoactive substances into five "schedules"; Table 1.2 provides the schedule classification of selected agents. Schedule I includes those substances that are considered to be of high abuse potential and have no accepted therapeutic use. The remainder have acceptable therapeutic use but also a potential for abuse, which declines from schedule II to schedule V. It should be noted that this is a *legal* classification, not medical, and that the two most important substances of abuse, tobacco and alcohol, are not included in this schedule. The proper prescribing of controlled substances is covered further in Chapter 14.

A NOTE ON TERMINOLOGY

The field of addiction is hampered by confusing and overlapping terminology: "drug abuse," "substance abuse/dependence," and "chemical dependence" are a few examples. This is further complicated by the fact that alcohol use disorders have their own parallel terminology: "alcoholism," "problem drinking," "hazardous drinking," "harmful drinking," and so on. Moreover, nicotine dependence (in the form of cigarette use) is generally referred to as "smoking" in the literature.

The DSM-IV recognizes two broad categories: "substance abuse" and "substance dependence" (6). Appendixes A and B provide the diagnostic criteria for each. In simplistic terms, "substance dependence" refers to a pattern of compulsive and persistent use of a substance despite significant physical, psychological, or social harm. While the development of "physical dependence"—tolerance to its effects and withdrawal symptoms with cessation—supports a diagnosis of "substance dependence," it is neither necessary nor sufficient to establish this diagnosis. For example, anyone who takes opioids chronically for pain will develop "physical dependence" but will not necessarily be "substance dependent" by DSM criteria. "Substance abuse," on the other hand, can be understood as a condition where an individual uses a substance in a manner that is harmful or dangerous to his or her health but does not meet the criteria for "substance dependence."

The term "addiction" has been largely replaced with "substance dependence," though some have argued that "addiction" should be resurrected as the preferred term, partly because "substance dependence" is easily confused with "physical dependence" on a substance (7). Furthermore, "addiction" is still used widely by the general public and many professional organizations. On the other hand, the term "addiction" is increasingly used to refer to other compulsive and harmful behaviors, such as gambling.

One could argue that "substance use disorders" would technically be a better description of the problems that we address in this handbook. We have chosen to favor "addiction" as a simple and straightforward term. We also, for the sake of brevity, sometimes refer to persons with this problem as "addicts" or "alcoholics" or "smokers"; this may seem derogatory to some, but it is analogous to referring to someone with diabetes as a "diabetic" and is often preferable to "substance-dependent person" or analogous terms.

REFERENCES

1. Miller, N. S., L. M. Sheppard, C. C. Colenda, and J. Magen. 2001. Why physicians are unprepared to treat patients who have alcohol- and drug-related disorders. *Acad. Med.* 76:410–418.
2. Coulehan, J. L., M. Zettler-Segal, M. Block, et al. 1987. Recognition of alcoholism and substance abuse in primary care patients. *Arch. Intern. Med.* 147:349–352.
3. Isaacson, J. H., M. Fleming, M. Kraus, et al. 2000. A national survey of training in substance use disorders in residency programs. *J. Stud. Alcohol.* 61:912–915.

4. McLellan, A. T., D. C. Lewis, C. P. O'Brien, and H. D. Kleber. 2000. Drug dependence, a chronic medical illness: Implications for treatment, insurance, and outcomes evaluation. *JAMA* 284:1689–1695.
5. Substance Abuse and Mental Health Services Administration. 2004. Results from the 2003 National Survey on Drug Use and Health: National Findings (Office of Applied Studies, NSDUH Series H-25, DHHS Publication No. SMA 04-3964). Rockville, MD.
6. American Psychiatric Association. 2000. *Diagnostic and statistical manual of mental disorders.* 4th ed. (text revision). Washington, DC: American Psychiatric Association.
7. Maddux, J. F., and D. P. Desmond. 2000. Addiction or dependence? *Addiction* 95:661–665.

2

Addiction from a Clinical Perspective

ADDICTION AND PRIMARY CARE

More than two-thirds of individuals with addiction see a primary care provider within a 6-month time frame (1). Thus, primary care providers have the opportunity to recognize, diagnose, and help most individuals with addiction. Unfortunately, many providers avoid issues related to addiction and often do not recognize this problem in their patients (2). This may be because they find it easier not to address addiction, they do not feel comfortable discussing the topic, they do not know how to help, or they have a perception that little can be done. However, the primary care setting offers a safe place for patients and providers to explore addiction problems, build rapport, develop treatment plans, and work together toward long-term abstinence. Moreover, studies suggest that addicts benefit from having a regular source of medical care (3) and from integration of addiction treatment with their primary medical care (4).

THE PHYSIOLOGY OF ADDICTION

Addiction is a chronic disorder in which individuals compulsively use drugs despite serious negative consequences (5). Drugs of addiction induce euphoria or relieve distress. Rapid onset and high intensity of drug effect increase abuse potential of drugs. Continued drug use causes changes in the central nervous system that lead to tolerance, dependence, and craving. Use is typically driven by craving for the pleasurable response initially but is often replaced by fear of—or aversion to—the withdrawal symptoms that arise with abstinence.

Addictive drugs act on the mesocorticolimbic dopamine systems, stimulating the release of dopamine into the nucleus accumbens, causing euphoria (6, 7). During drug withdrawal, there is a substantial decrease in dopamine levels in the nucleus accumbens (8). Addictive drugs can cause brain alterations that persist even after long periods of abstinence. These changes contribute to "priming" or "kindling"—the concept that reexposure to a formerly abused substance precipitates very rapid resumption of drug use at high levels. After only a few days, an individual who relapses to alcohol use can quickly drink large amounts of alcohol and when attempting to stop may have severe withdrawal.

The basis by which addiction develops in an individual is complex, and several models have been proposed to explain the origins or causes of addiction (9, 10). These models, although distinct, are not mutually exclusive, and most people fit into more than one model, illustrating the complexity of their disease. Theories about addiction have arisen from neurobiological evidence and studies of learned behavior.

Drugs that cause addiction have acute psychoactive effects that become reinforcing (Table 2.1). Eventually, environmental cues, even in the absence of the drug, cause a conditioned re-

Table 2.1. Categories of psychoactive drugs

CNS Depressants

Alcohol, benzodiazepines, barbiturates, meprobromate (Equanil or Miltown), carisprodol (Soma), gamma hydroxybutyrate (GHB)

Inhalants

Volatile organic compounds, volatile anesthetics, nitrites

Opioids

Morphine, hydromorphone (Dilaudid), heroin, oxycodone, meperidine (Demerol), codeine, methadone, fentanyl

Stimulants

Cocaine, amphetamines, methylphenidate (Ritalin), MDMA (Ecstasy), caffeine, nicotine, arecoline, phenmetrazine (Preludin)

Hallucinogens

Marijuana, LSD, mescaline, PCP, MDMA, belladonna alkaloids (atropine, scopolamine)

sponse—craving. Craving may overwhelm decision making and the ability to perceive the negative consequences of continued drug use. Personality traits and mental disorders are factors in drug addiction. Individuals with addiction tend to be risk takers and less concerned about the potential for negative impact from drug use (11). Addiction is often seen in individuals with psychiatric disorders ("dual diagnosis"), including bipolar disorder, schizophrenia, and attention deficit disorder, but no clear evidence shows a causal relationship (see Chapter 16).

DISEASE MODEL

Central to the disease model is the belief that an individual has a neurobiological susceptibility to drugs of abuse. The model applies only to individuals who meet the definitions of substance abuse or dependence and does not apply to those with social or experimental use of drugs. The disease model was originally proposed to counter adverse societal attitudes and judgmental views toward alcohol and drug abuse.

The disease model for addiction has generally been supported by self-help groups such as Alcoholics Anonymous and Narcotics Anonymous. The disease concept improves the public image of individuals with addiction and has likely increased public health resources for treatment and research in addiction.

Genetic factors contributing to addiction have been best studied for alcohol. Children of alcoholic parents adopted at birth by non-alcoholic parents have shown increased likelihood of alcoholism (12). Specific genes have been associated with alcohol dependence (13–16). A polymorphism of the gene for the mu opioid receptor has been associated with an increased risk of heroin abuse (17). Additional studies have found that changes in genes contribute to nicotine dependence (18) and drug dependence in general (19–21).

Independent of genetic factors, predisposition to addiction is still not well understood. For example, opiates produce predominantly euphoric effects in addicts, while producing mostly sedative effects in nonaddicts (22). Recent research has also examined the potential role of corticotropin-releasing factor (CRF) in mediating the effects of drugs of abuse (23). Brain CRF appears involved in relapse induced by environmental stressors, while hypothalamic CRF is involved in the reinforcing effects of alcohol and cocaine.

Although neurobiological models of addiction have explained craving and development of dependence, it is still often difficult to understand how individuals continue to use despite severe negative consequences. It is postulated that the frontal cortex of the brain, critical in inhibitory control over reward-related behavior, is dysfunctional in individuals with drug addiction (24–26). More studies of this hypothesis are needed.

Health care providers can use the disease model to take away blame from patients with addiction who commonly have low self-esteem, despair, and guilt. However, this must be balanced with the need to have patients take control of their lives and accept responsibility for treatment (27). There must be a message that genetics is not destiny and that change can happen, but this requires a carefully agreed-upon plan, often using multiple modalities of treatment. Some psychologists have viewed the effectiveness of self-help groups for treating addiction as evidence against the disease model. However, there are many other diseases in which nonpharmacologic therapies are effective.

MORAL FAILURE MODEL

This view attributes substance abuse to a failure by parents or parental surrogates (e.g., religious training, schools, movies, television, and music) to inculcate values. As a result, there is an absence of an ongoing morality that would prevent the use and abuse of drugs. From a public health viewpoint, this model is useful. However, when applied to an individual already dependent on drugs, this model is generally not useful, though a religious conversion experience or complete acceptance of the 12-step philosophy may motivate recovery.

PSYCHOSOCIAL MODEL

The psychosocial model sees addiction as the inadvertent effect of repeated self-medication by a vulnerable individual who is trying to relieve overwhelming anxiety or psychic pain resulting from hopelessness, boredom, depression, and fear. Drugs of abuse are potent and effective short-term alleviators of these symptoms. Vulnerability in this model is not a function of genetic predisposition, although this may enhance susceptibility. Addiction occurs because of youthful immaturity, socioeconomic disability, and the lack of responsible familial or peer support systems. Individuals have not developed the same array of behaviors that the greater part of society uses to cope with adversity. This model has the virtue of defining an at-risk population from among the young, the uneducated, and the socioeconomically disadvantaged that stereotypically describes many of those with addiction. The model also explains the potential for addiction in people who, although they may be socially and economically advantaged, may turn to self-medication with drugs of abuse in the face of losses, situational anxiety, demoralization, or physical pain. The psychosocial model avoids a simplistic expectation of cure by mere detoxification or by enforced abstinence if release back into the same environment occurs without change in the conditions of vulnerability. The model also relies on the use of support systems and self-help as a requirement of remission.

STAGES OF ADDICTION/RECOVERY

In a model described by Prochaska and DiClemente, individuals with addiction flow through stages as they attempt to achieve abstinence (Figure 2.1) (28). *Precontemplation* is the stage in which there is no plan for change and individuals lack insight into the problems arising from their addiction. Patients in precontemplation are reluctant to consider addressing their problem. It is fruitless for medical providers to try to initiate change in someone who is precontemplative. Instead, the goal should be to facilitate patient movement from precontemplation to contemplation.

Contemplation is the stage entered by an individual when family members, friends, coworkers, and health providers have

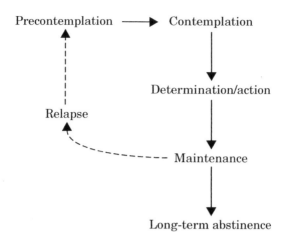

Figure 2.1.   Stages of change in addiction. Adapted from Prochaska, J. O., C. C. DiClemente, and J. C. Norcross. 1992. In search of how people change. Applications to addictive behaviors. *Am. Psychol.* **47:1102–1114.**

helped convince the individual that a problem exists. It is a stage that people often stay in for long periods of time. During this stage, patients are weighing the pros and cons (benefits and risks) of continued use of drugs.

This is followed by *preparation* or *determination* in which individuals have come to the conclusion that they want to change and are willing to set a plan. Some small behavioral changes may occur during this stage; for example, a smoker may decrease his smoking from two packs to one pack a day. However, the full step to attempted abstinence has not yet occurred.

Action is the stage in which individuals have taken the formal step to make a change. This may include changing environment, acquaintances, and activities, as well as ceasing use of a drug. This stage is generally regarded as lasting from 1 day up to 6 months. During this time, patients continue to attempt to strengthen strategies that have been helpful and define and overcome obstacles that make them vulnerable to relapse.

After the action stage, successful individuals enter the *maintenance* stage. During this stage, patients actively pursue continued abstinence. Continued efforts to stabilize people (family, friends, and acquaintances) and life circumstances (work and free time) are aimed at avoiding relapse. Optimally, the maintenance stage should not be viewed as static but rather as a continued stage of action.

When this model of change was first introduced, it contained only four stages. However, most individuals with addiction do not successfully maintain abstinence on their initial attempt. For example, most smokers attempt to stop three or four times before they are successful. *Relapse* is therefore an expected stage for most individuals with addiction, with the hope that with time, the amount of time spent in relapse gets shorter and periods of abstinence grow longer.

DEALING WITH RELAPSE

The relapse process generally begins long before the person actually uses the drug again (29). An analysis of 48 episodes of relapse revealed that most relapses were associated with three high-risk situations: (1) frustration and anger, (2) social pressure, and (3) interpersonal temptation (30). The relapse process often progresses in the following sequence: reactivation of denial, progressive isolation and defensiveness, building a crisis to justify symptom progression, immobilization, confusion and overreaction, depression, loss of control over behavior, recognition of loss of control, and finally relapse to drug use.

Although it should not be telegraphed to the patient, relapse is part of the natural history of successful recovery for most individuals with addiction. For example, in one cohort study, 90% of alcoholics had at least one relapse during a 4-year follow-up period (31). One should not become discouraged when relapse happens; instead, the patient should be immediately recruited back into treatment using the same motivational techniques employed initially. Relapse is a time for both patient and provider to learn from mistakes and to correct them by strengthening treatment.

REFERENCES

1. American Society of Addiction Medicine. Public policy statement on screening for addiction in primary care settings. Available at http://www.asam.org/ppol/screen.htm
2. Coulehan, J. L., M. Zettler-Segal, M. Block, et al. 1987. Recognition of alcoholism and substance abuse in primary care patients. *Arch. Intern. Med.* 147:349–352.
3. Laine, C., W. W. Hauck, M. N. Gourevitch, et al. 2001. Regular outpatient medical and drug abuse care and subsequent hospitalization of persons who use illicit drugs. *JAMA* 285:2355–2362. *Among Medicaid recipients in New York who were drug users, the adjusted odds of hospitalization was about 20–30% lower among those with regular medical care or drug abuse care (or both).*
4. Weisner, C., J. Mertens, S. Parthasarathy, et al. 2001. Integrating primary medical care with addiction treatment: A randomized controlled trial. *JAMA* 286:1715–1723. *Six hundred fifty-four adults with substance abuse or dependence were randomized to integrated or independent medical and addiction care; 592 (91%) completed 6-month follow-up and were included in the analyses. Overall, both groups had comparable improvements in addiction outcomes. Among those with substance abuse–related medical conditions, integrated care was associated with improved odds of achieving abstinence.*
5. Robinson, T. E., and K. C. Berridge. 2003. Addiction. *Ann. Rev. Psychol.* 54:25–53.
6. Cami, J., and M. Farre. 2003. Drug addiction. *N. Engl. J. Med.* 349:975–986.

7. Hyman, S. E., and R. C. Malenka. 2001. Addiction and the brain: The neurobiology of compulsion and its persistence. *Nat. Rev. Neurosci.* 2:695–703.

8. Nestler, E. J. 2001. Molecular basis of long-term plasticity underlying addiction. *Nat. Rev. Neurosci.* 2:119–128.

9. Koob, G. F., and M. Le Moal. 1997. Drug abuse: Hedonic homeostatic dysregulation. *Science* 278:52–58.

10. Everitt, B. J., A. Dickinson, and T. W. Robbins. 2001. The neuropsychological basis of addictive behaviour. *Brain Research* 36:129–138.

11. Conway, K. P., R. J. Kane, S. A. Ball, et al. 2003. Personality, substance of choice, and polysubstance involvement among substance dependent patients. *Drug Alcohol Depend.* 71:65–75.

12. Crabbe, J. C. 2002. Genetic contributions to addiction. *Annu. Rev. Psychol.* 53:435–462.

13. Blum, K., E. P. Noble, P. J. Sheridan, et al. 1990. Allelic association of human dopamine D2 receptor gene in alcoholism. *JAMA* 263:2055–2060. *In an analysis of 70 brain samples of alcoholics and non-alcoholics, the presence of A1 allele of the dopamine D2 receptor gene correctly classified 77% of alcoholics, and its absence 72% of non alcoholics.*

14. Lappalainen, J., H. R. Kranzler, R. Malison, et al. 2002. A functional neuropeptide Y Leu7Pro polymorphism associated with alcohol dependence in a large population sample from the United States. *Arch. Gen. Psychiatry* 59:825–831.

15. Nestler, E. J., and G. K. Aghajanian. 1997. Molecular and cellular basis of addiction. *Science* 278:58–63.

16. Schuckit, M. A., H. J. Edenberg, J. Kalmijn, et al. 2001. A genome-wide search for genes that relate to a low level of response to alcohol. *Alcohol Clin. Exp. Res.* 25:323–329.

17. Kreek, M. J. 2001. Drug addictions: Molecular and cellular endpoints. *Ann. NY Acad. Sci.* 937:27–49.

18. Rao, Y., E. Hoffmann, M. Zia, et al. 2000. Duplications and defects in the CYP2A6 gene: Identification, genotyping, and in vivo effects on smoking. *Mol. Pharmacol.* 58:747–755.

19. Noble, E. P. 2003. D2 dopamine receptor gene in psychiatric and neurologic disorders and its phenotypes. *Am. J. Med. Genet.* 116:103–125.

20. Sipe, J. C., K. Chiang, A. L. Gerber, et al. 2002. A missense mutation in human fatty acid amide hydrolase associated with problem drug use. *Proc. Natl. Acad. Sci. USA* 99:8394–8399.

21. Uhl, G. R., Q. R. Liu, and D. Naiman. 2002. Substance abuse vulnerability loci: Converging genome scanning data. *Trends Genet.* 18:420–425.

22. Smith, G. M., and H. K. Beecher. 1962. Subjective effects of heroin and morphine in normal subjects. *J. Pharmacol. Exp. Ther.* 136:47–52.

23. Sarnyai, Z., Y. Shaham, and S. C. Heinrichs. 2001. The role of corticotropin-releasing factor in drug addiction. *Pharmacol. Rev.* 53:209–243.

24. Lubman, D. I., M. Yucel, and C. Pantelis. 2004. Addiction, a condition of compulsive behavior? Neuroimaging and neuropsychological evidence of inhibitory dysregulation. *Addiction* 99:1491–1502.

25. Franklin, T. R., P. D. Acton, J. A. Maldjian, et al. 2002. Decreased gray matter concentration in the insular, or-

bitofrontal, cingulate, and temporal cortices of cocaine patients. *Biol. Psychiatry* 51:134–142.

26. Goldstein, R. Z., and N. D. Volkow. 2002. Drug addiction and its underlying neurobiological basis: Neuroimaging evidence for the involvement of the frontal cortex. *Am. J. Psychiatry* 159:1642–1652.

27. Ford, G. G. 1996. An existential model for promoting life change. *J. Subst. Abuse Treat.* 13:151–158.

28. Prochaska, J. O., C. C. DiClemente, and J. C. Norcross. 1992. In search of how people change. Applications to addictive behaviors. *Am. Psychol.* 47:1102–1114.

29. Bradley, B. P., G. Phillips, L. Green, and M. Gossop. 1989. Circumstances surrounding the initial lapse to opiate use following detoxification. *Br. J. Psychiatry* 154:354–359.

30. Marlatt, G. A. 1978. Craving for alcohol, loss of control, and relapse: A cognitive-behavioral analysis. In *Alcoholism: New directions in behavioral research and treatment.* Edited by P. E. Nathan, G. A. Marlatt, and T. Loberg, 271–314. New York: Plenum Press.

31. Polich, J. M., D. J. Armor, and H. B. Braiker. 1981. Stability and change in drinking patterns. In *The course of alcoholism: Four years after treatment.* 159–200. New York: John Wiley & Sons.

3

The Medical Encounter: Screening, Confronting, and Motivating

BACKGROUND

Recognition of a substance abuse problem begins with screening for this problem, followed by consideration of the diagnosis based on history, symptoms, and physical exam findings. In some circumstances, recognition occurs because of a positive drug screen obtained through the workplace or legal setting. Although the stereotype of the drug abuser is of a young, unemployed, antisocial male who uses drugs to get high, the abuse of drugs also occurs commonly among middle- and upper-class Americans. Even highly educated and successful people are not immune to this problem. Moreover, the abuse of prescription opiates by people who are in the mainstream of American society has escalated over the past decade. Patients with chronic anxiety, insomnia, or pain are at risk of abusing medications used to treat those conditions.

For the patient with substance abuse, the role of the primary care provider is to (1) recognize the problem, (2) facilitate the patient's acceptance of the problem, (3) motivate the patient to accept treatment, (4) create a treatment plan, (5) provide ongoing care for the patient's medical problems, and (6) motivate the patient to remain in recovery. All these steps depend on skillful medical interviewing that builds rapport and trust between the provider and patient.

SCREENING FOR ADDICTION

When taking a substance abuse history, details related to substance use should be determined in the context of general medical history using a nonjudgmental approach. Questions should be direct, and qualified answers and rationalizations should be challenged. The style of questioning should be persistent, but empathic and friendly. With the patient's consent, it may be helpful to obtain information from a family member or close friend. Screening tools for alcohol are reviewed in Chapter 5 and screening for drug use in adolescents is discussed in Chapter 17.

DRUG TESTING

Urine testing can detect the presence of most substances of abuse. Although urine testing seems like an easy and objective way of "catching" someone in denial, urine testing for illicit drug abuse can prove problematic. Obviously, patients already know they are using the substances that are detected. Furthermore, finding a positive drug screen may not necessarily help a provider understand whether the patient truly has a problem related to substance use. If they do, it does not help motivate them to get the help they need. In fact, a drug test done without a patient's willing consent will likely foster mistrust in health care providers and encourage further efforts to hide the substance use. Urine testing should be done with the informed voluntary consent of any person 18 years of age or older, except in true emergencies, and should not be performed in the primary care setting without the patient's knowledge (1). Consequently, laboratory testing yields no more information than the patient is willing to provide by history. Testing at the request of an employer or school authority produces difficult ethical questions regarding patient autonomy and preserving the patient–provider relationship. Nevertheless, many employers now require drug testing, which may provide evidence of illicit drug use that the patient is not willing to share.

The most commonly used test method for screening urine for drugs of abuse is immunoassay. A number of single-use devices incorporating immunoassays and designed to be used outside of the traditional laboratory are also available; many nonmedical environments such as workplaces and halfway houses use these devices. In addition to urine drug testing, saliva, hair, or nail clippings may be used for drug screening. Saliva can reveal drug use earlier than urine can, while hair and nail analyses provide information about more distant substance use. In addition, breath testing is used to detect volatile substances such as alcohol, which are not reliably detected in urine.

All positive urine-screening tests for drugs should be confirmed, especially if severe consequences can result from the positive test. The accepted confirmatory test for all drugs is gas chromatography–mass spectrometry (GC-MS). GC-MS can identify the specific substance ingested by recognizing not only the molecular structure

Table 3.1.   Maximal detection times for urine drug testing

Drug	Maximal Detection Time (days)
Amphetamines	3
Benzodiazepines	7 (duration is generally related to half-life of specific benzodiazepine)
Cannabis	30 (heavy use) 7 (light use)
Cocaine	22 (heavy use) 3 (light use)
Heroin	3
LSD	4
PCP	14

of the original compound but also its pattern of metabolites. In this confirmatory test, the drugs in the urine sample are isolated on a small chromatographic column, eluted with an organic solvent, and injected into the gas chromatograph–mass spectrometer. The gas chromatograph separates the substances present, and then each substance is broken into molecular fragments by the mass spectrometer. Substances are identified by comparison with known fragmentation patterns. Detection times for drugs of abuse are shown in Table 3.1.

There are problems of sensitivity and specificity in using urine drug-screening tests to identify drug abusers. False-negative results occur because of deception in collection and insensitive testing. False-positive results occur because of errors in processing samples and testing error. They are less likely with the GC-MS test method. Additionally, some foods (poppy seeds) and prescribed medications may give false-positive results (see Table 3.2), and some opioids (e.g., oxycodone) in small amounts may not be detected by urine

Table 3.2.   Medications that may give false-positive results on drug screen*

False-Positive Result	Drugs
Opiates	Quinolone antibiotics, rifampin, quinine in tonic water, poppy seeds
Marijuana	Efavirenz (Sustiva), nonsteroidal anti-inflammatory drugs, dronabinol (Marinol)
Phencyclidine (PCP)	Dextromethorphan
Benzodiazepines	Sertraline (Zoloft)
Amphetamines	Bupropion (Wellbutrin), selegiline (Eldepryl), over-the-counter decongestants, trazodone, chlorpromazine, desipramine, ranitidine (Zantac), amantadine

* Some false positives are less likely with advanced testing methods.

drug screen. Recreational use of illicit substances is common (especially marijuana), so a positive test does not establish a diagnosis of abuse or dependence. It also does not necessarily provide evidence of intoxication or impairment. Parents and legal guardians can authorize drug testing of patients under the age of 18. However, such testing raises issues of patient rapport and trust.

In most instances, urine drug testing should be performed only within a treatment program. Avoiding urine testing in the primary care setting helps foster trust in the doctor–patient relationship. Patients who relapse will be more likely to be honest and show up for medical visits if they do not have to worry about urine testing.

MOTIVATIONAL INTERVIEWING

Brief intervention is a motivational process of assessing drug or alcohol use, giving feedback, setting goals, arriving at a strategy for change, and providing a plan for follow-up. The process was developed and validated in individuals with alcoholism, but it can be applied to all individuals with substance abuse (2). In many of the published clinical trials, someone other than the individual's primary care provider performed the brief intervention. When a primary provider who has a relationship and rapport with the patient delivers brief intervention, it may be even more effective. On the other hand, most primary care providers have not received specific training in this intervention.

Implicit in the motivational process is an emphasis on clear advice to change and acceptance on the part of the patient for responsibility to change. Therapeutic empathy describes the recommended counseling style. The goal of brief intervention may not be abstinence but rather reducing use in a nondependent drug user. Brief intervention procedures used in studies vary, but most involve one to six counseling sessions. Typical follow-up sessions are usually 15 minutes long. Even a single brief 5- to 10-minute intervention may have an impact (3).

Brief interventions have been found to be effective in reducing alcohol consumption (or achieving treatment referral) in problem drinkers in the primary care setting (4, 5, 6, 7, 8). Clinical trials have also examined the utility of brief intervention for alcohol use in pregnant women (9), for alcohol-abusing patients in an emergency department (10), for alcohol use in participants in a needle exchange program (11), and for alcohol and drug use in adolescents (12, 13). Even a single brief intervention in the primary care setting can help patients achieve abstinence from heroin and cocaine (14). Randomized clinical trials of the cost benefit of brief provider intervention for problem drinking have shown benefit at 12 months (15) and 48 months (16). Follow-up of brief intervention in at-risk alcohol drinkers has shown the effect to be long lasting with continued impact on alcohol intake at 9 years (17).

Patients appropriate for motivational interviewing are those who are ambivalent about making a change. Despite some understanding of the benefits of change, a patient may "enjoy" alcohol or drug effects and be fearful of increased anxiety from stopping use of drugs such as sedatives or alcohol; motivational interviewing should specifically address such issues. The six steps of motivational interviewing are shown in Figure 3.1; these

1. Feedback of personal risk (patient-focused review of the specific evidence for problems related to drug use)
2. Emphasis on personal Responsibility for change (empowering the patient to take control of the decision for change—"This is not your fault, but you must take responsibility for making things better")
3. Clear Advice for change ("Based on all we have discussed, you need to make a change")
4. Offering a Menu of alternative options ("Here are some ways you can make a change")
5. Therapeutic Empathy as an innate part of the intervention ("I know this may be difficult")
6. Enhancement of patient Self-efficacy ("This is not hopeless; with change, things will get better for you")

Figure 3.1.   The Six components of motivational interviewing—FRAMES.

can be remembered by the acronym FRAMES (feedback, responsibility, advice, menu, empathy, and self-efficacy).

DEALING WITH DENIAL

Denial, the direct or implied message that there is no problem, is present in most actively drinking alcoholics. It is less common in individuals abusing other drugs, as they may lack insight but usually recognize they have a problem. Denial is the major obstacle to a patient accepting treatment. Denial is complex and may be caused by (1) conscious lying, (2) an attempt to avoid shame, (3) an inability to overcome the problem, (4) euphoric recall of remembering only the good times experienced when drinking or using drugs, (5) the fact that no one points out problems related to substance abuse, or (6) toxic effects of drugs on information processing and memory. Denial presents as rationalizations ("I get high because it is the only way I can relax"), glibness ("I drink less than all my friends, are they alcoholics too?"), hostility ("I came to you about my stomach pain and I would appreciate it if you could stay out of my personal life"), comparison of oneself with a "real problem drinker" ("I have a family, a job that I enjoy. . . I have nothing in common with those people who have lost everything. . . those are your alcoholics"), reticence to discuss drinking or substance abuse, and the assertions that friends and family members do not perceive a problem. These responses are a source of frustration for providers during screening/diagnostic interviewing and during efforts to get the patient to accept the diagnosis and agree to treatment.

Three motivational techniques are fundamental for breaking down denial in patients and, if necessary, in their family members: confrontation, showing empathy, and offering hope. These techniques are equally important in the medical interview. Confrontation consists of telling the patient the evidence for a substance abuse problem. The patient usually denies the diagnosis and may even get angry. However, with persistent and non-judgmental confrontation, most patients eventually admit that they have a problem. It is important in confrontation to avoid arguing with a patient; instead, simply restate the facts and show care and concern. Specific details of confrontation are outlined below.

Statements that convey empathy and offer hope are important in diminishing a patient's denial. Empathy is conveyed by acknowledging the patient's feelings ("I can see this is upsetting you") and by conveying concern ("I am very concerned about you"). Offering hope is essential, and patients must be able to "hear" that there is a way to change and improve their lives. After a diagnosis of substance abuse has been made, the objectives of care are to have the patient accept the diagnosis and agree to treatment

CONFRONTATION

Figure 3.2 summarizes a recommended approach to confrontation. This approach may be incorporated into the interview at a single visit or into interviews at multiple visits. One must be directive in confronting a patient with substance abuse. It is important, however, to include questions that give the patient some sense of control during this rather one-sided interaction. Because many patients (especially those with alcoholism) have negative emotional responses (e.g., anger and disbelief) to being told their diagnosis, they may not internalize what is told to them. Therefore, brevity and directness are essential. Statements of concern, optimism, and support for the person are

---

1. State the diagnosis (e.g., "I think you have the disease alcoholism and I am very concerned about you").
2. Acknowledge the patient's reaction (e.g., "I know this is making you uncomfortable . . .").
3. Ask the patient his/her view of the situation.
4. Explain the evidence for the problem; avoid fault and offer hope.
5. Ask the patient what he/she knows about treatment.
6. Tell the patient about treatment options, including the likely need for abstinence.
7. Assign responsibility to the patient to make a change and accept treatment.
8. Get the patient to select a treatment plan.
9. Take action to initiate treatment plan.
10. Specifically establish your role as an ally with the patient and schedule follow-up in a short time interval, ideally a few days.

Figure 3.2. Recommended approach for confrontation of a patient in whom an addiction problem has been diagnosed.

indicated. Such statements help patients while they are hearing a diagnosis that often brings shame. It is also important to not simply blame their disease; patients need to be specifically told that they must accept responsibility for making a change and seeking treatment.

The first goal of treatment in individuals with dependence is abstinence. Patients must accept help in the difficult process of recovery, even though most will say, "I can do it on my own." In addition to regular follow-up by a supportive physician who believes the patient can recover, the most important elements are a plan for detoxification, participation in self-help groups (Alcoholics/Narcotics Anonymous) or group therapy, and family involvement. Possible treatment options should be explained to the patient and the family. If the patient is in a crisis and not enough time is available during the first visit, a return appointment should be scheduled within a few days or the patient should be immediately referred to a reliable treatment program.

Despite concerned families and health care providers, not all patients respond to efforts to motivate them to accept treatment. In this situation, the option of a formal intervention should be considered. The aim of the intervention is to present, in a formal meeting, the situation as a crisis that motivates the patient to accept treatment.

The intervention team is composed of as many people as possible that are emotionally important to the patient. Before the actual intervention, this team meets to discuss how best to convince the patient that there is a problem and that he or she needs treatment. The process is initiated by having each participant describe specific details of how the patient's addiction led to anger, fear, disappointment, sadness, embarrassment, or other negative impact on the participant. The team then rehearses their confrontation, even scripting the order of speaking. Each person begins their confrontation with an expression of concern for the patient; followed by statements related to the impact the patient's drug use has had on him or her. Each participant ends their confrontation with specific measures they will take if the patient does not agree to treatment (e.g., loss of job, no further visits, being forced out of their home). As part of a formal intervention, arrangements may be made in advance to have the person admitted for drug treatment. Financing of treatment, arranging for absence from work, and other details must all be worked out by the team ahead of the intervention.

For many patients, employment problems are an important trigger to seeking addiction treatment. Sometimes such treatment is coercive, with treatment required in order to maintain employment. Many employers have recognized the economic and human costs of substance abuse and have developed employee assistance programs to motivate and assist employees into treatment. Physicians asked to write work excuses can often ally with employee assistance programs to help patients get appropriate addiction treatment. This approach uses the strong motivation to keep a job as leverage for getting treatment and following through to recovery.

REFERENCES

1. Warner, E. A., R. M. Walker, and P. D. Friedmann. 2003. Should informed consent be required for laboratory testing for drugs of abuse in medical settings? *Am. J. Med.* 115:54–58.

2. Miller, W. R. 1996. Motivational interviewing: Research, practice and puzzles. *Addict. Behav.* 21:835–842.

3. Reiff-Hekking, S., J. K. Ockene, T. G. Hurley, and G. W. Reed. 2005. Brief physician and nurse practitioner-delivered counseling for high risk drinking. Results of a 12-month follow-up. *J. Gen. Intern. Med.* 20:7–13. *Five hundred thirty high-risk drinkers in four academic primary care practices were randomized to a single 5- to 10-minute special intervention (SI) or usual care (UC). At 12-month follow-up, after controlling for baseline differences in alcohol consumption, SI participants had significantly greater reduction in weekly alcohol intake (–5.7 vs. –3.1 drinks per week) and were more likely to maintain safe drinking at 12 months.*

4. Bien, T. H., W. R. Miller, and J. S. Tonigan. 1993. Brief interventions for alcohol problems: A review. *Addiction* 88:315–335.

5. Fleming, M. F., K. L. Barry, L. B. Manwell, et al. 1997. Brief physician advice for problem alcohol drinkers: A randomized controlled trial in community-based primary care practices. *JAMA* 277:1039–1045. *Four hundred eighty-two men and 292 women were randomized to two 10- to 15-minute counseling visits delivered by physicians (IG) or control (C) and followed for 12 months. At 12-month follow-up, the IG group had a significantly greater reduction in the mean number of drinks in previous 7 days (from a baseline of 19 drinks in both groups to 11.5 [IG] vs. 15.5 [C]; p < 0.001), as well as fewer binge-drinking episodes during previous 30 days (3.1 vs. 4.2, compared to a baseline of 5.5), and percentage days drinking excessively in previous 7 days (17.8% vs. 32.5%, compared to 48% at baseline).*

6. Wilk, A. I., N. M. Jensen, and T. C. Havighurst. 1997. Meta-analysis of randomized control trials addressing brief interventions in heavy alcohol drinkers. *J. Gen. Intern. Med.* 12:274–283.

7. Grossberg, P. M., D. D. Brown, and M. F. Fleming. 2004. Brief physician advice for high-risk drinking among young adults. *Ann. Fam. Med.* 2:474–480. *Two hundred twenty-six young adults (aged 18–30 years) were randomized to a brief intervention or usual care. During the 4 years of follow-up, the intervention group had significant reductions in number of persons drinking more than three drinks per day, average 7-day alcohol use, number of persons drinking six or more drinks per occasion, and number of binge-drinking episodes in the previous 30 days. They also had significantly fewer emergency department visits (103 vs. 177), motor vehicle crashes (9 vs. 20), total motor vehicle events (114 vs. 149), and arrests for controlled substance or liquor violation (0 vs. 8).*

8. Manwell, L. B., M. F. Fleming, M. P. Mundt, et al. 2000. Treatment of problem alcohol use in women of childbearing age: Results of a brief intervention trial. *Alcohol Clin. Exp. Res.* 10:1517–1524. *Two hundred five female patients (ages 18–40) with problem drinking were randomized to a brief intervention or a control group; 174 (85%) completed the 48-month follow-up. Those assigned to the intervention had significantly lower 7-day alcohol use and fewer binge-drinking*

*episodes, and those who became pregnant during the follow-up pe-
riod had the most dramatic decreases in alcohol use.*

9. Chang, G., L. Wilkins-Haug, S. Berman, and M. A. Goetz. 1999.
Brief intervention for alcohol use in pregnancy: A randomized
trial. *Addiction* 94:1499–1508. *Two hundred fifty-eight women
initiating prenatal care were randomized to assessment only
(AO) or a brief intervention (BI). Among those who reported prenatal alcohol consumption before assessment, there was no subsequent difference between groups, but among those who were
abstinent pre-assessment, those who received BI were more likely
to maintain abstinence (86% vs. 72%).*

10. Crawford, M. J., R. Patton, R. Touquet, et al. 2004. Screening and
referral for brief intervention of alcohol-misusing patients in an
emergency department: A pragmatic randomized controlled
trial. *Lancet* 364:1334–1339.

11. Stein, M. D., A. Charuvastra, J. Maksad, and B. J. Anderson.
2002. A randomized trial of a brief alcohol intervention for needle exchangers (BRAINE). *Addiction* 97:691–700. *One hundred
eighty-seven clients of a needle exchange program were randomized to motivational intervention (MI) for alcohol use (two 1-hour
sessions 1 month apart) or no intervention. MI group was more
likely to have 7 or more consecutive days abstinent (OR 2.61).*

12. Spirito, A., P. M. Monti, N. P. Barnett, et al. 2004. A randomized
clinical trial of a brief motivational intervention for alcohol-pos-
itive adolescents treated in an emergency department. *J. Pediatr.*
145:396–402. *One hundred fifty-two alcohol-using adolescents in
an emergency room were randomized to motivational intervention (MI) for alcohol use or standard intervention. MI produced
significant reduction in average number of drinking days per
month and frequency of high-volume drinking.*

13. McCambridge, J., and J. Strang. 2004. The efficacy of single session motivational interviewing in reducing drug consumption
and perceptions of drug-related risk and harm among young people: Results from a multi-site cluster randomized trial. *Addiction*
99:39–52.

14. Bernstein, J., E. Bernstein, K. Tassiopoulos, et al. 2005. Brief motivational intervention at a clinic visit reduces cocaine and
heroin use. *Drug Alcohol Depend.* 77:49–59. *One thousand one
hundred seventy-five patients in inner-city teaching hospital outpatient clinics were randomized to a single-session motivational
intervention (MI) for heroin and cocaine use or standard inter
vention. At 6 months follow-up, the MI group was more likely to
be abstinent than the control group for cocaine alone (22.3% vs.
16.9%, OR 1.51), heroin alone (40.2% vs. 30.6%, OR 1.57), and
both drugs (17.4% vs. 12.8%, OR 1.51).*

15. Fleming, M. F., M. P. Mundt, M. T. French, et al. 2000. Benefit-
cost analysis of brief physician advice with problem drinkers in
primary care settings. *Med. Care* 38:7–18. *Four hundred eighty-
two men and 292 women who reported drinking above a threshold limit were randomized to brief physician advice or control,
and at 6- and 12-month follow-up, outcomes examined included
alcohol use, emergency department visits, hospital days, legal
events, and motor vehicle accidents. The total economic benefit of
the brief intervention was estimated to be $423,519, composed of*

$195,448 in savings in emergency department and hospital use and $228,071 in avoided costs of crime and motor vehicle accidents. The average (per subject) benefit was $1151. The estimated total economic cost of the intervention was $80,210, or $205 per subject. The benefit-cost ratio was 5.6:1, or $56,263 in total benefit for every $10,000 invested.

16. Fleming, M. F., M. P. Mundt, M. T. French, et al. 2002. Brief physician advice for problem drinkers: Long-term efficacy and benefit-cost analysis. *Alcohol Clin. Exp. Res.* 26:36–43. *Four hundred eighty-two men and 292 women who reported drinking above a threshold limit were randomized to brief physician advice or control; at 48-month follow-up, subjects in the treatment group exhibited significant reductions in 7-day alcohol use, number of binge-drinking episodes, and frequency of excessive drinking as compared with the control group. The treatment sample also experienced fewer days of hospitalization (p = 0.05) and fewer emergency department visits (p = 0.08). Seven deaths occurred in the control group and three in the treatment group. Benefit-cost analysis showed a $43,000 reduction in future health care costs for every $10,000 invested in brief intervention for problem drinking.*

17. Nilssen, O. 2004. Long-term effect of brief intervention in at-risk alcohol drinkers: A 9-year follow-up study. *Alcohol Alcoholism* 39:548–551.

4

Overview of Addiction Treatment

BACKGROUND

There are a wide variety of treatment modalities used for addiction treatment. Despite the tremendous variation in substances that are used, there are common themes in addiction treatment and many similarities in the therapeutic approaches utilized for different substances. In this chapter we will address treatment setting and then briefly review types of treatment and their applications. References on their use can be found in the corresponding chapters on specific substances.

Most addiction treatment can be roughly divided into two types of modalities: (1) *psychosocial treatment,* which includes self-help groups, counseling, cognitive behavioral therapy, and analytic psychotherapy, and (2) *pharmacotherapy,* which includes drug antagonists or agonists and other agents. Of course, these treatments are not mutually exclusive and the best approach in many cases is a combination of therapeutic modalities. There are other treatments including *aversion therapy* (sometimes utilizing pharmacological agents) and a number of "alternative" therapies, such as acupuncture, that are utilized as well.

Unfortunately, much of the research on addiction treatment has serious limitations, though these are not unique to this field. At the end of this chapter we will briefly outline some of the common problems encountered in this research and the reasons why they are of concern.

TREATMENT SETTING

When treating an individual with a substance use disorder, one of the first decisions that needs to be made is the optimal treatment setting. This decision is often limited by availability, insurance, and patient preference. The American Society of Addiction Medicine (ASAM) has developed patient placement criteria to help guide this decision (1). Unfortunately, there is little data on the utility of these criteria. One observational study of alcoholics admitted to different levels of care reported that those who were *undertreated* (i.e., were placed at a lower level of care than would be recommended by placement criteria) did worse than those who were appropriately matched; moreover, *overtreatment* was not associated with better outcomes (2). However, another observational study reported that outcomes between "matched" and "mismatched" patients were not significantly different (3). Nevertheless, these criteria are widely used and many insurance companies use them to determine medical necessity. The ASAM placement criteria for adults divide patients into four general treatment levels: (I) outpatient treatment, (II) intensive outpatient treatment or partial hospitalization, (III) residential treatment, and (IV) medically managed intensive inpatient treatment; levels II and III are respectively subdivided into two and four further levels. The appropriate level is determined by the patient's status in six dimensions: (1) intoxication/potential for withdrawal, (2) biomedical conditions, (3) emotional/behavioral conditions, (4) treatment acceptance/resistance, (5) relapse/continued-use potential, and (6) recovery environment. The criteria can be summarized thus:

Level I (outpatient treatment) is appropriate for patients who (1) have minimal risk of severe withdrawal, (2/3) have no unstable biomedical or emotional conditions, (4) are cooperative, (5) have adequate coping skills, and (6) are in a supportive environment.

Level II (intensive outpatient or partial hospitalization) is appropriate for patients who (1) have minimal to moderate risk of severe withdrawal, (2/3) mild or manageable biomedical or emotional conditions, (4) are somewhat resistant to change, (5) have a high risk of relapse, and (6) are in an unsupportive environment. Level II is further subdivided into Level II.1 (intensive outpatient) and II.5 (partial hospitalization).

Level III (residential services) is appropriate for patients who (1) have minimal to moderate risk of withdrawal that can be managed at this level, (2/3) have medical or emotional conditions that require monitoring and structure (but not intensive treatment), (4) are resistant to treatment, (5) are unable to control their use, and (6) are in an environment that is dangerous for recovery. Level III is further subdivided into Level III.1 (clinically managed low-intensity residential), III.3 (medium intensity residential), III.5 (medium/high-intensity residential), and III.7 (medically monitored intensive inpatient).

Level IV (medically managed inpatient services) is appropriate for patients who (1) have a severe withdrawal risk or (2/3) require 24-hour medical or psychiatric and nursing care for medical or emotional conditions (dimensions 4 through 6 have no impact on determining this level).

PSYCHOSOCIAL TREATMENT

A variety of psychosocial modalities have been used in addiction treatment. Providing brief advice or counseling in primary care settings has been shown to be effective. Participation in self-help groups is associated with improved outcomes, and drug counseling (group or individual) may also be helpful. A number of behavioral approaches appear to be modestly effective, but analytically based psychotherapeutic approaches have not been shown to be effective.

Brief Advice

The simplest and most straightforward form of treatment is to screen patients for tobacco, alcohol, and other drug use and to counsel those in whom you believe this is a problem. This generally takes the form of giving advice on the health effects of the drug, assessing the patient's readiness for change, and providing information and assistance on treatment options. This can be done by physicians, nurse practitioners, nurses, or trained counselors and has been shown to be modestly effective for smokers, problem drinkers, and heroin and cocaine users.

Motivational Enhancement

For many individuals, lack of motivation to change appears to be an important barrier; for this reason, *motivational interviewing* and *motivational enhancement therapy* have been developed as treatment options. These treatments typically involve one to four patient-centered sessions in which the patient's goals and the role that addiction plays in the patient's life are explored and the negative consequences of this problem are discussed, followed by help and encouragement for further treatment. Strategies employed include expressing empathy for the patient and acceptance of his or her ambivalence for change, pointing out discrepancies between the patient's goals and his or her current situation, providing new perspectives when resistance is encountered, and expressing confidence in the patient's ability to change. A number of studies suggest that this approach is effective for some, though there is little data on its use in the primary care setting. This topic is covered in more detail in Chapter 3 on the medical interview.

Self-Help Groups

Self-help groups (also known as "mutual help groups" or "mutual self-help groups") are one of the oldest and most commonly used forms of addiction treatment. Alcoholics Anonymous (AA) is perhaps the best-known example of this approach; Narcotics Anonymous (NA) and Cocaine Anonymous (CA) are analogous groups for those addicted to opioids or stimulants. These groups are organized and led by recovering addicts, not treatment professionals, and many use a "12-step" approach (these are outlined in Chapter 5 on alcohol). The data on the effectiveness of these groups (primarily from observational studies) is limited but suggests that participation is associated with better outcomes. However, it is difficult to gauge the impact of this type of treatment from observational data, since it is likely that those who participate are a more motivated subset of addicts.

Drug Counseling

After self-help groups, drug counseling is probably the most commonly used treatment modality; this can be done in a group or individual setting. In contrast to self-help groups, group drug counseling sessions are typically led by trained drug counselors. However, the philosophy and approach of these groups are often quite similar, with a focus on the stages of recovery and providing a supportive atmosphere for maintaining abstinence and making lifestyle changes.

Individual drug counseling is a more intensive one-on-one treatment led by a trained counselor; like group counseling, it often focuses on stages of recovery and the development of tasks and goals based on the 12-step philosophy. Therapists often assist individuals with social, family, and legal problems. A number of studies suggest that both of these modalities are modestly effective in the short term (i.e., while individuals participate), but there is limited data on longer-term effectiveness.

Behavioral Therapy

There are a wide variety of behavioral approaches that appear to be effective for treating substance use disorders. In general, behavioral therapy focuses on particular behaviors that affect an individual's functioning (e.g., illicit drug use); the therapist works with the patient to find effective strategies to reduce these "target behaviors." A distorted perception of self and the world around one is thought to lead to negative thoughts and hopelessness that contribute to drug use. One strategy is to examine the thought process that underlies specific behaviors in order to help the individual recognize these "dysfunctional" patterns of thinking and develop strategies to counter them—this is referred to as *cognitive behavior therapy*. A variant of this approach is referred to as *coping skills therapy*, which tries to foster coping skills to reduce the risk of use; these include assertiveness training, focusing on the consequences of use, finding alternative behaviors, and learning ways to avoid or escape situations that lead to use. Another similar approach is sometimes referred to as *relapse prevention therapy*; this uses a variety of cognitive and coping strategies to deal with high-risk situations and early signs of impending relapse. Addicts are encouraged to find healthy activities that decrease their need for substances and to prepare for possible lapses in abstinence in order to prevent these from developing into a full-blown relapse. *Network therapy* utilizes behavioral techniques and enlists family members and friends to reinforce compliance and undermine denial.

Yet another behavioral strategy is to provide rewards for desirable behaviors or punishment for undesirable ones; this is often referred to as *contingency management*. Most studies of contingency management use vouchers as a reward for drug-free urine toxicology screens, often in the setting of methadone maintenance programs. Another treatment modality attempts to promote "alternate reinforcers" and a healthier lifestyle by combining cognitive behavior therapy with vocational rehabilitation, as well as contingency management and other behavioral modalities; this is sometimes referred to as *community reinforcement*. These approaches appear to be modestly effective while in place, but the effect seems to dissipate once the rewards and other external factors are removed.

Drug Courts

"Drug courts" have recently become—in the United States, at least—a common way of dealing with illicit drug users who break the law. This approach is quite similar to contingency management with an emphasis on sanctions rather than rewards. Typically, offenders in these programs are required to enter an addiction treatment program, undergo frequent testing (generally urinalyses) to verify abstinence, and appear frequently in court to be monitored by judges; those who do not comply with the program requirements face the threat of sanctions, including imprisonment. Studies (generally observational) suggest that these programs do reduce drug use and recidivism, at least while participants are under court supervision. However, evidence of long-term effectiveness is lacking.

Analytic Psychotherapy

Analytic psychotherapy utilizes a variety of strategies to help individuals deal with their problems (including addiction). While behavioral therapy focuses on problem behaviors, analytic psychotherapy focuses on understanding the thoughts and feelings that lead to these behaviors. *Expressive-supportive therapy* is one such analytically based treatment modality. In the expressive mode, the patient focuses on interpersonal relationships and transference to others; in the supportive mode, the patient forms a therapeutic alliance and tries to strengthen coping skills and defenses to reestablish equilibrium. Techniques that are utilized include confrontation, clarification, partial interpretation, and suggestion (advice); in contrast to traditional psychoanalysis, there is limited free association and less focus on interpretation and developing insight into origins of a problem. *Interpersonal psychotherapy* is a time-limited treatment that focuses on current events and problems and tries to alleviate symptoms and social dysfunction. In general, this type of approach has not been shown to be effective for addiction treatment but may offer some benefits, especially for those with a co-occurring psychiatric disorder.

Residential Treatment

Residential programs are another heterogeneous treatment modality that can range from halfway houses that are little more than a place to stay to more intensive treatment facilities. In general, observational data suggests that most individuals who enter this type of treatment do not complete it, but those who stay tend to have better outcomes.

Therapeutic communities are a variant of residential treatment; they are typically organized and led by recovering addicts, though many employ professional staff—who are often recovering addicts themselves. In these communities, the focus is on members' behaviors, and their lives are often tightly controlled and monitored by the group; in general, contact outside of the community is very limited. Older members serve as role models and undesirable behaviors are sanctioned, often through peer confrontation. These types of programs are probably more effective than their less-structured counterparts, but they typically have high attrition rates.

Modified therapeutic communities are a more recently developed model of care; they are less intense and more flexible, and they focus more on individualized treatment. These programs emphasize positive reinforcement and conflict resolution instead of confrontation and sanctions. There is some research that supports their effectiveness, particularly for mentally ill substance abusers.

PHARMACOTHERAPY

Drug Antagonists

The use of specific agents to block the effect of an abused substance is an attractive option that has been long pursued in search of an effective treatment for addiction. So far, this approach has largely failed. The best-studied example is the use of opioid antagonists, such as naltrexone, to block the effect of opioids. While opioid antagonists are very effective for treatment of acute overdose, these agents have not been found to be effective for addiction treatment in general—except perhaps in a subset of highly motivated opioid addicts. This is probably because opioid antagonists do not lessen drug craving.

An analogous approach is to use a drug that antagonizes some of the CNS effects of a substance, such as using dopamine antagonists (for example, olanzapine) for treatment of stimulant (specifically cocaine) addiction; this has not been found to be effective. However, the search for effective drug antagonists has not been abandoned; injectable or implantable long-acting formulations of opioid antagonists may prove to be effective, and there is active research into the development of antibodies to specific drugs.

Drug Agonists

In contrast to drug antagonists, drug agonists have been shown to be effective in addiction treatment. These agents have been utilized for treatment of addiction to a variety of substances in two ways: (1) for detoxification and (2) for maintenance therapy. The benzodiazepine sedative-hypnotics are effective treatment for alcohol withdrawal. Likewise, methadone, an opioid agonist, and buprenorphine, a partial agonist and antagonist, are effective for treating the symptoms of opioid withdrawal. Nicotine replacement is yet another agonist approach and has been shown to help smokers quit.

Maintenance therapy has become an important treatment modality for opioid dependence. Methadone and buprenorphine maintenance treatment are both effective at reducing illicit opioid use and the risk of complications (especially overdose). Long-acting stimulants may likewise help reduce illicit cocaine (and methamphetamine) use, but there is much less experience with this approach. Using alternative nicotine-delivery systems, such as a type of chewing tobacco called "Snus," has been proposed as a way to reduce the morbidity and mortality associated with smoking.

Other Agents

A wide variety of other agents have been studied for addiction treatment, and a few have been modestly effective or show promise. The antidepressants bupropion and nortriptyline have been found to help smokers quit (but other antidepressants do not). Naltrexone and acamprosate appear to be modestly effective for alcoholism. The antiepileptic agent topiramate may prove to be effective for alcoholism and cocaine dependence. Disulfiram, initially utilized as a treatment for alcoholism, has shown promise as a treatment for cocaine addiction.

AVERSION THERAPY

Another treatment strategy is to pair an unpleasant stimulus with the use of a particular substance; this is referred to as "aversion therapy" or "aversive conditioning." The best-studied example of this is the use of disulfiram (Antabuse), which causes an unpleasant reaction when combined with alcohol use. A variety of aversive treatments have been tried to help smokers quit, including rapid puffing, smoke-holding, excessive smoking, and silver acetate. Unfortunately, this therapeutic approach has not been shown to be effective.

ALTERNATIVE THERAPIES

There are a number of so-called alternative therapies that are utilized for addiction treatment. The one that has been studied best is acupuncture (specifically for smoking and cocaine dependence); this has not been shown to be effective. Hypnotherapy is a popular treatment for smoking cessation and has also been used for other addictions; like acupuncture, there is no evidence that it

is effective. Other proposed treatment modalities include meditation, biofeedback, and relaxation therapy. The research in this
area of therapy is still in its infancy, and there may yet prove to
be a role for them in the treatment of substance use disorders.

ADDICTION TREATMENT RESEARCH LIMITATIONS

Performing high-quality research on addicts is a difficult task.
This problem is compounded by the relatively low priority that
is given to research in this area, despite its importance. A number of issues limit the strength of many of the available research
studies (4); these are not unique to addiction research but must
be taken into account. Table 4.1 offers some general guidelines
for evaluating therapeutic studies. We will offer a brief overview
of some of these issues and why they are important. Many read-
ers will already be familiar with these general principles from
evidence-based medicine, but it may be helpful to review them in
the context of addiction treatment research.

Lack of Control Group (Observational Data)

Many research studies on addiction treatment are observational studies and lack a control group for comparison. These
often take the form of a "before and after" analysis where the
subjects' drug use (or other measures) after a specific treatment
is compared with their "baseline" status before treatment to establish the effectiveness of an intervention. While finding an improvement in a particular outcome measure (such as drug use)
during or after a certain treatment is certainly evidence in support of that intervention, it is very limited at best. Given the
cyclical nature of addiction, if one were to take a group of addicts
who wished to stop or cut down on their use and followed them
over time (without any intervention), it is likely that you would
observe a relative improvement. This is further reinforced by the
observation that when studies do have a control group, there is
often a significant improvement from baseline in that group (5).
Without a comparable control group (preferably selected by ran-
domization), it is impossible to know whether the treatment was
really effective, and if it is effective, to what extent.

**Table 4.1.   Suggested guidelines for assessing treatment
studies**

Was the assignment of patients to treatments randomized?
Were all patients who entered the study accounted for at its conclusion?
Was the analysis performed on an intention-to-treat basis?
Were the study patients recognizably similar to my own?
Were all clinically relevant outcomes reported?
Were both statistical and clinical significance considered?
Is the treatment feasible in my practice setting?

Adapted from Sackett, D. L., R. B. Haynes, G. H. Guyatt, et al. 1991. *Clinical
epidemiology: A basic science for clinical medicine.* 2nd ed. Boston: Little,
Brown.

Exclusion of Dropouts

Even when a clinical trial utilizes a randomly assigned control group for comparison, the study is often limited by dropouts; this problem weakens the ability of a trial to detect a significant difference and tends to dilute the measured effect of a treatment (if there is one). This is a particular problem in addiction research since these studies typically have high dropout rates. There are two general ways of dealing with this problem (6). One is to include everyone enrolled in the study—even those who did not remain in treatment—in the analysis of the outcomes and to count all of those for whom you do not have outcome data as treatment failures; this is called "intention-to-treat analysis" and is the most rigorous way of analyzing the data. If a study can demonstrate a benefit even when utilizing intention-to-treat analysis, this is strong evidence in support of that treatment. Unfortunately, this is hard to do and many studies of addiction treatment exclude those who drop out and rely on an "as-treated analysis." This may introduce a bias because those who drop out are typically different in many ways from those who stay in treatment; furthermore, even if the treatment is truly effective (for those who remain), this type of analysis tends to make the treatment appear to be more effective than it really is (for all those who enter treatment).

Limited Generalizability

When evaluating the relevance of a clinical trial to one's own practice, it is important to carefully look at who the subjects were and whether they are comparable to the individuals you are caring for. Many addiction research studies are conducted on relatively healthy and motivated volunteers. Individuals with polysubstance dependence or serious medical or psychiatric co-morbidities are often excluded (7). This makes it difficult to generalize the results and apply them to the many individuals who do not fit this profile. One way to gauge this is to look at the number of subjects who were screened to find those who were included in the trial; unfortunately, many reports do not give this information.

Varied Outcome Measures

What is the goal of addiction treatment? Long-term abstinence is the simplest and most obvious answer to this question, but "cure" is rarely achieved in practice and there are many other benefits of addiction treatment. These potential benefits include reducing substance misuse, preventing medical complications of addiction, and ameliorating its societal impact (crime, homelessness, unemployment, etc.). The individual's own satisfaction and sense of well-being are also important outcomes. Moreover, there are numerous ways to measure each of these outcomes, and it is not unusual for a study to use multiple measures for each (8). The wide variety of possible outcome measures speaks to the importance of addiction but also creates problems for researchers and those evaluating their research. It is only natural that researchers will tend to emphasize those measures in which positive outcomes were found—especially in the abstracts of their articles—but this obviously is fertile ground for the introduction of bias (9). The wide variety of outcome measures also makes it difficult to compare one study with another. Some have developed composite measures of addiction; a commonly used example is the Addiction Severity Index (ASI), which includes questions on medical and psychiatric status, employment status, drug/alcohol use, legal status, and family/social relationships, but these measures are not consistently used.

Questionable Clinical Significance

Even when a well-designed study shows a *statistically* significant improvement in an outcome measure, the clinician must always ask whether this difference is *clinically* significant. It is not unusual for studies to report statistically significant but relatively modest changes in substance use associated with a specific treatment. Furthermore, many trials look at treatment outcomes over a relatively short period of time (typically 12 to 24 weeks), and it is impossible to determine the long-term significance of their findings. Clinicians need to keep this in mind when deciding whether to utilize a treatment for a specific patient. On the other hand, there is always a range of responses, so even when the average response is not impressive, there will be some individuals who may have a clinically significant response to a specific treatment (as well as those who do not respond at all).

Limited Applicability

Last (but not least), practitioners must ask whether the treatment can be applied where they practice. Most addiction treatment studies are not conducted in office-based practices and may not be feasible in that setting. For example, there are many studies of different treatment strategies in the setting of methadone maintenance programs, which take advantage of having a "captive audience" and probably could not be employed in the typical primary care office.

REFERENCES

1. Mee-Lee, D., G. Shulman, and L. Gartner. 2000. *ASAM patient placement criteria for the treatment of psychoactive substance-related disorders*. 2nd ed. Chevy Chase, MD: American Society of Addiction Medicine.
2. Magura, S., G. Staines, N. Kosanke, et al. 2003. Predictive validity of the ASAM patient placement criteria for naturalistically matched vs. mismatched alcoholism patients. *Am. J. Addict.* 12:386–397.
3. McKay, J. R., J. S. Cacciola, A. T. McLellan, et al. 1997. An initial evaluation of the psychosocial dimensions of the American Society for Addiction Medicine criteria for inpatient versus intensive outpatient substance abuse rehabilitation. *J. Stud. Alcohol.* 58:239–252.
4. Moyer, A., J. W. Finney, and C. E. Swearingen. 2002. Methodological characteristics and quality of alcohol treatment outcome studies, 1970–98: An expanded evaluation. *Addiction* 97:253–263.
5. Moyer, A., and J. W. Finney. 2002. Outcomes for untreated individuals involved in randomized trials of alcohol treatment. *J. Subst. Abuse Treat.* 23:247–252.

6. Nich, C., and K. M. Carroll. 2002. Intention-to-treat meets missing data: Implications of alternate strategies for analyzing clinical trials data. *Drug Alcohol Depend.* 68:121–130.
7. Humphreys, K., and C. Weisner. 2000. Use of exclusion criteria in selecting research subjects and its effect on the generalizability of alcohol treatment outcome studies. *Am. J. Psychiatry* 157:588–594.
8. Finney, J. W., A. Moyer, and C. E. Swearingen. 2003. Outcome variables and their assessment in alcohol treatment studies: 1968–1998. *Alcohol Clin. Exp. Res.* 27:1671–1679.
9. Chan, A. W., and D. G. Altman. 2005. Identifying outcome reporting bias in randomised trials in PubMed: Review of publications and survey of authors. *BMJ* 330:753–756.

5

Alcohol

BACKGROUND

The use of alcoholic beverages dates back thousands of years to a biblical reference to Noah drinking wine and getting drunk.

Table 5.1. Common alcohol containers: volume and number of drinks

Type of Alcohol	Container	Volume (Metric)	Approximate Drinks*
Beer	12 oz bottle/can	340 ml	1
(3–5% alcohol)	22 oz	620 ml	2
	40 oz	1133 ml	3–4
Wine	Glass	140 ml	1
(10–15% alcohol)	Standard bottle	750 ml	5–6
Distilled alcohol	Shot	30 ml	1
(40–50% alcohol)	Miniature	50 ml	2
	Half-pint	237 ml	8–9
	Pint	473 ml	16–18
	Fifth	757 ml	25–30
	Quart	946 ml	31–37
	Half-gallon	1892 ml	63–73

One drink contains approximately 12 grams of alcohol
* Actual conversion will depend on alcohol content.

Distillation of alcohol into whiskey started during the Middle Ages when alcohol was first used for medicinal reasons as an anxiolytic. Not long after that, the detrimental effects of alcohol were first recognized.

Alcoholic beverages are fermented (wine and beer) or distilled. The concentration of alcohol (ethanol) in wine ranges from 10 to 22% by volume, while most beer contains 4 to 5% alcohol by volume. Distilled alcoholic beverages (e.g., whiskey, brandy, rum, gin, and vodka) contain a higher percentage of alcohol. "Proof" (in the United States) is double the percentage of alcohol by volume—for example, 90 proof is equivalent to 45% alcohol by volume. One drink of distilled alcohol (1 fluid oz), one glass of wine (4 oz), and one beer (12 oz) contain approximately 12 grams of alcohol. Table 5.1 lists common alcohol containers and approximate equivalence in drinks.

EPIDEMIOLOGY

An estimated 119 million Americans (half of all Americans over the age of 12) were current drinkers in a 2003 survey (1). In the same survey, 16.1 million Americans (6.8% of population) were classified as heavy drinkers (five or more drinks on the same occasion on at least 5 out of the past 30 days). Additionally, 13.6% of the population drove under the influence at least once in the 12 months previous to the survey. Binge drinking (consuming five or more drinks on one occasion) has steadily increased in the United States with 1.5 billion episodes in 2001 (2). Rates of binge drinking are greatest for those aged 18–25, with resultant high rates of motor vehicle accidents in this population. Along with cardiovascular disease and cancer, alcoholism ranks among the top three causes of death and disability in the United States. The estimated cost of alcoholism to society in 1998 was $184.6 billion (3).

The causes of alcoholism are multifactorial and poorly under-stood (4, 5). Genetic predisposition to alcoholism appears to be present in at least half of all alcoholics (6, 7). Social conditioning, enabling behavior by others close to the individual, and being a child in a dysfunctional family are important nongenetic factors. Other psychiatric disorders (antisocial personality disorder, pri-mary abuse of other substances, or an affective disorder) may also play a role. For elderly alcoholics, isolation is often associ-ated with the onset of problem drinking.

DRUG EFFECTS

Acute Effects

On average, 1 ounce of distilled alcohol (or the equivalent of beer or wine) produces a peak blood alcohol level (BAL) of ap-proximately 25 mg/dl within 30 minutes of ingestion. Approximately 15 mg/dl is metabolized per hour. A BAL of 100 mg/dl is equivalent to 0.08% on a breathalyzer, the units com-monly used by law enforcement to indicate driving impairment. Thus, to reach this level an individual must consume at least four drinks.

The distribution of alcohol throughout the body is uniform, with equivalent plasma and central nervous system concentra-tions. At the cellular level, ethanol is a depressant, similar to anesthetics. At low levels, alcohol preferentially depresses neu-rons that are inhibitory, resulting in a stimulatory effect on be-havior. However, this same inhibition accounts for the decline in coordination and reaction time that occurs with even small doses of alcohol. At higher doses of ethanol, memory lapses and changes in mood occur. There is great individual variance in re-gard to the euphoria-producing and hallucinogenic effects of al-cohol. Some become dysphoric at even low doses of alcohol. For all individuals, the depressant/sedative effects of alcohol pre-dominate at higher doses. Women may have greater sedation than men do at equivalent blood alcohol levels (8).

Overdose

Alcohol overdose or intoxication is characterized by an initial period of excitement and euphoria followed by depression and sleep, or possibly coma. Other symptoms may include impaired coordination, loudness, lowered inhibitions, poor memory and judgment, labile mood, slurred speech, nausea, and vomiting. The duration and magnitude of intoxication depend on the amount and the rapidity with which the alcohol was consumed and whether the patient drank on an empty stomach (enhancing the rate of absorption). Tolerance is also a significant factor, as an alcoholic may acquire the capacity to increase the rate of al-cohol metabolism. Individuals may develop substantial central tolerance, appearing sober at blood alcohol levels of 150 mg/dl or more, while most people without tolerance become intoxicated at levels between 100 and 200 mg/dl. Levels over 400 mg/dl may be lethal, with death resulting from depressed respiration or aspi-ration of vomit.

Blackouts and amnesia for events that occurred during over-dose are common. Alcohol idiosyncratic intoxication (pathologic intoxication) is an uncommon syndrome characterized by an aggressive or violent reaction to drinking alcohol, followed by amnesia for the episode.

Withdrawal

The four major manifestations of alcohol withdrawal are tremors, seizures, hallucinosis, and delirium tremens (9). Many ambulatory alcoholic patients who stop drinking develop none of the four major manifestations of withdrawal. Tremulousness usually begins 8 to 12 hours after the patient's last drink and peaks in 24 to 36 hours. Withdrawal seizures occur most commonly within 8 to 24 hours of the last drink and may occur without other manifestations of alcohol withdrawal. Both seizures and tremulousness can occur before the blood alcohol level has reached zero.

Alcohol withdrawal hallucinations may also occur without other signs of withdrawal. In a series of 50 consecutive patients, 58% of hallucinations were purely visual, 16% were purely auditory, and 26% were mixed (10). Hallucinations usually appear in the first 48 hours but may begin up to several days after the patient stops or markedly reduces alcohol use. Typically, alcoholic hallucinosis lasts from minutes to days (usually less than 1 week), but in a very small percentage of patients, hallucinosis may continue for weeks or months and, rarely, as a persistent symptom.

Delirium tremens is a late manifestation of withdrawal, occurring anytime from 48 hours to 14 days after cessation of drinking (11). It is most likely to occur in someone who has had this before with abstinence and is more common in older alcoholics (uncommon in patients under the age of 30). It may begin after the patient has shown signs of improvement from the early manifestations of withdrawal. Patients become agitated and delirious. Increased sympathetic tone results in tachycardia, systolic hypertension, and diaphoresis. Patients startle easily, have difficulty concentrating, and crave alcohol. Treatment of delirium tremens is a medical emergency and these patients often require high doses of sedatives; this should generally be done in a closely monitored setting (such as an intensive care unit) because of the risk of respiratory depression and other complications.

DIAGNOSIS

The diagnosis of alcoholism requires skillful interviewing and careful evaluation (12). A useful, broad definition of alcoholism is a condition in which drinking alcohol leads to recurring trouble in one or more of several domains—interpersonal (family and friends), educational, legal, financial, medical, or occupational. Physiological manifestations related to dependence—tolerance (the need for increased amounts of a substance to achieve intoxication or desired effect) and withdrawal—might occur late.

In 1992, a multidisciplinary committee of the National Council on Alcoholism and Drug Dependence and the American Society of Addiction Medicine issued its current definition of alcoholism: "Alcoholism is a primary, chronic disease with genetic, psychosocial, and environmental factors influencing its development and manifestations. The disease is often progressive and fatal. It is characterized by impaired control over drinking, preoccupation with the drug alcohol despite adverse consequences, and distortions in thinking, most notably denial. Each of these symptoms may be continuous or periodic" (13). Unlike previous definitions, this one specifically included denial as a key element of the definition of alcoholism.

The American Psychiatric Association (APA) considers alcoholism under the category "Substance-Related Use Disorders" (14). In its subclassification for these disorders, the APA has criteria for *substance abuse* (abnormal use, with unwanted consequences) and *substance dependence* (more intensive abuse patterns or physiological manifestations of addiction)—see Appendixes A and B for the DSM-IV diagnostic criteria. Continuous inability to control the use of alcohol is not always present. The National Institute on Alcohol Abuse and Alcoholism defines "at-risk drinking" as more than 14 drinks per week or more than 4 drinks per occasion for men and more than 7 drinks per week or more than 3 drinks per occasion for women (15). More recently, the terms "alcohol use disorder," "problem drinking," "hazardous drinking," and "unhealthy alcohol use" have also been used in the literature. These terms aim to include individuals who do not meet DSM-IV criteria for alcohol abuse or dependence but who may be at increased risk for alcohol-related problems or have had isolated problems related to drinking alcohol, such as a DUI. These individuals do not necessarily need alcohol treatment but may benefit from primary care intervention to prevent negative consequences from drinking.

Diagnostic Tools

Alcoholism and problem alcohol use are common and the evidence for them is often not volunteered, and therefore all patients should be screened; this recommendation is supported by the United States Preventive Services Task Force (16). The goal of screening is to be confident that one has ruled out alcoholism, has detected definite alcoholism, or must continue to consider alcoholism as a possible diagnosis, as well as to detect alcohol misuse.

There are a number of ways to screen for the cardinal features of alcoholism. The approach outlined in Figure 5.1 incorporates the four CAGE questions into the interview (17). In this approach, inquiry about the use of alcoholic beverages follows discussion about other habits. Inquiry begins with an open-ended question that prompts patients to respond with more than a simple yes or no or with a quantitative reply. In patients who report current use of alcohol, discomfort or glibness increases the likelihood that a problem exists (18). CAGE questions must be interpreted within a recent time frame, as someone now in his fifties may have gotten into trouble while in college and not had a problem since. In a study of adult outpatients in an urban university clinic, a CAGE score of 2 or more was associated with a sensitivity and specificity of 74% and 91%, respectively (19). Probabilities of an alcohol problem were 7%, 46%, 72%, 88%, and 99% for CAGE scores 0 through 4. A positive "C" answer is the

1. Integrate alcohol use inquiry into interview so that it follows inquiry about less sensitive habits:

    "We have talked about your usual diet and your smoking. Can you tell me how you use alcoholic beverages?"

2. For patients who report present or past use of alcohol, screen for evidence of alcoholism:

    "Has your use of alcohol caused any kinds of problems for you?" or "Have you ever been concerned about your drinking?"

3. CAGE Questions: If the patient has not disclosed a problem with drinking, use these four focused questions and probe for clarification of positive or ambivalent responses.

    "I would like to ask you a few more questions about alcohol that I ask all of my patients..."

    C "Have you ever felt you ought to CUT DOWN on your drinking?"

    A "Have people ANNOYED you by criticizing your drinking?"

    G "Have you ever felt bad or GUILTY about your drinking?"

    E "Have you ever had a drink first thing in the morning (EYE OPENER) to steady your nerves or got rid of a hangover?"

Figure 5.1.   Using the CAGE questionnaire.

most sensitive (i.e., lowest false-negative rate), while a positive "E" answer is the most specific (i.e., lowest false-positive rate). In clinical practice, one positive answer should always lead to further probing, both on the initial visit and on subsequent visits.

Lengthier than the CAGE, the Michigan Alcoholism Screening Test (MAST) is a 24-question standardized instrument that has been used extensively for alcoholism screening for study purposes (Figure 5.2) (20). The questions in the MAST may be helpful when one is attempting to uncover occult alcoholism. The questions are best used to gather additional information within the flow of obtaining a history related to drinking, complementing and adding information to positive CAGE answers. The CAGE questions have the advantage of being simple to incorporate into an office interview and being phrased in a nonthreatening way. Another screening tool, the 10-item AUDIT, developed by the World Health Organization, focuses on alcohol consumption and as such can be regarded as a screening tool for problem drinking (Figure 5.3) (21). It is important to note that in many studies evaluating the lengthier screening tools, such as the AUDIT and MAST, the questions were asked by research assistants, not by actual providers as part of the clinical interview. A shorter variant of the AUDIT, incorporating only its first three questions, is called the AUDIT-C (**22**). Some studies have suggested the AUDIT is a better tool than the CAGE in specific populations such as women (23, 24) and minorities (25). Two other screening tests, the TWEAK (developed for screening for alcohol use in pregnant women) and the CRAFFT (developed for screening for drug use in adolescents), are discussed in Chapter 17. Although quantitative inquiry may be helpful for identifying an occasional

Question	Points
1. Do you feel you are a normal drinker?	2
2. Have you ever awakened the morning after some drinking the night before and found that you could not remember a part of the evening before?	2
3. Does either of your parents, a family member, spouse, or partner ever worry or complain about your drinking?	1
4. Can you stop drinking without a struggle after one or two drinks?	2
5. Do you ever feel bad or guilty about your drinking?	1
6. Do friends or relatives think you are a normal drinker?	2
7. Are you always able to stop drinking when you want to?	2
8. Have you ever attended a meeting of Alcoholics Anonymous (AA)?	5
9. Have you gotten into fights when drinking?	1
10. Has your drinking ever created problems between you and family or friends?	2
11. Has your spouse (or other family member) ever gone to anyone for help related to your drinking?	2
12. Have you ever lost friends because of drinking?	2
13. Have you ever gotten into trouble at work because of drinking?	2
14. Have you ever lost a job because of drinking?	2
15. Have you ever neglected your obligations, your family, or your work for 2 or more days in a row because you were drinking?	2
16. Do you ever drink before noon?	1
17. Have you ever been told you have liver trouble? Cirrhosis?	2
18. Have you ever had delirium tremens (DTs), had severe shaking, heard voices, or seen things that were not there after heavy drinking?	2
19. Have you ever gone to anyone for help about your drinking?	5
20. Have you ever been in a hospital because of drinking?	5
21. Have you ever been a patient in a psychiatric hospital or on a psychiatric ward of a general hospital where drinking was part of the problem?	2
22. Have you ever been seen at a psychiatric or mental health clinic or gone to a doctor, social worker, or clergyman for help with an emotional problem in which drinking played a part?	2
23. Have you ever been arrested, even for a few hours, because of drunken behavior?	2
24. Have you ever been arrested for drunk driving or driving after drinking?	2

Score points for negative answers to questions 1, 4, 6, and 7 and positive answers to all other questions. A score of 5 or more points is indicative of alcoholism.

Figure 5.2.   Michigan alcoholism screening test (MAST).

1. **How often do you have a drink containing alcohol?**
    (0) Never   (1) Monthly or less   (2) Two to four times a month
    (3) Two to three times a week   (4) Four or more times a week
2. **How many drinks containing alcohol do you have on a typical day when you are drinking? [Code number of standard drinks.]**
    (0) 1 or 2   (1) 3 or 4   (2) 5 or 6   (3) 7 to 9   (4) 10 or more
3. **How often do you have six or more drinks on one occasion?**
    (0) Never   (1) Less than monthly   (2) Monthly   (3) Weekly
    (4) Daily or almost daily
4. **How often during the last year have you found that you were not able to stop drinking once you had started?**
    (0) Never   (1) Less than monthly   (2) Monthly   (3) Weekly
    (4) Daily or almost daily
5. **How often during the last year have you failed to do what was normally expected from you because of drinking?**
    (0) Never   (1) Less than daily   (2) Monthly   (3) Weekly
    (4) Daily or almost daily
6. **How often during the last year have you needed a first drink in the morning to get yourself going after a heavy drinking session?**
    (0) Never   (1) Less than monthly   (2) Monthly   (3) Weekly
    (4) Daily or almost daily
7. **How often during the last year have you had a feeling of guilt or remorse after drinking?**
    (0) Never   (1) Less than monthly   (2) Monthly   (3) Weekly
    (4) Daily or almost daily
8. **How often during the last year have you been unable to remember what happened the night before because you had been drinking?**
    (0) Never   (1) Less than monthly   (2) Monthly   (3) Weekly
    (4) Daily or almost daily
9. **Have you or someone else been injured as a result of your drinking?**
    (0) No   (2) Yes, but not in the last year   (4) Yes, during the last year
10. **Has a relative or friend or a doctor or other health worker been concerned about your drinking or suggested you cut down?**
    (0) No   (2) Yes, but not in the last year   (4) Yes, during the last year

A score of 8 or more indicates a strong likelihood of harmful alcohol consumption.

Figure 5-3.   The AUDIT questionnaire.

patient who is ready to discuss problems associated with drinking, its disadvantages are that it does not focus on inability to control use or on adverse consequences of drinking.

Findings on history, physical exam, and laboratory testing that may aid in the diagnosis of alcoholism are found in Table 5.2. The CAGE questions are superior to laboratory tests (gamma-glutamyl transpeptidase (GGT), other liver function tests, and red blood cell mean corpuscular volume) in diagnosing alcoholism (**26**). However, abnormalities in these tests may be helpful in supporting persistent inquiry and in confrontation of the suspected alcoholic. A recently developed blood test, carbohydrate-deficient transferrin (CDT), helps identify heavy alcohol intake and may help monitor a male alcoholic's abstinence (**27**). It is not useful in women or individuals

Table 5.2. Findings on history, physical examination, and laboratory testing suggestive (unmarked to *) to highly suggestive (to ***) or diagnostic (****) of alcoholism**

Presenting History

****	Drinking problem, recurring	* Legal problem
***	Blackouts with drinking	* Noncompliance in treatment
***	Spouse/other complains of patient's drinking	* School learning problem
***	Driving while intoxicated (DWI) record	* Hypertension
**	Gastrointestinal bleeding, especially upper	Headache
**	Traumatic injuries	Palpitations
**	Parent, grandparent, or relative alcoholic	Abdominal pain
**	Friends alcoholic or other chemical dependence	Amenorrhea
**	Family or other violence	Weight loss
**	First seizure in an adult	Vague complaints
**	Job performance problem	Insomnia
*	Unexplained syncope	Anxiety
*	Depression	Marital discord
*	Suicide attempt	Financial problem
*	Sexual dysfunction	

continued

Table 5.2. *Continued*

Past Medical History

****	Hepatitis, alcoholic	**	Attempted suicide
***	Pancreatitis, acute or chronic	**	Gastritis
***	Cirrhosis	**	Refractory hypertension
***	Portal hypertension	**	Cerebellar degeneration
***	Wernicke-Korsakoff syndrome	**	Peripheral neuropathy
***	Frequent trauma	**	Aspiration pneumonia
***	Cold injury	*	Gout
***	Nose and throat cancer	*	Cardiomyopathy
**	Other chemical dependence	*	Tuberculosis
**	Near drownings	*	Anxiety
**	Burns, especially third-degree	*	Depression
**	Leaves hospital against medical advice	*	Marital discord or family problem

Physical Examination

***	Odor of beverage alcohol on breath	*	Borderline tachycardia
***	Parotid gland enlargement, bilateral	*	Splenomegaly
***	Spider nevi or angioma	*	Hypertension
***	Tremulousness, hallucinosis		Diaphoresis
**	Breath mints odor		Alopecia

continued

Table 5.2.   *Continued*

Physical Examination

**	Hepatomegaly
**	Gynecomastia
**	Small testicles
**	Unexplained bruises, abrasions, or cuts
	Abdominal tenderness
	Cerebellar signs (e.g., nystagmus)

Laboratory Abnormalities

****	Blood alcohol level >300 mg/100 ml
***	Blood alcohol level >100 mg/100 ml without impairment
***	High serum ammonia
***	Gamma-glutamyl transpeptidase elevation
**	Blood alcohol level positive, any amount
**	High amylase (nonspecific for pancreas)
**	Abnormal liver function tests (especially AST > ALT)
**	Anemia, macrocytic or megaloblastic, microcytic, or mixed
**	Hyperuricemia
*	Creatine kinase elevation
*	Hypophosphatemia
	Hypomagnesemia
	Hyponatremia
	Hypokalemia
	Thrombocytopenia
	Hyperlipoproteinemia, type 4 or 5

with significant liver disease. As such, it has not yet been shown to be useful in screening general medical patients for alcoholism.

MEDICAL COMPLICATIONS

Recent studies suggest that moderate alcohol consumption may reduce the risk of heart disease (28), cerebrovascular disease (29), and kidney disease (30). However, these benefits are generally lost at higher levels of alcohol consumption. Prospective studies show that alcoholics have higher rates of mortality and medical morbidity than do matched controls (31). The most common causes of early death in alcoholics are cirrhosis of the liver, cancers of the respiratory and gastrointestinal tracts, accidents, suicide, and ischemic heart disease. Most alcoholics smoke and, in fact, lung cancer is the most common cancer diagnosed in alcoholics (32). Links between alcohol and cancers of the breast (33) and colon (34) have also been reported. Alcohol-related traffic accidents are the leading cause of death for teenagers and young adults (1). Importantly, alcoholic men who achieve long-term abstinence do not differ from nonalcoholic men in mortality rate (35). However, relapse significantly impacts on mortality.

Pulmonary Complications

Most of the pulmonary complications seen in individuals with alcoholism are related to the fact that virtually all such patients also smoke. Besides lung cancer, patients who drink and smoke have high rates of chronic obstructive lung disease and emphysema. Individuals who drink to intoxication are at high risk for aspiration pneumonia. Finally, alcoholism and homelessness/incarceration increase the risk for tuberculosis. Chronic cough should always be evaluated with a chest X-ray to evaluate for the presence of any of these possible diagnoses.

Cardiovascular Complications

An association between hypertension and heavy alcohol consumption has been found in physiological (36) and clinical studies (37). Hypertension may also increase the risk of stroke in alcoholics, although there may be an increased independent risk of stroke in heavy drinkers (38). Drinking also makes hypertension more difficult to treat, as medication noncompliance is common. Most reported studies of alcohol's role in hypertension are cohort studies, and in many of these studies, individuals become normotensive with abstinence (39). Clinical guidelines for treatment of hypertension include consideration of alcohol intake as a contributing factor for hypertension (40).

An association between alcoholism and dilated cardiomyopathy has been reported with anecdotal reports of the reversal of cardiomyopathy with abstinence. Most reported cases of alcoholic cardiomyopathy occur in individuals who have been drinking for decades (41). However, a recently published large cohort study of the Framingham population found no association between heart failure and alcohol intake (42). As risk factors for ischemic cardiomyopathy (hypertension and smoking) are also present in many alcoholics, patients with symptoms of heart failure should be evaluated for the presence of coronary artery disease.

Arrhythmias (most commonly atrial fibrillation) are commonly seen after an alcohol binge ("holiday heart") (**43**). The risk of developing atrial fibrillation appears to be especially associated with alcohol in men (**44**). Alcohol-associated atrial fibrillation may spontaneously revert to sinus rhythm without the need for medication or cardioversion.

Gastrointestinal Complications

Alcohol affects the digestive system from the oropharynx to the rectum. Poor oral hygiene is common in alcoholics, resulting in both dental and gum disease, with potential risk of consequent bacteremia. Glossitis, cheilitis, and parotid gland enlargement are generally associated with malnutrition and/or liver disease.

Alcohol lowers esophageal sphincter pressure, contributing to symptoms of reflux. In the long term, this increases the risk of developing Barrett's esophagus. Vomiting from alcohol intoxication puts patients at risk for Mallory-Weiss tears. Alcohol causes mucosal changes in the stomach causing gastritis and increases the risk for ulcer disease. In the small intestine, absorption is affected, contributing to malabsorption of vitamins and diarrhea.

Pancreatitis from alcohol occurs with varying incidences in different populations. The mechanism by which alcohol induces pancreatic inflammation is unknown, as most alcoholics, even those who develop cirrhosis, are never diagnosed with pancreatitis. Abdominal pain from pancreatitis typically is midepigastric and radiates to the back, laboratory testing reveals elevation in amylase and lipase, and imaging shows evidence of pancreatic inflammation. Management consists of withholding oral feeding and narcotic pain medication until signs and symptoms improve. Continued drinking after recovery from an episode of pancreatitis may result in chronic pancreatitis, with endocrine (hyperglycemia) and exocrine abnormalities (malabsorption).

Liver disease from alcohol use is largely related to amount and duration of use. The risk of cirrhosis is greater for women (**45**), with cirrhosis occurring at lower amounts of alcohol intake and at an earlier age (46). Hepatic steatosis (fatty liver) is the earliest effect of alcohol on the liver, and it can occur even with moderate drinking. Patients are most often asymptomatic, but on exam they have enlarged livers. On laboratory evaluation, aminotransferases are normal or mildly elevated. With continued drinking, hepatic steatosis progresses to hepatitis in most individuals.

Alcoholic hepatitis is a histological diagnosis with hepatocellular necrosis, inflammatory exudates, fibrosis, and Mallory bodies present on biopsy. Patients may be asymptomatic or present acutely with jaundice and ascites. Hepatomegaly is present in most individuals. Laboratory testing reveals elevation in bilirubin, aminotransferases, and alkaline phosphatase, suggesting cholestasis. Anemia, thrombocytopenia, and coagulopathy are markers of more severe disease. Patients with alcoholic hepatitis should also be assessed for presence of hepatitis C virus; in cohort studies up to 25% of alcoholics test positive for hepatitis C infection (47). Therapy for alcoholic hepatitis is generally supportive, with abstinence from alcohol imperative. Therapies investigated without clear benefit include propylthiouracil (48), pentoxifylline (49), androgens (50), etanercept (51), and infliximab (52). The data from studies of corticosteroids are mixed with some clinical trials showing benefit (53, 54) and others showing no benefit (55, 56). Even meta-analyses of these studies provide conflicting answers, mostly related to the large difference in patient populations in the studies (57–59). Nevertheless, the American College of Gastroenterology guideline for the treatment of alcoholic hepatitis recommends the use of corticosteroids (prednisolone 40 mg/day for 4 weeks, followed by a taper) in patients with encephalopathy or "discriminant function" over 32. The discriminant function is calculated by multiplying the number of seconds the prothrombin time is above control by 4.6 and then adding the total bilirubin (mg/dl) (60). Therapy is not recommended for individuals with active infection, renal failure, pancreatitis, or gastrointestinal bleeding.

Cirrhosis occurs in up to one-third of chronic alcoholics. Liver biopsy shows fibrosis, scarring with regenerating nodules, and necrosis. Radiographic imaging shows a small, shrunken liver. These pathologic changes cause portal hypertension and hepatocellular dysfunction. Nonspecific symptoms include weakness, anorexia, and fatigue; specific symptoms and signs related to hepatic dysfunction include jaundice, ascites, confusion (hepatic encephalopathy), spider angiomata, hemorrhoids, palmar erythema, gynecomastia, testicular atrophy, and impotence. Laboratory studies show impairment in hepatic synthetic function with elevation in prothrombin time and decreased albumin. Colchicine has been studied for the treatment of alcoholic cirrhosis without clear evidence of benefit (61, 62). Cirrhosis also puts individuals at risk for hepatocellular carcinoma. Most patients progress to liver failure, and the only effective treatment option is liver transplantation. Most programs require sobriety of at least 6 months before transplantation is considered. Posttransplant outcomes in patients who undergo transplantation for alcoholic liver disease are comparable to those who undergo transplantation for other causes of endstage liver disease (63).

Renal Complications

Electrolyte abnormalities (hypokalemia, hypomagnesemia, and hypophosphatemia) are common in patients with alcoholism. Most abnormalities are related to poor nutrition, but renal tubular disorders may contribute. Treatment is electrolyte repletion, either orally or intravenously. Hyponatremia typically occurs in beer drinkers who have large-volume intake of high-calorie, low-sodium beer, accompanied by little other oral intake. The term "beer potomania" is often used to describe this syndrome.

Alcoholic ketoacidosis is an uncommon complication of alcoholism and typically occurs when susceptible individuals have prolonged vomiting and anorexia after drinking heavily (64). In these individuals, liver metabolites acetaldehyde and acetate trigger liver production of beta-hydroxybutyrate and acetoacetate, resulting in acidosis. Treatment is intravenous saline and glucose.

Acute renal failure may occur in the setting of rhabdomyolysis, discussed below. In the setting of cirrhosis with liver failure, the hepatorenal syndrome may occur. Histologically the kidneys appear normal. Renal insufficiency in this disorder is likely related to splanchnic vasodilatation and renal vasoconstriction (65). There is no clear treatment, except liver transplantation.

Neuromuscular Complications

Wernicke's encephalopathy, a syndrome of global confusion, ataxia, and impaired eye movement (lateral gaze nystagmus and lateral rectus muscle paralysis most commonly), is caused by thiamine (vitamin B1) deficiency. The condition does not occur if dietary thiamine intake is adequate. Korsakoff's psychosis is the term associated with the confabulatory and amnesia components of the encephalopathy. Acute Wernicke's encephalopathy is a medical emergency. Treatment with parenteral thiamine (100 mg) may improve ocular symptoms within a few hours. Magnesium should also be repleted, as it is a cofactor for thiamine transketolase, an enzyme necessary for glucose metabolism. With abstinence from alcohol and good nutrition for several months, some patients recover entirely (66). However, many individuals remain impaired and may require institutional care.

Confusion may also be caused by hepatic encephalopathy occurring in the setting of liver failure. Ammonia and gamma-aminobutyric acid are generated by the action of bacteria in the gut and are normally metabolized by the liver. In the setting of cirrhosis, these two compounds enter the systemic circulation in high amounts causing confusion, disorientation, and coma. Treatment includes lactulose, which acidifies stool, preventing back diffusion of ammonia, and neomycin, which reduces colonic bacteria levels.

Cerebellar degeneration, independent from Wernicke's encephalopathy, may result in ataxia with a wide-based gait. Nutritional factors and direct toxic effects of alcohol have been implicated as causes. With abstinence and nutritional support, patients may improve.

Peripheral neuropathy can be the result of trauma or B vitamin (thiamine, pyridoxine, and pantothenic acid) deficiency. When peripheral neuropathy is due to nutritional deficiency, lower extremity involvement is more common. Symptoms, which usually include pain, paresthesia, and weakness, are distal and symmetric. Treatment consists of abstinence and B-complex vitamin replacement. There are no randomized trials examining the use of anticonvulsants or tricyclic antidepressants (medications often used for diabetic peripheral neuropathy) for the relief of the pain associated with alcohol-related peripheral neuropathy.

Although alcohol-related seizures have traditionally been thought of as occurring during withdrawal, it appears that alcoholics are at increased risk of seizures at any time in the cycle of drinking, not just during the withdrawal period (67). Alcohol-related seizures are typically grand mal, but status epilepticus is very rare. Patients with new seizures should be evaluated with computerized tomography and EEG, as the etiology could be related to trauma or an intracranial bleed (68). Management of seizures is discussed later in this chapter, under treatment of withdrawal.

Acute alcohol myopathy or rhabdomyolysis occurs most commonly in the setting of binge drinking, without history of trauma.

Multiple muscle groups are tender and painful. The etiology is unknown, but hypophosphatemia is present in many cases. Rhabdomyolysis may also occur in the setting of intoxication as a result of focal muscle trauma. Treatment in both instances is hydration, correction of metabolic abnormalities, and monitoring for renal damage. A chronic form of alcoholic myopathy may occur in patients with alcoholic polyneuropathy. This myopathy is painless and progresses with significant muscle atrophy.

Psychiatric Complications

Among patients with chronic mental illness, especially depression and anxiety, alcoholism is common. In many patients, alcoholism is the primary problem and treatment of depressive symptoms is not successful unless alcoholism treatment is initiated first (69). This topic is covered further in Chapter 16.

Other Medical Complications

Accidents and trauma, including burns, are highly associated with alcoholism. In the majority of patients with severe trauma, alcohol or other psychoactive drug use can be detected. Alcohol-related traffic accidents are the leading cause of death for teenagers and young adults (3). Osteonecrosis of the femoral head is associated with alcoholism for unclear reasons (70). Hip replacement is often required. Alcohol also impacts on bone metabolism, with an increased risk of osteoporosis in alcoholic men (71), while moderate amounts of alcohol intake in women appear to actually improve bone density (72).

Hematologic abnormalities (elevated mean corpuscular volume of red blood cells, anemia, thrombocytopenia) are related to nutritional deficiencies (B vitamins) as well as direct toxic effects of alcohol on the gut (malabsorption and/or mucosal injury) and bone marrow. Alcohol-induced hypogonadism results in decreased libido and impotence. Dermatologic disorders common in alcoholics include sunburn (with increased risk for skin cancer), rosacea (classically the large red nose), and porphyria cutanea tarda.

Gout has long been associated with alcohol intake without definitive data. A recent large study of a cohort of men found that those who drank beer, but not wine, were at increased risk for having an episode of gout (73).

Pregnancy

Morphologic abnormalities (especially of the face), low birth weight, and developmental and cognitive impairment manifest the fetal alcohol spectrum disorder (74). This syndrome is a consequence of alcohol ingestion during pregnancy. The risk of minor abnormalities (e.g., low birth weight) begins with the consumption of one drink per day; this risk increases with increasingly larger amounts of alcohol consumption. A further discussion of alcohol and pregnancy can be found in Chapter 17.

TREATMENT

The goal of treatment in patients with alcoholism or alcohol dependence is the achievement of abstinence (or progressively longer periods of abstinence from alcohol) with improved life functioning for patients and their families. For individuals with alcohol abuse or problem drinking (without dependence), a decision of abstinence versus decreased drinking must be made.

Brief Advice

Primary care providers through a brief intervention can help patients reduce their alcohol consumption (75). The details of brief intervention are covered in Chapter 3.

Detoxification/Abstinence

Many alcoholics can be detoxified from alcohol as outpatients (76). The decision between inpatient and outpatient detoxification should be based on comorbid medical conditions and severity of alcohol withdrawal symptoms. A history of severe withdrawal, systolic hypertension, and comorbid medical conditions are identified risk factors for severe alcohol withdrawal (**77**). Indications for referring a withdrawing alcoholic patient for inpatient detoxification are listed in Table 5.3. Inpatient detoxification provides careful 24-hour monitoring and treatment of withdrawal, evaluation of intercurrent medical problems, and removal of patients from the environment that has facilitated their drinking. If medically stable, patients participate in group therapy, attend Alcoholics Anonymous (AA), and receive individual counseling.

For mildly symptomatic patients with a stable home environment and supportive family and friends, outpatient detoxification supervised at daily visits to a treatment program or physician's office is as effective as inpatient detoxification. Patients may contract to attend an AA meeting daily with a friend or family member. For moderately sick patients, the choice of outpatient versus inpatient detoxification should be based on what programs are

Table 5.3.   Indications for inpatient detoxification

Evidence of hallucinations, severe tachycardia, severe tremor, fever, extreme agitation

History of severe withdrawal symptoms

History of seizure disorder

Presence of ataxia, nystagmus, confusion, or ophthalmoplegia, which may be indicative of Wernicke's encephalopathy

Severe nausea and vomiting that would prevent the ingestion of medication

Evidence of acute or chronic liver disease that may alter the metabolism of drugs used in the treatment of withdrawal

Presence of cardiovascular disease such as severe hypertension, ischemic heart disease, or arrhythmia, for which increased sympathetic output during withdrawal poses particular risk

Pregnancy

Presence of associated medical or surgical condition requiring treatment

Lack of medical or social support system to allow outpatient detoxification available. Some outpatient detoxification programs are intensive, requiring patients to spend entire days being monitored, with patients receiving medication as needed and participating in group counseling but going home to sleep. Other outpatient detoxification programs consist of only brief daily visits with assessment of withdrawal, administration of medication for withdrawal, and supplies of take-home medications for use later in the day.

Using Drugs in Detoxification

A useful tool for making decisions about pharmacological treatment of alcohol withdrawal is the Clinical Institute Withdrawal Assessment for Alcohol (CIWA-A) (see Figure 5.4) (78). Pharmacological therapy is generally not indicated for a score less than 10. For scores of 10 to 20, clinical judgment should determine the need for pharmacological treatment. For scores greater than 20, treatment with medications is indicated and should be administered on either an outpatient or an inpatient basis. For scores of 20 to 40, a score can be repeated after administering a dose of medication. Patients without improvement need more intensive monitoring as inpatients. Notably, pulse and blood pressure are not part of the CIWA scale. Although elevations of these two measures occur in alcohol withdrawal, the symptoms in the CIWA scale are more reliable in the assessment of severity of withdrawal.

Detoxification using orally administered psychoactive drugs is most effective when treatment is given early. The safest and most effective drugs for this purpose are the benzodiazepines (79). All of the benzodiazepines are effective. Diazepam has an advantage of having a rapid onset of action and long half-life. Its long half-life permits loading on the first day—5 to 10 mg every 1 to 4 hours until severe symptoms dissipate. This approach will reduce or perhaps eliminate the need for further dosing on subsequent days. Lorazepam (Ativan) does not require hepatic metabolism and is safer in patients with severe liver disease (i.e., prolonged prothrombin time). Additionally, patients should receive 100 mg of thiamine, 1 mg of folate, and a multivitamin daily. These vitamins should be continued for the first month or more of recovery.

Patient response to a dose of benzodiazepine is not necessarily related to the amount of drinking. Patients should be monitored for response after initial dosing to make an assessment of indicated dosage and dosing interval. Dosing should be titrated to effect. Essential to management is early recognition of withdrawal, early treatment, frequent monitoring, and continual treatment. Low dosages of sedative-hypnotic drugs should be tried first for most patients (Table 5.4). High dosages of these drugs may be indicated when the low dosage does not suppress or prevent symptoms in the first few hours or when there is a history of a patient requiring high doses in the past. In the setting of alcohol withdrawal delirium, control of agitation should be with benzodiazepines and not neuroleptic agents (80).

The aim of drug treatment is to alleviate the most severe symptoms and signs of withdrawal and to prevent seizures. Symptom-driven therapy, compared to fixed-schedule therapy, has been shown to decrease treatment duration and the amount of benzodiazepine used (81). Benzodiazepines should be given

NAUSEA AND VOMITING—Ask "Do you feel sick to your stomach? Have you vomited?" Observation.
0 no nausea and no vomiting
1 mild nausea with no vomiting
2
3
4 intermittent nausea with dry heaves
5
6
7 constant nausea, frequent dry heaves and vomiting

TREMOR—Arms extended and fingers spread apart. Observation.
0 no tremor
1 not visible, but can be felt fingertip to fingertip
2
3
4 moderate, with patient's arms extended
5
6
7 severe, even with arms not extended

PAROXYSMAL SWEATS—Observation.
0 no sweat visible
1 barely perceptible sweating, palms moist
2
3
4 beads of sweat obvious on forehead
5
6
7 drenching sweats

ANXIETY—Ask "Do you feel nervous?" Observation.
0 no anxiety, at ease
1 mildly anxious
2
3
4 moderately anxious, or guarded, so anxiety is inferred
5
6
7 equivalent to acute panic states, as seen in severe delirium or acute schizophrenic reactions

AGITATION—Observation.
0 normal activity
1 somewhat more than normal activity
2
3
4 moderately fidgety and restless
5
6
7 paces back and forth during most of the interview, or constantly thrashes about

Total CIWA-A Score _____ (Maximum Possible Score 67)

Patients with scores less than 10 can generally be followed without medication and scores greater than 20 generally require pharmacological treatment. Patients with scores between 10 and 20 should be followed closely for possible worsening of withdrawal.

Figure 5.4.   Addiction research foundation clinical institute withdrawal assessment for alcohol (CIWA-Ar).

TACTILE DISTURBANCES—Ask "Have you any itching, pins and needles sensations, any burning, any numbness, or do you feel bugs crawling on or under your skin?" Observation.

0 none
1 very mild itching, pins and needles, burning or numbness
2 mild itching, pins and needles, burning or numbness
3 moderate itching, pins and needles, burning or numbness
4 moderately severe hallucinations
5 severe hallucinations
6 extremely severe hallucinations
7 continuous hallucinations

AUDITORY DISTURBANCES—Ask "Are you more aware of sounds around you? Are they harsh? Do they frighten you? Are you hearing anything that is disturbing you? Are you hearing things you know are not there?" Observation.

0 not present
1 very mild harshness or ability to frighten
2 mild harshness or ability to frighten
3 moderate harshness or ability to frighten
4 moderately severe hallucinations
5 severe hallucinations
6 extremely severe hallucinations
7 continuous hallucinations

VISUAL DISTURBANCES—Ask "Does the light appear to be too bright? Is its color different? Does it hurt your eyes? Are you seeing anything that is disturbing to you? Are you seeing things you know are not there?" Observation.

0 not present
1 very mild sensitivity
2 mild sensitivity
3 moderate sensitivity
4 moderately severe hallucinations
5 severe hallucinations
6 extremely severe hallucinations
7 continuous hallucinations

HEADACHE, FULLNESS IN HEAD—Ask "Does your head feel different? Does it feel like there is a band around your head?" Do not rate for dizziness or lightheadedness. Otherwise, rate severity.

0 not present
1 very mild
2 mild
3 moderate
4 moderately severe
5 severe
6 very severe
7 extremely severe

ORIENTATION AND CLOUDING OF SENSORIUM—Ask "What day is this? Where are you? Who am I?"

0 oriented and can do serial additions
1 cannot do serial additions or is uncertain about date
2 disoriented for date by no more than 2 calendar days
3 disoriented for date by more than 2 calendar days
4 disoriented for place and/or person

Table 5.4. Benzodiazepines in the treatment of alcohol withdrawal

	Onset of Action	Rate of Metabolism	Liver Metabolized	Low Dosage (mg/6 hr)	High Dosage (mg/2–4 hr)
Chlordiazepoxide	Intermediate	Long	Yes	25	100
Diazepam	Fast	Long	Yes	2–5	10–20
Lorazepam	Intermediate	Intermediate	No	No	0.5 2
Oxazepam	Slow	Short	No	10–15	30

such that withdrawal symptoms are improved without over sedating the patient. If the patient is being treated as an outpatient, each day's medication should be entrusted to a family
member or friend who will be staying with the patient. Most patients need to be medicated for only 24 to 72 hours.

Two classes of antihypertensive have been studied for use in
the management of alcohol withdrawal—centrally acting alpha
agonists (i.e., clonidine) (**82**) and beta-blockers (83–85). These
drugs effectively alleviate the sympathetic markers of withdrawal (hypertension and tachycardia) but do little for the more
severe aspects of withdrawal (seizures and hallucinosis).

Other drugs studied in the treatment of alcohol withdrawal include the anticonvulsants gabapentin, valproate, and carbamazepine.
Carbamazepine was effective in treating patients with mild to moderate alcohol withdrawal in three studies (86–**88**). Valproate reduced the severity of alcohol withdrawal in one study, but patients
still required treatment with a benzodiazepine (89). Gabapentin has
not been found to be effective (**90**). One small study of acupuncture
in treating alcohol withdrawal found no benefit (**91**).

Prevention of Withdrawal Seizures

There is no consensus about whether phenytoin (Dilantin)
should be included in the detoxification of patients with a history of withdrawal seizures. In one study, phenytoin at a dosage
of 300 mg/day for 5 days appeared to prevent most withdrawal
seizures, even though therapeutic plasma levels of phenytoin are
not reached (92). However, in another study, when patients received an intravenous load of phenytoin or placebo within 6
hours of a first alcohol withdrawal seizure, phenytoin provided
no benefit in preventing further seizures (**93**).

There is evidence that a high-dosage benzodiazepine regimen
for withdrawal can prevent seizures (94). Additionally, benzodiazepines can prevent recurrent seizures in someone who has already had a seizure related to alcohol withdrawal (**95**). Therefore,
patients who are significantly symptomatic and receiving sufficient pharmacological therapy with a benzodiazepine do not require phenytoin. However, for mildly symptomatic patients with a
history of a withdrawal seizure who are not going to be treated
with a benzodiazepine, prophylactic phenytoin may be considered,
especially since a seizure may occur in the absence of other manifestations of alcohol withdrawal (67).

Treatment after Detoxification

Overview

Treatment consists of motivating the patient toward change, initiating a treatment plan, and providing regular follow-up.
Treatment options differ mostly based on environment and include
outpatient alcohol counseling (individual and group), residential
treatment, and halfway/recovery house. Effective treatment programs are abstinence-oriented, use AA or group therapy as a main-
stay of treatment, avoid the use of psychoactive drugs in long-term
treatment, involve the family, and provide close follow-up. Whether
to use pharmacotherapy as an adjunct must be decided. Table 5.5 is
a summary of alcohol abuse and dependence treatment studies.

Table 5.5.   Summary of alcohol abuse and dependence treatment studies

Intervention	Studies	Outcomes
Psychosocial		
Brief advice	RCTs Meta-analysis	Effective for reducing alcohol use among problem drinkers
Self-help groups	Observational	Participation is associated with better outcomes
Counseling	RCTs	Effective (in some studies)
Cognitive behavioral therapy (CBT)	RCTs Meta-analysis	Effective (in some studies)
Residential treatment	Observational	Participation is associated with better outcomes (in some studies)
Detoxification		
Benzodiazepines	RCTs Meta-analysis	Effective; as-needed treatment as effective as fixed-dose
Carbamazepine	RCTs	Effective for mild-moderate withdrawal
Pharmacotherapy		
Disulfiram	RCTs Meta-analysis	Not shown to be effective overall, but may be beneficial for selected individuals
Naltrexone	RCTs Meta-analysis	Effective in short-term (3–6 months)
Acamprosate	RCTs Meta-analysis	Effective in short-term (3–6 months)
Topiramate	RCT	Effective in one 12-week RCT
Ondansetron	RCT	Effective in a subgroup of early-onset alcoholics in one RCT

See text for references and more details.
RCT: randomized controlled trial.

Primary care providers should reinforce patient participation in their treatment program at all follow-up visits.

Self-Help Groups

Self-help groups potentially break down the denial process and deal with the associated guilt and shame through a combination of nonjudgmental acceptance and support. Alcoholics should be encouraged to attend Alcoholics Anonymous (AA) regularly. The Process of AA is shown in Figure 5.5. Regular AA attendance is correlated with long-term recovery and improved functioning, though experimental evidence of its effectiveness

Meetings

AA meetings are held daily in most communities in the United States and in most other countries. Meetings are either open or closed (most are open and most welcome nonalcoholics interested in treating alcoholism). A published directory of meetings, places, and times is available via the Internet. By contacting AA, an alcoholic can almost always arrange to be taken to a meeting in his or her community. Most AA members attend meetings several times a week and early in recovery attend at least one meeting per day. Lifelong activity in AA is the basis for maintaining health for many recovering alcoholics.

Meetings are usually 1 hour in length. Most are held in the evening, although there are many daytime meetings, especially early morning and lunchtime. Meetings begin with a recitation by a member of the Twelve Steps and the Twelve Traditions. Personal experiences related to alcoholism and the steps toward recovery are then described by a number of members.

The 12 Steps

1. We admitted we were powerless over alcohol, that our lives had become unmanageable.
2. Came to believe that a power greater than ourselves could restore us to sanity.
3. Made a decision to turn our will and our lives over to the care of God as we understood Him.
4. Made a searching and fearless moral inventory of ourselves.
5. Admitted to God, to ourselves, and to another human being the exact nature of our wrongs.
6. Were entirely ready to have God remove all these defects of character.
7. Humbly asked Him to remove our shortcomings.
8. Made a list of all persons we had harmed, and became willing to make amends to them all.
9. Made direct amends to such people wherever possible, except when to do so would injure them or others.
10. Continued to take personal inventory, and when we were wrong promptly admitted it.
11. Sought through prayer and meditation to improve our conscious contact with God, as we understood Him, praying only for knowledge of His will for us and the power to carry that out.
12. Having had a spiritual awakening as the result of the Steps, we tried to carry this message to alcoholics and to practice these principles in all our affairs.

The 12 Traditions

1. Our common welfare should come first; personal recovery depends on AA unity.
2. For our group purpose there is but one ultimate authority—a loving God as He may express Himself in our group conscience. Our leaders are but trusted servants; they do not govern.
3. The only requirement for AA membership is a desire to stop drinking.
4. Each group should be autonomous except in matters affecting other groups or AA as a whole.
5. Each group has but one primary purpose—to carry out its message to the alcoholic who still suffers.
6. An AA group ought never endorse, finance, or lend the AA name to any related facility or outside enterprise, lest problems of money, property, and prestige divert us from our primary purpose.
7. Every AA group ought to be fully self-supporting, declining outside contributions.
8. Alcoholics Anonymous should remain forever nonprofessional, but our service centers may employ special workers.
9. AA, as such, ought never to be organized, but we may create service boards or committees directly responsible to those they serve.
10. Alcoholics Anonymous has no opinion on outside issues; hence the AA name ought never be drawn into public controversy.
11. Our public relations policy is based on attraction rather than promotion; we need always maintain personal anonymity at the level of press, radio, and films.
12. Anonymity is the spiritual foundation of our Traditions, ever reminding us to place principles before personalities.

Figure 5.5. The process of Alcoholics Anonymous.

(i.e., clinical trials) is lacking (5, **96**). Nonetheless, patients who continue to attend AA after inpatient treatment have improved outcomes (97).

Many patients are reluctant to attend AA or a therapy group. When referring a patient to AA, it is important to convey familiarity with how AA works and that one has confidence in the program. Immediate action, taken while the patient is in the office, may consist of having the patient contact a family member or friend who is active in AA or telephoning the local AA office and having the patient request a contact to take him or her to a convenient AA meeting. The best way for providers to learn about these programs is to attend one or more AA meeting and, if available, open group therapy meetings. To locate such meetings, one can call the local AA office or look on the Internet at www.alcoholics-anonymous.org.

Counseling and Psychotherapy

Counseling or psychotherapy, in group or individual setting, is probably the most common form of alcohol treatment after self-help groups. Some groups are little more than self-help groups that are led by a trained counselor. Others use more structured psychotherapeutic approaches, particularly cognitive behavioral therapy and its variants (coping skills therapy, relapse prevention, etc.). More information on these approaches can be found in Chapter 4.

The evidence for the effectiveness of these psychosocial interventions is mixed, probably at least partly due to the heterogeneity of the programs. A study that compared alcoholics who attended a 6-week program of twice-weekly group counseling sessions with those who received a single confrontational interview did not find significant differences in alcohol use (98). On the other hand, a study comparing "standard treatment" of group and individual counseling with "minimal treatment" (an educational movie) found that the counseling was superior to minimal treatment (99).

Another study comparing advice with "extended therapy" (mainly in the form of group cognitive therapy; half also received inpatient treatment) found that the extended therapy was associated with improvement in alcohol-related problems after 1 year (**100**). A variant of cognitive behavioral therapy known as "relapse prevention" was judged to be effective in a meta-analysis that included nine studies of its use for alcoholics (**101**). However, some randomized controlled trials of cognitive behavioral therapy have failed to show a significant effect (102), even when it is targeted to individuals who are thought to benefit most (103). Furthermore, some studies of pharmacotherapy (i.e., naltrexone and acamprosate) suggest that these agents are just as effective when not accompanied by conventional psychotherapeutic interventions (104, 105).

Inpatient Rehabilitation

Treatment outcomes for alcoholism tend to be similar, regardless of setting (106). However, inpatient rehabilitation for 2 to 6 weeks may be especially helpful for some patients

(**107**). Indications for inpatient rehabilitation include unsuccessful or too slow recovery despite adequate outpatient treatment; weak support systems; danger to self or others; severe medical, psychiatric, or other problems related to the alcoholism; and possibly patient's desire for inpatient treatment (108). There is little data on the effectiveness of longer-term residential treatment, which can range from unstructured halfway houses to highly structured therapeutic communities.

Although treatment goals among inpatient rehabilitation programs vary, goals include breaking down denial, educating about alcoholism, providing an introduction to group treatment (self-help groups and group therapy), learning how to ask for help, learning how to communicate directly and honestly, learning how to enjoy life while abstinent, beginning the healing of relationships, and developing a specific, structured long-term recovery program.

Pharmacological Treatment of Alcohol Dependence

Pharmacological treatment for alcohol dependence should be considered in individuals who relapse despite being able to achieve sobriety for periods of time and who are active in behavioral therapy. Pharmacotherapy should be considered as an adjunct to treatment, rather than the focus of treatment. In the United States, three drugs are approved for use in the treatment of alcoholism—disulfiram, naltrexone, and acamprosate.

DISULFIRAM (ANTABUSE). Although controlled studies have not shown that it increases duration of sobriety (**109, 110**), the use of disulfiram to prevent drinking should be considered for some patients. Patients who are motivated to succeed in recovery and who have experienced relapse or dread the likelihood of relapse are candidates for disulfiram. Because disulfiram is taken once daily, it is a constant reminder that one cannot drink. Additionally, the decision not to drink has to be made only once a day. Patients must be in active recovery, including AA and individual or group therapy. Disulfiram is available, as Antabuse, in the form of scored tablets containing 250 or 500 mg.

Alcohol is initially metabolized by the hepatic enzyme alcohol dehydrogenase to acetaldehyde, and disulfiram inhibits acetaldehyde oxidation by interfering with aldehyde dehydrogenase. This effect may persist for up to 2 weeks after cessation of disulfiram. The symptoms of the alcohol–disulfiram reaction are the result of elevated acetaldehyde levels. Some individuals have typical symptoms after drinking only small amounts of alcohol. A small percentage of patients are able to drink despite taking disulfiram without significant symptoms. An alcohol–disulfiram reaction usually begins within 10 minutes of drinking and may last for up to several hours. Symptoms include flushing, headaches, anxiety, sweating, nausea, vomiting, dizziness, palpitations, hyperventilation, and confusion.

Disulfiram at recommended dosages of 250–500 mg/day is well tolerated by most patients. Contraindications for the use of disulfiram include diabetes, emphysema, seizures, significant liver or renal disease, coronary artery disease, pregnancy, or a history of drinking while taking disulfiram. If alcohol-related liver disease is present, prescribing of disulfiram should be delayed until the levels of serum aspartate aminotransferase (AST) and serum alanine aminotransferase (ALT) are less than three times the normal range. Disulfiram may impair the metabolism and potentiate the effects of caffeine, warfarin, ritonavir, and phenytoin, and it may worsen the neurological side effects of isoniazid (ataxia, psychosis). It should be used with caution in conjunction with alpha- or beta-adrenergic antagonists, vasodilators, sympathomimetic amines, monoamine oxidase inhibitors, tricyclic antidepressants, and neuroleptics. Patients on Antabuse should carefully avoid medications (cough syrups) and foods (e.g., salad dressings) that may contain alcohol.

NALTREXONE.   The opioid antagonist naltrexone (Revia) is potentially useful as an adjunct to a formal treatment program for individuals with alcohol dependence. Unlike disulfiram, patients do not become ill if they drink while taking naltrexone. Naltrexone may reduce alcohol craving and as a result may be useful in preventing relapse in motivated patients. Additionally, when patients relapse they tend to drink smaller amounts. A number of studies suggest that it is effective at reducing alcohol use in the short term (111, **112**). There is no data supporting naltrexone assisting in long-term abstinence; most studies have been small and have followed patients for only 3 to 6 months. A large multicenter study of alcoholic veterans did not find a benefit from using naltrexone over 1 year (**113**). Nevertheless, a recent Cochrane review of the use of opioid antagonists for alcoholism concluded that the evidence supports the use of naltrexone as a "short-term treatment for alcoholism" (114).

Naltrexone is an opiate antagonist and therefore it cannot be prescribed to patients on opioid analgesics, and patients maintained on naltrexone will not obtain pain relief if prescribed an opiate. Naltrexone is well tolerated, with nausea as its main side effect. Patients should be prescribed 25 mg (half tablet) a day for 2 days and 50 mg/day thereafter. Naltrexone can be used in combination with disulfiram. Although there is no clear evidence of hepatotoxicity, the manufacturers of naltrexone advise monitoring of liver function tests (initially at monthly intervals and then less frequently). If naltrexone is tolerated and is successful in diminishing drinking, the recommended initial course of treatment is 3 months. Naltrexone does not cause physical dependence and can be stopped at any time without withdrawal symptoms. If a patient is going to have elective surgery, naltrexone should be stopped at least 72 hours beforehand to allow the use of opiate analgesia.

ACAMPROSATE.   In 2004, the FDA approved acamprosate (calcium acetylhomotaurinate) as a treatment for chronic alcoholism. It has been available outside the United States for over a decade. Compliance is often a challenge, as acamprosate must be taken as 666 mg (two pills) three times a day. Most studies of acamprosate examine its utility in patients who have just completed detoxification. Results of studies are mixed with at best a modest benefit (**115–117**). One study of the combined use of acamprosate and naltrexone in relapse prevention had a dropout rate of over 50%, limiting the interpretation of its findings (118). Nevertheless, a recent meta-analysis of acamprosate concluded that it is an effective adjuvant therapy for alcoholism and significantly improves abstinence rate (119).

OTHER DRUGS. Many other pharmacological agents, including carbamazepine (120), have been studied in nonrandomized trials or in trials with small numbers of subjects. Agents not found useful include fluoxetine (121), buspirone (122), and lithium (123). However, several agents have been recently studied in randomized clinical trials with promising results. Topiramate, in a 12-week study of alcoholics, improved abstinence rates and reduced the amount of alcohol consumed among those who drank (**124**). Further studies are needed to confirm these findings. Side effects, including paresthesias, psychomotor slowing, and weight loss, are a barrier to its use. Ondansetron, a selective 5-HT3 serotonin receptor antagonist, has been reported to be effective (in one study) in a subgroup of subjects with early-onset alcoholism, increasing days of abstinence (125). This finding has not been confirmed in other randomized controlled trials, and the high cost of ondansetron has limited its use.

Although many alcoholics have symptoms such as anxiety, insomnia, and tremors, the use of sedatives should be avoided, as they interfere with successful recovery. All sedatives are cross-tolerant with alcohol and may trigger relapse. Additionally, combining sedatives with alcohol increases risk of respiratory depression, and the inability to control consumption, a key feature of alcoholism, occurs with prescribed sedative drugs too.

PREVENTION AND MANAGEMENT OF RELAPSE

After denial and motivating the patient to change, follow-up is the most difficult part of treatment. Patients often have a honeymoon period during which they feel and look so good that one is lulled into believing that regular follow-up is unnecessary. During the first 6 weeks after stopping drinking, patients need a great deal of support, as this is the time when they are at highest risk to relapse. Weekly patient phone contact is indicated for this time, with a gradually decreasing frequency thereafter. High-risk times for relapse include special days and occasions such as vacations, holidays, business trips, birthdays, anniversaries, or crises such as separation, divorce, death of a close person, or illness in the family.

The relapse process begins before the person drinks. This process often progresses in a predictable manner: reactivation of denial, progressive isolation and defensiveness, building a crisis to justify symptom progression, depressed mood, loss of control over behavior, and finally relapse to drinking. Relapse is part of the natural history of recovery and should not cause shame. Instead, one should immediately recruit the patient back into treatment using the same motivational techniques used initially. Relapse is a time to learn from mistakes and correct them by strengthening treatment.

REFERENCES

1. Substance Abuse and Mental Health Services Administration. 2004. *Results from the 2003 National Survey on Drug Use and Health: National Findings* (Office of Applied Studies, NSDUH Series H-25, DHHS Publication No. SMA 04-3964). Rockville, MD.
2. Naimi, T. S., R. D. Brewer, A. Mokdad, et al. 2003. Binge drinking among US adults. *JAMA* 289:70–75.
3. Secretary of Health and Human Services. 2000, June. *Tenth special report to the U.S. Congress on alcohol and health.* Washington, DC: U.S. Department of Health and Human Services.
4. Jellinek, E. M. 1952. Phases of alcohol addiction. *Q. J. Stud. Alcohol.* 13:673–684.
5. Vaillant, G. E., ed. 1996. *The natural history of alcoholism, revisited.* Cambridge, MA: Harvard University Press.
6. Blum, K., E. P. Noble, P. J. Sheridan, et al. 1990. Allelic association of human dopamine D2 receptor gene in alcoholism. *JAMA* 263:2055–2060.
7. Conneally, P. M. 1991. Association between the D2 dopamine receptor gene and alcoholism: A continuing controversy. *Arch. Gen. Psychiatry* 48:757–759.
8. Ammon, E., C. Schafer, U. Hofmann, and U. Klotz. 1996. Disposition and first-pass metabolism of ethanol in humans: Is it gastric or hepatic and does it depend on gender? *Clin. Pharmacol. Ther.* 59:503–513.
9. Turner, R. C., P. R. Lichstein, J. G. Peden, Jr., et al. 1989. Alcohol withdrawal syndromes: A review of pathophysiology, clinical presentation, and treatment. *J. Gen. Intern. Med.* 4:432–434.
10. Victor, M., and J. M. Hope. 1958. The phenomenon of auditory hallucinations in chronic alcoholism. *J. Nerv. Ment. Dis.* 126:451–481.
11. Saunders, J. B. 2000. Delirium tremens: Its aetiology, natural history and treatment. *Curr. Opin. Psych.* 13:629–633.
12. Johnson, B., and W. Clark. 1989. Alcoholism: A challenging physician–patient encounter. *J. Gen. Intern. Med.* 4:445–452.
13. Morse, R. M., and D. K. Flavin. 1992. The definition of alcoholism. *JAMA* 268:1012–1014.
14. American Psychiatric Association. 2000. *Diagnostic and statistical manual of mental disorders.* 4th ed. (DSM IV-TR). Washington, DC: American Psychiatric Association.
15. National Institute on Alcohol Abuse and Alcoholism. 1995. *The physician's guide to helping patients with alcohol problems* (NIH publication no. 95-3769). Washington, DC: Government Printing Office.
16. U.S. Preventive Services Task Force. 2004. Screening and behavioral counseling interventions in primary care to reduce alcohol misuse: Recommendation statement. *Ann. Intern. Med.* 140:554–556.
17. Mayfield, D. G., G. McLeod, and P. Hall. 1974. The CAGE questionnaire: Validation of a new alcoholism screening instrument. *Am. J. Psychiatry* 131:1121–1123.
18. Cyr, M. G., and S. A. Wartman. 1988. The effectiveness of routine screening questions in the detection of alcoholism. *JAMA* 259:51–54.

19. Buchsbaum, D. G., R. G. Buchanan, R. M. Centor, et al. 1991. Screening for alcohol abuse using CAGE scores and likelihood ratios. *Ann. Intern. Med.* 115:774–777.

20. Powers, J. S., and A. Spickard. 1984. Michigan Alcoholism Screening Test to diagnose early alcoholism in a general practice. *South. Med. J.* 77:852–856.

21. Saunders, J. B. 1993. Development of the Alcohol Use Disorders Identification Test (AUDIT). *Addiction* 88:791–804.

22. Bush, K., D. R. Kivlahan, M. B. McDonell, et al. 1998. The AUDIT alcohol consumption questions (AUDIT-C): An effective brief screening test for problem drinking. *Arch. Internal Med.* 158:1789–1795. *Among 243 male veterans, the three-item AUDIT-C, with a cutoff of 3, had a sensitivity of 90% and a specificity of 60% for alcohol dependence.*

23. Bradley, K. A., K. R. Bush, A. J. Epler, et al. 2003. Two brief screening tests from the Alcohol Use Disorders Identification Test (AUDIT). *Arch. Intern. Med.* 163:821–829.

24. Bradley, K. A., J. Boyd-Wickizer, S. H. Powell, and M. L. Burman. 1998. Alcohol screening questionnaires in women. A critical review. *JAMA* 280;166–171.

25. Steinbauer, J. R., S. B. Cantor, C. E. Holzer, and R. J. Volk. 1998. Ethnic and sex bias in primary care screening tests for alcohol use disorders. *Ann. Intern. Med.* 128:353–362.

26. Beresford, T. P., F. C. Blow, E. Hill, et al. 1990. Comparison of CAGE questionnaire and computer assisted laboratory profiles in screening for covert alcoholism. *Lancet* 336:482–485. *Nine hundred fifteen adults were studied; 244 were alcohol dependent. The CAGE (≥2 positive answers) was 76% sensitive and 94% specific with a positive predictive value of 87%. No laboratory value had a significant predictive value.*

27. Huseby, N. E., O. Nilssen, A. Erfurth, et al. 1997. Carbohydrate-deficient transferrin and alcohol dependency: Variation in response to alcohol intake among different groups of patients. *Alcoholism Clin. Exp. Res.* 21.201–205. *Sensitivity of carbohydrate-deficient transferrin (CDT) was 75% for patients admitted for alcohol detoxification but less than 50% for alcoholics admitted for surgery. In both groups, sensitivity was worse for women and patients under age 35.*

28. Murkamal, K. J., K. M. Conigrave, M. A. Mittleman, et al. 2003. Role of drinking pattern and type of alcohol consumed in coronary heart disease in men. *N. Engl. J. Med.* 348.109–118.

29. Hart, R. G., L. A. Pearce, R. McBride, et al. 1999. Factors associated with ischemic stroke during aspirin therapy in atrial fibrillation: Analysis of 2012 participants in the SPAF I-III clinical trials. *Stroke* 30:1223–1229.

30. Schaeffner, E. S., T. Kurth, P. E. de Jong, et al. 2005. Alcohol consumption and the risk of renal dysfunction in apparently healthy men. *Arch. Intern. Med.* 165:1048–1053.

31. Klatsky, A. L., M. A. Armstrong, and G. D. Friedman. 1992. Alcohol and mortality. *Ann. Intern. Med.* 117:646–654. *In this prospective cohort study of 128,934 Californians comparing those who drank more than six drinks per day with nondrinkers, the relative risk of death from noncardiovascular causes was 1.6. For women, the relative risk was 2.2, and for those aged under 50, 1.9.*

32. Hurt, R. D., K. P. Offord, I. T. Croghan, et al. 1996. Mortality following inpatient addictions treatment. Role of tobacco use in a community based cohort. *JAMA* 275:1097–1103.

33. Singletary, K. W., and S. M. Gapstur. 2001. Alcohol and breast cancer: Review of epidemiologic and experimental evidence and potential mechanisms. *JAMA* 286:2143–2151. *Review of epidemiologic data, with emphasis on 26 papers (case-control and cohort) published since 1995. Relative risk ranged from 0.6 to 4.0. Taking into account differences in study design, there appears to be increased risk for breast cancer in women who consume more than three drinks per day.*

34. Cho, E., S. A. Smith-Warner, J. Ritz, et al. 2004. Alcohol intake and colorectal cancer: A pooled analysis of 8 cohort studies. *Ann. Intern. Med.* 140:603–613. *Pooled analysis of eight cohorts in North America and Europe, n = 489,979; multivariate relative risk for colorectal CA was increased in those who drank more than 2 drinks per day—1.16 for those who consumed 2–2.5 drinks per day and 1.41 for those who drank more than 2.5 drinks per day.*

35. Bullock, K. D., R. J. Reed, and I. Grant. 1992. Reduced mortality risk in alcoholics who achieve long-term abstinence. *JAMA* 267:668–672. *Eleven-year follow-up of cohort of 199 alcoholic veterans—101 relapsed and 98 stayed abstinent. Standardized mortality ratios were 4.96 for relapsed group and 1.25 for abstinent group.*

36. Randin, D., P. Vollenweider, L. Tappy, et al. 1995. Suppression of alcohol-induced hypertension by dexamethasone. *N. Engl. J. Med.* 332:1733–1737. *Nine normal subjects received infusions of alcohol following the infusion of placebo or dexamethasone. Alcohol caused a mean increase of 10±5 mm Hg in the placebo group with no change in dexamethasone group. Sympathetic–nerve action potentials also increased significantly in the placebo group, suggesting that alcohol causes pressor effects through a centrally mediated mechanism.*

37. Puddey, I. B., L. J. Beilin, and R. Vandongen. 1987. Regular alcohol use raises blood pressure in treated hypertensive subjects: A randomized controlled trial. *Lancet* 1:647–651.

38. Reynolds, K., L. B. Lewis, J. D. L. Nolen, et al. 2003. Alcohol consumption and risk of stroke—A meta-analysis. *JAMA* 289:579–588. *Meta-analysis of 35 cohort or case-control studies showed that consumption of approximately 60 grams of alcohol (4–5 drinks/day) was associated with an increased relative risk of total stroke (1.64), ischemic stroke (1.69), and hemorrhagic stroke (2.18).*

39. Minami, J., M. Yoshii, M. Todooki, et al. 2002. Effects of alcohol restriction on ambulatory blood pressure, heart rate and heart rate variability in Japanese men. *Am. J. Hypertens.* 15:125–129. *Randomized crossover study of 33 men, who drank more than 30 ml/day of alcohol (average 70). After 3 weeks of maintaining alcohol intake, participants either continued or reduced intake by at least 50% for 3 weeks. Systolic blood pressure decreased 4 mm in reduced-alcohol period.*

40. Seventh Report of the Joint National Committee on Prevention, Detection, Evaluation, and Treatment of High Blood Pressure. 2003. *Hypertension* 42:1206–1252.

41. McKenna, C. J., M. B. Codd, H. A. McCann, and D. D. Sugrue. 1998. Alcohol consumption and idiopathic dilated cardiomyopathy: A case control study. *Am. Heart J.* 135:833–837.

42. Walsh, C. R., M. G. Larson, and J. C. Evans. 2002. Alcohol consumption and risk for congestive heart failure in the Framingham Study. *Ann. Intern. Med.* 136:181–191. *Follow-up of 26,035 person-years in men and 35,563 person-years in women showing no increased risk for congestive heart failure in men who drink more than 15 drinks per week and women who drink more than 8. This study was not designed to look at risk in patients with alcoholism who drink far more than these amounts.*

43. Djousse, L., D. Levy, E. J. Benjamin, et al. 2004. Long-term alcohol consumption and the risk of atrial fibrillation in the Framingham Study. *Am. J. Cardiol.* 93:710–713. *Of those who drank more than three drinks per day, the relative risk of having an episode of atrial fibrillation was 1.34. There was no increase in risk with lesser amounts of alcohol intake.*

44. Frost, L., and P. Vestergaard. 2004. Alcohol and risk of atrial fibrillation or flutter. *Arch. Intern. Med.* 164:1993–1998. *In this study of 49,949 participants followed for almost 6 years (mean age 56), men in the highest quintile of alcohol intake had adjusted hazard ratio of 1.46 for developing atrial fibrillation/flutter, but there was no increased risk for women at any level of alcohol intake.*

45. Becker, U., A. Deis, T. I. Sorenseon, et al. 1996. Prediction of risk of liver disease by alcohol intake, sex and age: A prospective population study. *Hepatology* 23:1025–1029. *Over 12 years, women who consumed 28 to 40 drinks per week had a relative risk for cirrhosis of 17, compared to 7 in men.*

46. Norton, R., R. Batey, T. Dwyer, and S. MacMahon. 1987. Alcohol consumption and the risk of alcohol-related cirrhosis in women. *BMJ* 295:80–82.

47. Fingerhood, M. I., J. T. Sullivan, and D. R. Jasinski. 1993. Prevalence of hepatitis C in a chemical dependence population. *Arch. Intern. Med.* 153:2025–2030.

48. Orrego, H., J. E. Blake, L. M. Blendis, et al. 1987. Long-term treatment of alcoholic liver disease with propylthiouracil. *N. Engl. J. Med.* 317:1421–1427. *Three hundred ten patients with alcoholic liver disease were randomized to propylthiouracil (PTU, 300 mg/day) or placebo for 2 years. Dropout rates were high—68% in PTU group and 60% on placebo. Those receiving PTU had a lower mortality rate (13% vs. 25%; p < 0.05), but the benefit was limited to those who were abstinent from alcohol.*

49. Akriviadis, E., R. Botla, W. Briggs, et al. 2000. Pentoxifylline improves short-term survival in severe acute alcoholic hepatitis: A double-blind, placebo-controlled trial. *Gastroenterology* 119:1637–1648. *One hundred one patients hospitalized with severe alcoholic hepatitis were randomized to pentoxifylline (400 mg, 3 times/day) or placebo; those on treatment had reduced in-hospital mortality (25% vs. 46%).*

50. Rambaldi, A., G. Iaquinto, and C. Gluud. 2002. Anabolic-androgenic steroids for alcoholic liver disease: A Cochrane review. *Am. J. Gastroenterol.* 97:1674–1681. *Meta-analysis of five randomized clinical trials comparing anabolic androgens and placebo;*

there were no differences in mortality or other outcome measures between the groups.

51. Menon, K. V., L. Stadheim, P. S. Kamath, et al. 2004. A pilot study of the safety and tolerability of etanercept in patients with alcoholic hepatitis. *Am. J. Gastroenterol.* 99:255–260. *Thirteen patients with moderate or severe alcoholic hepatitis were given etanercept (32 mg/m² intravenously on day 1, followed by 25 mg subcutaneously on days 4, 8, and 12); 30-day survival was 92% (12/13). Three patients dropped out due to decompensation or bleeding.*

52. Naveau, S., S. Chollet-Martin, S. Dharancy, et al. 2004. A double-blind randomized controlled trial of infliximab associated with prednisolone in acute hepatitis. *Hepatology* 39:1390–1397. *Thirty-six alcoholics with acute hepatitis were randomized to infliximab with prednisolone or placebo with prednisolone. The study was stopped because of a high rate of infection and death in the infliximab group.*

53. Carithers, R. L., Jr., H. F. Herlong, A. M. Diehl, et al. 1989. Methylprednisolone therapy in patients with severe alcoholic hepatitis. A randomized multicenter trial. *Ann. Intern. Med.* 110:685–690. *Sixty-six patients hospitalized with severe alcoholic hepatitis were randomized to methylprednisolone (32 mg/day for 28 days followed by 12-day taper) or placebo; 28-day mortality was 11/31 for placebo group and 2/35 for treatment group (p = 0.006). Among those with hepatic encephalopathy, mortality was 9/19 on placebo and 1/14 on treatment (p = 0.02).*

54. Ramond, M. J., T. Poynard, B. Rueff, et al. 1992. A randomized trial of prednisolone in patients with severe alcoholic hepatitis. *N. Engl. J. Med.* 326:507–512. *Sixty-four alcoholics with biopsy-proven alcoholic hepatitis and either encephalopathy (n = 19) or discriminant-function score greater than 32 were randomized to prednisolone (40 mg/day for 28 days) or placebo. Mortality at 66 days was lower among those on prednisolone (13% vs. 50%).*

55. Mendenhall, C. L., S. Anderson, P. Garcia-Pont, et al. 1984. Short-term and long-term survival in patients with alcoholic hepatitis treated with oxandrolone and prednisolone. *N. Engl. J. Med.* 311:1464–1470. *Two hundred sixty-three patients with alcoholic hepatitis were randomized to 30 days of treatment with oxandrolone, prednisolone, or placebo; there was no difference in 30-day mortality for either treatment group when compared to placebo.*

56. Cabre, E., P. Rodriguez-Iglesias, and J. Caballeria. 2000. Short- and long-term outcome of severe alcohol-induced hepatitis treated with steroids or enteral nutrition: A multicenter randomized trial. *Hepatology* 32:36–42. *Seventy-one patients were randomized to prednisolone 40 mg/day or enteral feeding at 2000 kcal/day for 28 days; 80% had cirrhosis. There was no difference in mortality: 9/36 in steroid group and 11/35 in enteral feeding group.*

57. Imperiale, T. F., and A. J. McCullough. 1990. Do corticosteroids reduce mortality from alcoholic hepatitis? A meta-analysis of the randomized trials. *Ann. Intern. Med.* 113:299–307. *Analysis of 11 studies (10 placebo-controlled) showed a 37% reduction in mortality with corticosteroids. However, among those without hepatic*

encephalopathy, no study showed benefit, and patients with gas-
trointestinal bleeding were almost uniformly excluded.

58. Christensen, E., and C. Gluud. 1995. Glucocorticoids are ineffec-
tive in alcoholic hepatitis. A meta-analysis adjusting for confounding variables. *Gut* 37:113–118.

59. Mathurin, P., C. L. Mendenall, R. L. Carithers, et al. 2002.
Corticosteroids improve short-term survival in patients with severe alcoholic hepatitis (AH): Individual data analysis of the last
three randomized placebo-controlled trials of corticosteroids in
severe AH. *J. Hepatology* 36:480–487. *Meta-analysis of three
studies of 215 patients with severe alcoholic hepatitis treated
with corticosteroids or placebo; 28-day survival was higher in the
treated group (84.6% vs. 65.1%; p = 0.001).*

60. McCullough, A. J., and J. F. O'Connor. 1998. Alcoholic liver disease: Proposed recommendations for the American College of
Gastroenterology. *Am. J. Gastroenterol.* 93:2022–2036.

61. Kershenobich, D., F. Vargas, G. Garcia-Tsao, et al. 1988.
Colchicine in the treatment of cirrhosis of the liver. *N. Engl. J.
Med.* 318:1709–1713. *One hundred patients with cirrhosis were
randomized to colchicine (1 mg/day, 5 days/week) or placebo; 54
had alcoholic cirrhosis (no separate analysis of these). Median
survival was longer in the colchicine group (11 vs. 3.5 years; p <
.001). Colchicine was well tolerated.*

62. Cortez-Pinto, H., P. Alexandrino, M. E. Camilo, et al. 2002. Lack
of effect of colchicine in alcoholic cirrhosis: Final results of a double blind randomized trial. *Eur. J. Gastroenterol. Hepatol.*
14:377–381. *Fifty-five patients with alcoholic cirrhosis were randomized to colchicine (1 mg/day for 5 days/week) or placebo;
there was no significant difference in 3-year survival.*

63. The U.S. Organ Procurement and Transplantation Network
and the Scientific Registry of Transplant Recipients.
Transplant statistics: 2003 annual report. Available at http://
www.ustransplant.org

64. Levy, L. J., J. Duga, M. Girgis, and E. E. Gordon. 1973.
Ketoacidosis associated with alcoholism in non diabetic sub
jects. *Ann. Intern. Med.* 78:213–219.

65. Arroyo, V., M. Guevara, and P. Gines. 2002. Hepatorenal syndrome
in cirrhosis: Pathogenesis and treatment. *Gastroenterology*
122:1658–1676.

66. Meyer, J. S., N. Tanahashi, Y. Ishikawa, et al. 1985. Cerebral at
rophy and hypoperfusion improve during treatment of
Wernicke-Korsakoff syndrome. *J. Cereb. Blood Flow Metab.*
5:376–385.

67. Ng, S. K., W. A. Hauser, J. C. Brust, et al. 1988. Alcohol consumption and withdrawal in new onset seizures. *N. Engl. J. Med.*
319:666–673.

68. Earnest, M. P., H. Feldman, J. A. Marx, et al. 1988. Intracranial
lesions shown by CT scans in 259 cases of first alcohol-related
seizures. *Neurology* 38:1561–1565.

69. Nunes, E. V., and F. R. Levin. 2004. Treatment of depression in
patients with alcohol or other drug dependence. A meta-analysis. *JAMA* 291:1887–1896.

70. Matsuo, K., T. Hirohata, Y. Sugioka, et al. 1988. Influence of alcohol
intake, cigarette smoking, and occupational status on idiopathic

osteonecrosis of the femoral head. *Clin. Orthoped.* 234:115–123. *Comparison of 112 patients with idiopathic osteonecrosis with 168 matched hospital controls. Regular drinkers had elevated risk for osteonecrosis (RR = 7.8, p < .001) with linear effect—RRs were 3.3, 9.8, and 17.9 for drinking 0–400, 400–1000, and >1000 ml/week of alcohol, respectively.*

71. Kelepouris, N., K. D. Harper, F. Gannon, et al. 1995. Severe osteoporosis in men. *Ann. Intern. Med.* 123:452–460.

72. Felson, D. T., Y. Zhanh, M. T. Hannan, et al. 1995. Alcohol intake and bone mineral density in elderly men and women. The Framingham study. *Am. J. Epidemiol.* 142:485–492. *Among 1154 Framingham participants, women who drank at least 7 ounces of alcohol per week had higher bone densities at most sites (mean 7.7%) when compared to women who drank less than 1 ounce per week.*

73. Choi, H. K., K. Atkinson, E. W. Karlson, et al. 2004. Alcohol intake and risk of incident gout in men: A prospective study. *Lancet* 363:1277–1281. *Forty-seven thousand one hundred fifty men with 730 cases of gout were followed over 12 years. Relative risk of gout compared to nondrinkers was 1.96 for those who consumed 1–2 drinks per day and 2.53 for more than 2 drinks per day. Beer consumption had the highest risk and wine the least, with no increased risk in those who drank one glass of wine per day.*

74. Sokol, R. J., V. Delaney-Black, and B. Nordstrom. 2003. Fetal alcohol spectrum disorder. *JAMA* 290:2996–2999.

75. Bertholet, N., J. B. Daeppen, V. Wietlisbach, et al. 2005. Reduction of alcohol consumption by brief alcohol intervention in primary care: Systematic review and meta-analysis. *Arch. Intern. Med.* 165:986–995.

76. Hayashida, M., A. I. Alterman, T. McLellan, et al. 1989. Comparative effectiveness and costs of inpatient and outpatient detoxification of patients with mild to moderate alcohol withdrawal syndrome. *N. Engl. J. Med.* 320:358–365.

77. Fiellin, D. A., P. G. O'Connor, E. S. Holboe, and R. I. Horwitz. 2002. Risk for delirium tremens in patients with alcohol withdrawal syndrome. *Subst. Abuse* 23:83–94. *Fifteen patients with delirium tremens (DT) were compared with 45 uncomplicated alcohol withdrawal controls. Cases were more likely to report prior complicated withdrawal (DT or alcohol withdrawal seizure) (53% vs. 27%; OR 3.1), have a systolic blood pressure greater than 145 mm Hg on admission (60% vs. 27%; OR 4.1), and have comorbidity scores of at least 1 (60% vs. 18%; OR 6.9).*

78. Sullivan, J. T., K. Sykora, J. Schneiderman, et al. 1989. Assessment of alcohol withdrawal: The revised clinical institute withdrawal assessment for alcohol scale (CIWA Ar). *Br. J. Addict.* 84:1353–1357.

79. Mayo-Smith, M. F., for the American Society of Addiction Medicine Workshop Group on Pharmacologic Management of Alcohol Withdrawal. 1997. Pharmacologic management of alcohol withdrawal. A meta-analysis and evidence-based medicine practice guideline. *JAMA* 278:144–151.

80. Mayo-Smith, M. F., L. H. Beecher, T. L. Fischer, et al. 2004. Management of alcohol withdrawal delirium. An evidence-based

practice guideline. *Arch. Intern. Med.* 164:1405–1412. *Meta-analysis of nine prospective controlled trials; neuroleptics, when used in setting of alcohol withdrawal delirium, carry a relative risk of death of 6.6 compared to benzodiazepines. There were no deaths in any study using benzodiazepines.*

81. Saitz, R., M. F. Mayo Smith, M. S. Roberts, et al. 1994. Individualized treatment for alcohol withdrawal. A randomized double-blind controlled trial. *JAMA* 272:519–523. *One hundred one consecutive admissions for inpatient treatment of alcohol withdrawal were randomized to chlordiazepoxide in response to symptoms or every 6 hours (50 mg doses × 4 and 25 mg doses × 8). The symptom-triggered group received less medication than the fixed-dose (mean of 100 mg vs. 425 mg; p < 0.001).*

82. Robinson, B. J., G. M. Robinson, T. J. Maling, and R. H. Johnson. 1989. Is clonidine useful in the treatment of alcohol withdrawal? *Alcohol Clin. Exp. Res.* 13:95–98. *Thirty-two patients were randomized to clonidine or chlormethiazole for treatment of alcohol withdrawal. There were no complications in chlormethiazole group, but clonidine group had 8 patient failures—2 seizures, 2 hallucinosis, 3 hypotension, and 1 drowsiness.*

83. Kraus, M. L., L. D. Gottlieb, R. I. Horwitz, and M. Anscher. 1985. Randomized clinical trial of atenolol in patients with alcohol withdrawal. *N. Engl. J. Med.* 313:905–909.

84. Horwitz, R. I., L. D. Gottlieb, and M. L. Kraus. 1989. The efficacy of atenolol in the outpatient management of the alcohol withdrawal syndrome: Results of a randomized clinical trial. *Arch. Intern. Med.* 149:1089–1093.

85. Worner, T. M. 1994. Propranolol versus diazepam in the management of the alcohol withdrawal syndrome: Double-blind controlled trial. *Am. J. Drug Alcohol Abuse* 20:114–124.

86. Malcolm, R., J. C. Ballenger, E. T. Sturgis, and R. Anton. 1989. Double-blind controlled trial comparing carbamazepine to oxazepam treatment of alcohol withdrawal. *Am. J. Psychiatry* 146:617–621.

87. Stuppaeck, C. H., R. Pycha, C. Miller, et al. 1992. Carbamazepine versus oxazepam in the treatment of alcohol withdrawal: A double-blind study. *Alcohol Alcohol.* 27:153–158.

88. Malcolm, R., H. Myrick, J. Roberts, et al. 2002. The effects of carbamazepine and lorazepam on single versus multiple previous alcohol withdrawals in an outpatient randomized trial. *J. Gen Intern. Med.* 17:349–355. *One hundred thirty-six alcoholics were stratified by number of previous detoxifications and randomized to a 5-day taper beginning with (1) carbamazepine 600–800 mg/day or (2) lorazepam 6–8 mg/day. The two were equally effective for symptoms of withdrawal; patients assigned to carbamazepine had fewer rebound symptoms and drank less in the week after treatment.*

89. Reoux, J. P., A. J. Saxon, C. A. Malte, et al. 2001. Divalproex sodium in alcohol withdrawal: A randomized double-blind placebo-controlled clinical trial. *Alcohol Clin. Exp. Res.* 23:1324–1329.

90. Bonnet, U., M. Banger, M. Lewek, et al. 2003. Treatment of acute alcohol withdrawal with gabapentin: Results from a controlled two-center trial. *J. Clin. Psychopharmacol.* 23:514–519. *Sixty-*

one patients were randomized to gabapentin 400 mg four times per day or placebo, in addition to symptom-driven clomethiazole. There was no difference in consumption of clomethiazole or in alleviating withdrawal symptoms.

91. Trumpler, F., S. Oez, P. Stahli, et al. 2003. Acupuncture for alcohol withdrawal: A randomized controlled trial. *Alcohol Alcohol.* 38:369–375. *Forty-eight inpatients undergoing alcohol withdrawal were randomized to laser acupuncture, needle acupuncture, or sham laser acupuncture; there were no differences in intensity or duration of withdrawal or in use of medication.*

92. Sampliner, R., and F. Iber. 1974. Diphenylhydantoin control of alcohol withdrawal seizures. *JAMA* 230:1430–1432.

93. Alldredge, B. K., D. H. Lowenstein, and R. P. Simon. 1989. Placebo-controlled trial of intravenous diphenylhydantoin for short-term treatment of alcohol withdrawal seizures. *Am. J. Med.* 87:645–648. *Ninety patients who had an alcohol withdrawal seizure within 6 hours of presentation were randomized to intravenous infusion of placebo or 1 g diphenylhydantoin. After 12 hours of observation, 6/45 patients in each group had a seizure.*

94. Sellers, E. M., C. A. Naranjo, M. Harrison, et al. 1983. Diazepam loading: Simplified treatment of alcohol withdrawal. *Clin. Pharmacol. Ther.* 34:822–826.

95. D'Onofrio, G., N. K. Rathlev, A. S. Ulrich, et al. 1999. Lorazepam for the prevention of recurrent seizures related to alcohol. *N. Engl. J. Med.* 340:915–919. *One hundred eighty-six inpatients after alcohol withdrawal seizure were randomized to 2 mg lorazepam intravenously or placebo. In subsequent 6 hours, those in the lorazepam group had a lower rate of recurrent seizure (3% vs. 24%; odds ratio of 10.4).*

96. Hoffmann, N. G., P. A. Harrison, and C. A. Belille. 1983. Alcoholics Anonymous after treatment: Attendance and abstinence. *Int. J. Addict.* 18:311–318. *In a cohort of 900 alcoholics who completed inpatient detoxification, at 6 months, 73% of those who attended AA at least once per week were abstinent, compared to 33% of those who attended less than once per week.*

97. Gossop, M., J. Harris, D. Best, et al. 2003. Is attendance at alcoholics anonymous meetings after inpatient treatment related to improved outcomes? A 6-month follow-up study. *Alcohol Alcohol.* 38:421–426.

98. Chapman, P. L. H., and I. Huygens. 1988. An evaluation of three treatment programmes for alcoholism: An experimental study with 6- and 18-month follow-ups. *Br. J. Addict.* 83:67–81.

99. Davis, W. T., L. Campbell, J. Tax, and C. S. Lieber. 2002. A trial of "standard" outpatient alcoholism treatment vs. a minimal treatment control. *J. Subst. Abuse Treat.* 23:9–19.

100. Chick, J., B. Ritson, J. Connaughton, et al. 1988. Advice versus extended treatment for alcoholism: A controlled trial. *Br. J. Addict.* 83:159–170. *One hundred fifty-two alcoholics were stratified by severity of dependence and marital status and randomized to (1) brief advice (5 min), (2) amplified advice (30–60 min), or (3) extended treatment (advice plus detox if needed, and group therapy). After 1 year the extended treatment group had significantly fewer alcohol-related problems, but not reduced al-*

cohol consumption; however, the 21% in the advice arms who severely deteriorated were given more intensive treatment.

101. Irvin, J. E., C. A. Bowers, M. E. Dunn, and M. C. Wang. 1999. Efficacy of relapse prevention: A meta-analytic review. *J. Consult. Clin. Psychol.* 67:563–570. *Twenty-six studies with 9504 subjects were included; 9 studies were of alcoholics. Relapse prevention was found to be effective for alcoholics.*

102. Burtscheidt, W., W. Wolwer, R. Schwarz, et al. 2002. Out-patient behaviour therapy in alcoholism: Treatment outcome after 2 years. *Acta Psychiatr. Scand.* 106:227–232.

103. Kadden, R. M., M. D. Litt, N. L. Cooney, et al. 2001. Prospective matching of alcoholic clients to cognitive-behavioral or interactional group therapy. *J. Stud. Alcohol.* 62:359–369.

104. O'Malley, S. S., B. J. Rounsaville, C. Farren, et al. 2003. Initial maintenance naltrexone treatment for alcohol dependence using primary care vs. specialty care: A nested sequence of 3 randomized trials. *Arch. Intern. Med.* 163:1695–1704.

105. De Wildt, W. A. J. M., G. M. Schippers, W. Van den Brink, et al. 2002. Does psychosocial treatment enhance the efficacy of acamprosate in patients with alcohol problems? *Alcohol Alcohol.* 37:375–382.

106. Longabaugh, R., B. McCrady, E. Fink, et al. 1983. Cost effectiveness of alcoholism treatment in partial vs. inpatient settings. Six-month outcomes. *J. Stud. Alcohol.* 44:1049–1071.

107. Walsh, D. C., R. W. Hingson, D. M. Merrigan, et al. 1991. A randomized trial of treatment options for alcohol abusing workers. *N. Engl. J. Med.* 325:775–782. *Two hundred twenty-seven workers identified by an employee assistance program as needing treatment for alcohol abuse were randomized to (1) inpatient treatment, (2) Alcoholics Anonymous (AA) meetings, or (3) their choice of treatment. All three groups improved, with no difference in job-related outcomes, but the inpatient group was less likely to need further inpatient treatment in follow-up—23% vs. 38% of the choice group and 63% of the AA group.*

108. Finney, J. W., A. C. Hahn, and R. H. Moos. 1996. The effectiveness of inpatient and outpatient treatment for alcohol abuse: The need to focus on mediators and moderators of setting effects. *Addiction* 91:1773–1796.

109. Fuller, R. K., and H. P. Roth. 1979. Disulfiram for the treatment of alcoholism: An evaluation of 128 men. *Ann. Intern. Med.* 90:901–904. *One hundred twenty-eight alcoholic men were randomized to (1) disulfiram 250 mg/day, (2) disulfiram 1 mg/day, or (3) no medication. There was no significant difference in abstinence rates by intention-to-treat; however, abstinence rates were higher among those who took the disulfiram than among those who did not.*

110. Fuller, R. K., L. Branchey, D. R. Brightwell, et al. 1986. Disulfiram treatment of alcoholism. A Veterans Administration cooperative study. *JAMA* 256:1449–1455. *Six hundred five men were randomized to disulfiram 250 mg/day, placebo, or no medication (all received behavioral counseling); there was no difference in total abstinence or time to first drink.*

111. O'Connor, P. G., C. K. Farren, B. J. Rounsanville, and S. S. O'Mallory. 1997. A preliminary investigation of the management

of alcohol dependence with naltrexone by primary care providers. *Am. J. Med.* 103:477–482.

112. Volpicelli, J. R., A. I. Alterman, M. Hayashida, et al. 1992. Naltrexone in the treatment of alcohol dependence. *Arch. Gen. Psychiatry* 49:876–880. *Seventy patients who completed alcohol detoxification were randomized to naltrexone (50 mg/day) or placebo and treated for 12 weeks; 14/35 on placebo and 11/35 on naltrexone did not finish the study. Among those who did complete the study, fewer on naltrexone relapsed (11% vs. 54%), but the study did not have sufficient power to show significance.*

113. Krystal, J. H., J. A. Cramer, W. F. Krol, et al. 2001. Naltrexone in the treatment of alcohol dependence. *N. Engl. J. Med.* 345:1734–1739. *Six hundred twenty-seven veterans (97% male) were randomized to 12 months of naltrexone (50 mg daily), 3 months of naltrexone followed by 9 months of placebo, or 12 months of placebo. All were offered individual counseling and were encouraged to attend AA meetings. At 13 weeks, there were no differences in days to relapse, and at 52 weeks, there were no differences in drinking days or number of drinks per drinking day.*

114. Srisurapanont, M., and N. Jarusuraisin. 2005. Opioid antagonists for alcohol dependence. *The Cochrane Database of Systematic Reviews.* Issue 1. Art. No.: CD001867.

115. Tempesta, E., L. Janiri, A. Bignamini, et al. 2000. Acamprosate and relapse prevention in the treatment of alcohol dependence: A placebo-controlled study. *Alcohol Alcohol.* 35:202–209. *Three hundred thirty alcoholics after detoxification were randomized to acamprosate 666 mg three times per day or placebo; all received counseling. At 6 months, abstinence rate was higher in the acamprosate group (58% vs. 45%). Three months after the end of the study (with no medication), there was no difference between the groups.*

116. Gual, A., and P. Lehert. 2001. Acamprosate during and after acute alcohol withdrawal: A double-blind placebo-controlled study in Spain. *Alcohol Alcohol.* 36:413–418. *Two hundred ninety-six alcoholics after detoxification were randomized to acamprosate (666 mg 3x/day) or placebo for 180 days; all received counseling. One hundred ten patients dropped out of the study. With intent-to-treat analysis, mean abstinence duration was longer for the acamprosate group (93 vs. 74 days; p = 0.006). Full abstinence was achieved by more individuals in the acamprosate group (53 vs. 26; p = 0.068).*

117. Chick, J., H. Howlett, M. Y. Morgan, et al. 2000. United Kingdom multicentre acamprosate study: A 6-month prospective study of acamprosate versus placebo in preventing relapse after withdrawal from alcohol. *Alcohol Alcohol.* 35:176–187. *Five hundred eighty-one alcoholics were randomized to acamprosate (666 mg 3x/day) or placebo; all received counseling. Treatment was initiated on average 24 days after detoxification. Compliance was poor with only 57% of patients taking at least 90% of pills by week 2. There was no difference in outcomes between groups, with complete abstinence rates of 12% for acamprosate group versus 11% on placebo.*

118. Kiefer, F., H. Jahn, and T. Tarnaske. 2003. Comparing and combining naltrexone and acamprosate in relapse prevention of alcoholism. *Arch. Gen. Psychiatry* 60:92–99.

119. Bouza, C., M. Angeles, A. Munoz, and J. M. Amate. 2004. Efficacy and safety of naltrexone and acamprosate in the treatment of alcohol dependence: A systematic review. *Addiction* 99:811–828.

120. Mueller, T. I., R. L. Stout, S. Rudden, et al. 1997. A double-blind placebo-controlled study of carbamezepine for the treatment of alcohol dependence. *Alcohol Clin. Exp. Res.* 21:86–92.

121. Kranzler, H. R., J. A. Burleson, P. Korner, et al. 1995. Placebo-controlled trial of fluoxetine as an adjunct to relapse prevention in alcoholics. *Am. J. Psychiatry* 152:391–397.

122. Malec, E., T. Malec, M. A. Gagne, and M. Dongier. 1996. Buspirone in the treatment of alcohol dependence: A placebo-controlled trial. *Alcohol Clin. Exp. Res.* 20:307–312.

123. Dorus, W., D. G. Ostrow, R. Anton, et al. 1989. Lithium treatment of depressed and non-depressed alcoholics. *JAMA* 262:1646–1652.

124. Johnson, B. A., N Ait-Daoud, C, L. Bowden, et al. 2003. Oral topiramate for treatment of alcohol dependence: A randomised controlled trial. *Lancet* 361:1677–1685. *One hundred fifty alcoholics were randomized to topiramate at escalating doses of 25–300 mg/day or placebo. Those on topiramate had significantly fewer drinks per day, fewer drinks per drinking day, and more days abstinent (44.2% vs. 18.0%).*

125. Johnson, B. A., J. D. Roache, M. A. Javors, et al. 2000. Ondansetron for reduction of drinking among biologically predisposed alcoholic patients: A randomized controlled trial. *JAMA* 284:963–971. *Three hundred twenty-one alcoholics were enrolled and 271 randomized to 11 weeks of ondansetron 1, 4, or 16 μg/kg twice daily or placebo. There was no improvement among those with late-onset alcoholism, but at all three doses, those with early-onset alcoholism on ondansetron had fewer drinks per day and fewer drinks per drinking day; only the 4 μg/kg group had significantly fewer drinking days when compared to placebo (50% vs. 70%).*

6

Sedative-Hypnotics

BACKGROUND

The sedative-hypnotics are central nervous system (CNS) depressants and include benzodiazepine, barbiturates, and other agents. Table 6.1 shows a list of commonly used non-benzodiazepine sedative-hypnotics; the benzodiazepines are listed in Table 6.2. These agents are used therapeutically at low doses for treatment of anxiety, panic disorder, and insomnia and at higher doses for sedation or anesthesia. Sedative-hypnotics are also used for treating status epilepticus (benzodiazepines) and preventing seizures (barbiturates). Butalbital, an intermediate-acting barbiturate, is an ingredient of the migraine medicines Fiorinal and Fioricet. The proper prescribing of sedative-hypnotics and avoidance of abuse is discussed in Chapter 14.

Table 6.1.   Non-benzodiazepine sedative-hypnotic drugs*

Generic	Brand
Barbiturates	
Amobarbital	Amytal
Butabarbital	Sarisol
Butalbital	Fiorinal†
Pentobarbital	Nembutal
Phenobarbital	Many‡
Secobarbital	Seconal
Others	
Carisoprodol	Soma
Chloral hydrate	Noctec, Somnote
Eszopiclone	Lunesta
Gamma-hydroxybutyrate	Xyrem
Meprobamate	Miltown, Equanil
Zaleplon	Sonata
Zolpidem	Ambien

* Benzodiazepines are listed in Table 6-2.
† Combination with aspirin and caffeine.
‡ Found in many different combination products.

Table 6.2.   Comparison of benzodiazepines

Generic Name	Brand Name (U.S.)	Equipotent Oral Dose*
High Potency/Short Acting		
Alprazolam	Xanax	1 mg
Flunitrazepam	Rohypnol†	1 mg
Lorazepam	Ativan	2 mg
Triazolam	Halcion	0.5 mg
High Potency/Long Acting		
Clonazepam	Klonopin	1 mg
Low Potency/Short Acting		
Oxazepam	Serax	30 mg
Temazepam	Restoril	30 mg
Low Potency/Long Acting		
Chlordiazepoxide	Librium	25 mg
Clorazepate	Tranxene	15 mg
Diazepam	Valium	10 mg
Flurazepam	Dalmane	30 mg

* Approximately equivalent to 30 mg of phenobarbital.
† Not available by prescription in the United States.

Bromides, introduced in 1826, were the first sedative-hypnotic drugs, followed by barbital (the first barbiturate) in 1903, chloral hydrate in 1932, and meprobamate in 1955. Chlordiazepoxide (Librium), introduced in 1961, was the first benzodiazepine. Benzodiazepines quickly surpassed barbiturates as the most prescribed sedative-hypnotic, since they were able to decrease anxiety with less sedation and risk for respiratory depression.

All barbiturates are derived from barbituric acid. They are classified into three groups based on duration of action. The short-acting barbiturates are used to induce anesthesia and are generally administered intravenously. The intermediate-acting barbiturates are prescribed as oral sedative-hypnotics and are the group most commonly abused. The long-acting barbiturates are prescribed for oral use as anticonvulsants.

When first introduced, benzodiazepines were thought to have low risk for abuse and were not classified as scheduled drugs. Subsequently, abuse liability studies in animals and humans of benzodiazepines showed them to be drugs that may lead to abuse and addiction (1, 2). However, relative to medically legitimate use, the incidence of benzodiazepine abuse is modest (3). Most individuals who abuse benzodiazepines abuse other drugs as well (4).

Benzodiazepines can be divided into three groups: those that have active metabolites (chlordiazepoxide, diazepam, flurazepam, flunitrazepam, clorazepate), those that do not produce active metabolites (lorazepam, oxazepam), and a group that produces an active metabolite with little clinical activity (alprazolam, triazolam). A classification of benzodiazepines based on potency, onset of action, and half-life is shown in Table 6.2. Abuse liability is greatest for drugs with rapid onset of action (5–7).

Three new sedative-hypnotics—zolpidem (Ambien), eszopiclone (Lunesta), and zaleplon (Sonata)—are used for insomnia and are chemically distinct from the benzodiazepines, but they bind to the same receptors (8). Other prescribed sedative-hypnotics include chloral hydrate, prescribed short-term for the treatment of insomnia; meprobamate (Miltown or Equanil), an anxiolytic with high abuse potential; carisoprodol (Soma), a muscle relaxant not currently classified as a controlled substance, whose metabolite is meprobamate; and γ-hydroxybutyrate (GHB). GHB is therapeutically used for the treatment of narcolepsy. Abused GHB is produced illicitly and is used recreationally at raves. Two drugs related to GHB, 1,4-butanediol (used to clean electronic equipment) and γ-butyrolactone, are metabolized to GHB. GHB is easily manufactured in illicit laboratories as a powder that is dissolved in water and often mixed in alcoholic beverages.

For individuals with substance abuse, and especially those on methadone maintenance, abuse of benzodiazepines is common (9–11). Patients with alcoholism are also at greater risk for benzodiazepine abuse (12–14). The most commonly abused benzodiazepines are alprazolam (Xanax), clonazepam (Klonopin), and diazepam (Valium) (15). Flunitrazepam (Rohypnol) has recently gained attention for abuse as "the date rape drug" (16, 17). It is not licensed in the United States but is sold illicitly on the street. Some users grind flunitrazepam into a powder and then snort it. Flunitrazepam may cause paradoxical agitation and is not detectable by routine urine toxicology.

EPIDEMIOLOGY

In a national survey between 1990 and 1992, the lifetime prevalence of self-reported sedative dependence was 0.5% (18). Of these individuals, 7.1% reported nonprescribed use. The 2003 United States National Survey on Drug Use and Health estimated that 1.8 million Americans were current users of sedatives taken without prescription and 20.2 million Americans had taken a sedative without a prescription at least once (19). In 2002, 100,784 emergency room visits in the United States were related to benzodiazepines, with nearly half of these the result of suicide attempts (20). Patients age 26–44 had the highest rate of benzodiazepine-related emergency room visits. Rates of benzodiazepine abuse appear particularly high among injection drug users (21–23). In 2002, there were 3330 GHB-related emergency room visits in the United States (20).

Reported abuse of zolpidem and zaleplon is rare, with only 36 cases reported in the literature; most cases occur in individuals who abuse other drugs as well (24). Carisoprodol abuse is only recently being recognized. In a 6-month study at a university hospital in San Diego, 19 of 4245 urine samples had positive drug screens for carisoprodol (25). All of the 19 patients had clinical complications thought related to carisoprodol, with most patients lethargic or obtunded, and several presenting with seizures

DRUG EFFECTS

Acute Drug Effects

Sedative-hypnotics interact at the gamma-aminobutyric acid (GABA) receptor. GABA is an inhibitory transmitter in the central nervous system. Benzodiazepines do not directly bind to GABA receptors but rather potentiate the actions of GABA by causing GABA to bind more tightly to receptors, enhancing CNS inhibitory tone. Barbiturates bind to the GABA receptor complex and prolong opening of chloride channels, inhibiting excitable cells in the central nervous system. There is some evidence that there is a specific barbiturate receptor site, with a correlation between binding affinity and drug effect (26). Carisoprodol and its active metabolite meprobamate also act directly at the GABA receptor complex.

Sedatives cause intoxication similar to that seen with alcohol. They produce a depression of cortical function and relax social and personal inhibitions. Mood is elevated and anxiety is reduced. Barbiturates are more likely than benzodiazepines to cause motor incoordination, slurred speech, and respiratory depression. While reinforcing effects of benzodiazepines are variable, barbiturates have consistently demonstrated high abuse liability. Patients, including those with anxiety disorders, do not necessarily find the effects of benzodiazepines pleasurable or reinforcing. Used for sleep, sedative-hypnotic drugs decrease sleep latency and temporarily diminish awakenings from sleep.

Effects on sleep diminish with chronic use. Additionally, REM sleep (restful sleep) is actually diminished. Benzodiazepines also cause acute amnesia after high-dose intravenous administration, an effect used therapeutically for medical procedures.

Carisoprodol has clinical effects similar to the benzodiazepines but may also cause tachycardia, involuntary movements, hand tremor, and horizontal gaze nystagmus (27). GHB has clinical effects 15–30 minutes after oral ingestion, producing an initial euphoria, followed by dizziness, hypersalivation, drowsiness, and amnesia.

Overdose

Overdose from sedative-hypnotics leads to slurred speech, impaired judgment, and unsteady gait. At the extreme, overdose may lead to stupor, coma, respiratory depression, vasomotor collapse, and death. Benzodiazepines do not impair motor coordination as much as barbiturates and almost never cause death when taken alone, even in large doses, unless given rapidly by intravenous route (e.g., midazolam or diazepam). However, the combination of alcohol and benzodiazepines can be lethal. Barbiturate overdose is a life-threatening occurrence that should be treated in an emergency department. There is one case report of a near-fatal overdose of carisoprodol (28).

For benzodiazepine overdose, flumazenil, a specific benzodiazepine antagonist, should be administered—0.2 mg intravenously followed by 0.3 mg in 30 seconds and another 0.5 mg every 60 seconds for up to six doses. For benzodiazepine-dependent patients, flumazenil may cause symptoms of withdrawal. Flumazenil may also be effective in the treatment of carisoprodol intoxication (29).

Severe intoxication with GHB may produce coma and apnea (30). Overdose is common as the strength of street GHB can vary greatly. Agitation, myoclonus, and seizures are common. In addition, GHB overdose may result in bradycardia or hypothermia in about a third of individuals (31, 32). Intoxication with 1,4-butanediol produces more prolonged symptoms, especially sedation (33). Treatment of GHB overdose is supportive. Bradycardia does not usually produce hemodynamic instability. Endotracheal intubation may be temporarily necessary in individuals with severely depressed mental status. Fomepizole, an alcohol dehydrogenase inhibitor, may be useful in 1,4-butanediol overdose, but clinical data is still pending (34). This agent is already approved for use in ethylene glycol and methanol intoxication.

Withdrawal

Because of physiological dependence, patients who use sedative drugs are at risk of serious withdrawal symptoms, including agitation, restlessness, insomnia, anxiety, and seizures (35). Table 6.3 shows a list of sedative withdrawal symptoms. The onset of withdrawal symptoms is related to drug half-life, with cessation of shorter-acting drugs causing the onset of withdrawal symptoms in 24–48 hours and cessation of longer-acting drugs typically causing withdrawal in 48–96 hours. Most withdrawal seizures occur 24–72 hours after cessation of

Table 6.3.   Characteristics of sedative-hypnotic withdrawal

Anxiety
Hallucinations
Delusions/paranoia
Myoclonic jerks
Ataxia
Confusion/delirium
Mood changes—irritability, emotional depression, dysphoria, apathy
Tremor
Nausea and vomiting
Weakness
Orthostatic hypotension
Hypersensitivity to external stimuli
Impaired memory/concentration
Insomnia
Seizures

use. From a clinical point of view, it is important to recognize that many patients with physical dependence to sedative-hypnotics also abuse other drugs concurrently. Seizures are more likely to occur in individuals who also abuse or are dependent on alcohol.

Although chronic use may create the risk of withdrawal symptoms, there is evidence that patients may use benzodiazepines on a chronic basis without developing tolerance to the anxiolytic effects of the medication (36–38). Physical dependence on benzodiazepines and the potential for major withdrawal symptoms may occur in as little as 2 months if dosages substantially above therapeutic levels are used. Withdrawal symptoms occur in patients taking therapeutic dosages daily for several weeks or more (39). For individuals taking a short-acting benzodiazepine only at night for insomnia, withdrawal symptoms will likely be limited to reemergence and heightening of their insomnia.

A rare but serious complication of benzodiazepine withdrawal is nonconvulsive status epilepticus. Individuals with this syndrome often exhibit bizarre behavior and respond rapidly to benzodiazepines. The diagnosis can be made with electroencephalogram (EEG) (40).

Barbiturate withdrawal tends to be particularly severe with a high risk for seizures. Severe barbiturate withdrawal can occur in migraine patients who abruptly stop butalbital-containing medications (41).

Signs and symptoms of GHB withdrawal include tremor, tachycardia, anxiety, hallucinations (auditory, tactile, and visual), paranoia, delusions, delirium, diaphoresis, hypertension, and nausea. There has been one reported death (42). Withdrawal usually starts 24–48 hours after last use and may last several days.

Carisoprodol withdrawal has been reported in patients taking seven tablets or more per day (tablets are 350 mg each) for at least 1 year, with symptoms of insomnia, anxiety, headache, and irritability (43, 44). Withdrawal symptoms usually peak 2–3 days after cessation of use.

DIAGNOSIS

Chronic use of benzodiazepines may go undetected until confusion, irritability, slurred speech, and ataxia are recognized as signs of sedative toxicity. Physical examination may include ecchymoses from injuries sustained. Urine drug screen will be positive for detecting barbiturates and most benzodiazepines, with the exception of flunitrazepam. Other sedative-hypnotics are not detected by urine drug screen but may be detected by full urine toxicology testing.

MEDICAL COMPLICATIONS

Virtually all of the literature on medical complications of sedative-hypnotic use is specific to the benzodiazepines. Memory impairment may occur in some individuals using benzodiazepines chronically (45–47). This effect appears more prevalent in the elderly and in individuals using high-potency, short-half-life benzodiazepines (48). One study showed sustained cognitive impairment 6 months after patients were withdrawn from long-term benzodiazepine use (49). However, elderly patients who discontinue chronic benzodiazepine use may see improvement in memory and cognitive functioning (50, 51). Because alcohol is known to produce brain atrophy, several studies have examined whether chronic benzodiazepines use contributes to pathological changes also. While some studies show some effect (52, 53), other studies do not (54, 55).

Benzodiazepine use may increase the risk of accidental injury (**56**). Additionally, in a study of older adults, an elevated rate of automobile accident was found in benzodiazepine users (57). Several epidemiological studies have shown that benzodiazepines and other sedative-hypnotics increase the risk of falls (58–61) and hip fractures in the elderly (**62**–65). One study found an increased risk of incurring an accidental injury within 6 months of receiving a prescription for a benzodiazepine (66). There are no good studies showing an increased risk of suicide in benzodiazepine users. However, one study did show an increased risk of suicide attempt in benzodiazepine users with borderline personality disorder (67).

TREATMENT

Detoxification from benzodiazepines in patients receiving them therapeutically can be managed by tapering the prescribed benzodiazepine (68) or by switching to a benzodiazepine with a longer half-life and tapering it over several weeks (69). Typically, the dose can be reduced 50% within a few days, the next 25% over a week or two, and the last 25% over a few weeks. The final 25% is most often the most difficult stage for patients (70). Inpatient treatment is often required for high-dose abuse and can be managed using phenobarbital, which has a long half-life (80 to 100 hours) and provides the pharmacokinetic umbrella to prevent withdrawal symptoms, including seizures. Table 6.2 shows milligram equivalents between the benzodiazepines, with conversion doses for treating benzodiazepine withdrawal with phenobarbital. For patients abusing benzodiazepines, self-report of daily use is likely not reliable. We have had success treating benzodiazepine withdrawal in hundreds of patients using phenobarbital according to the fixed schedule shown in Table 6.4. Doses are withheld for sedation or unsteady gait. Phenobarbital can also be used for treating barbiturate withdrawal with evidence of successful treatment in patients withdrawing from butalbital-containing headache medications (71).

Recent clinical trials have reported on the use of topiramate (a single case successfully treated) (72) and captodiamine (73) (not available in the United States, but potentially useful once further studies are performed) in the treatment of benzodiazepine withdrawal. Ondansetron (74) and paroxetine (75) have been found to not be useful. Other drugs (propranolol [76], clonidine, carbamazepine, and buspirone) used anecdotally as adjuncts in the treatment of sedative-hypnotic withdrawal have insufficient clinical trial data to support their use.

GHB withdrawal can be managed similarly to alcohol withdrawal using benzodiazepines as outlined in Chapter 5 (42). There is also one report of using diazepam in the treatment of zolpidem withdrawal in an individual using over 400 mg/day of zolpidem (77).

Even in patients prescribed benzodiazepines, self-reported improvements in quality of life are reported after treatment for benzodiazepine dependence (78). Studies have not shown cognitive behavioral therapy to be a useful adjunct to the pharmacological treatment of benzodiazepine dependence (68, 79). Following successful cessation of benzodiazepine use, individuals continue to have high rates of morbidity, including high rates of depression and suicide (80–82). Comorbid mental illness requires ongoing psychiatric care. For the many individuals with addiction to other drugs besides sedatives, treatment options are outlined in Chapter 4. Many methadone programs have clear contingency management plans for patients who abuse sedatives.

Table 6.4.   Phenobarbital dosing protocol for treatment of benzodiazepine withdrawal

Phenobarbital 200 mg orally, then
Phenobarbital 100 mg orally every 4 hours times five doses, then
Phenobarbital 60 mg orally every 4 hours times four doses, then
Phenobarbital 60 mg orally every 8 hours times three doses

Note—Hold dose if patient is sedated.

REFERENCES

1. Ator, N. A, and R. R. Griffiths. 1987. Self-administration of barbiturates and benzodiazepines: A review. *Pharmacol. Biochem. Behav.* 27:391–398.
2. DuPont, R. L. 1988. Abuse of benzodiazepines: The problems and the solutions. *Am. J. Drug Alcohol Abuse* 14:S1–S69.
3. Griffiths, R. R., and E. M. Weerts. 1997. Benzodiazepine self-administration in humans and laboratory animals—Implications for problems of long-term use and abuse. *Psychopharmacology* 134:1–37.
4. Busto, U. E., M. K. Romach, and E. M. Sellers. 1996. Multiple drug use and psychiatric comorbidity in patients admitted to the hospital with severe benzodiazepine dependence. *J. Clin. Psychopharmacol.* 16:51–57.
5. Bergman, U., and R. R. Griffiths. 1986. Relative abuse of diazepam and oxazepam: Prescription forgeries and theft/loss reports in Sweden. *Drug Alcohol Depend.* 16:293–301.
6. Griffiths, R. R., D. R. McLeod, G. E. Bigelow, et al. 1984. Relative abuse liability of diazepam and oxazepam: Behavioral and subjective dose effects. *Psychopharmacology* 84:147–154.
7. Griffiths, R. R., and B. Wolf. 1990. Relative abuse liability of different benzodiazepines in drug abusers. *J. Clin. Psychopharmacol.* 10:237–243.
8. Hajak, G., W. E. Muller, H. U. Wittchen, et al. 2002. Abuse and dependence potential for the non-benzodiazepine hypnotics zolpidem and zopiclone: A review of case reports and epidemiologic data. *Addiction* 98:1371–1378.
9. Barnas, C., M. Rossmann, H. Roessler, et al. 1992. Benzodiazepines and other psychotropic drugs abused by patients in a methadone maintenance program: Familiarity and preference. *J. Clin. Psychopharmacol.* 12:397–402.
10. Iguchi, M. Y., L. Handelsman, W. K. Bickel, and R. R. Griffiths. 1993. Benzodiazepine and sedative use/abuse by methadone maintenance clients. *Drug Alcohol Depend.* 32:257–266.
11. Darke, S., W. Swift, W. Hall, and M. Ross. 1993. Drug use, HIV risk-taking and psychosocial correlates of benzodiazepine use among methadone maintenance clients. *Drug Alcohol Depend.* 34:67–70.
12. Ciraulo, D. A., B. F. Sands, and R. I. Shader. 1988. Critical review of liability for benzodiazepine abuse among alcoholics. *Am. J. Psychiatry* 145:1501–1506.
13. Ciraulo, D. A., J. G. Barnhill, D. J. Greenblatt, et al. 1988. Abuse liability and clinical pharmacokinetics of alprazolam in alcoholic men. *J. Clin. Psychiatry* 49:333–337.
14. Ross, H. E. 1993. Benzodiazepine use and anxiolytic abuse and dependence in treated alcoholics. *Addiction* 88:209–218.
15. National Institute on Drug Abuse. *Prescription drugs: Abuse and addiction—CNS depressants.* Research report series. Available at http://www.drugabuse.gov
16. Druid, H., P. Holmgren, and J. Ahlner. 2001. Flunitrazepam: An evaluation of use, abuse and toxicity. *Forens. Sci. Int.* 122:136–141.
17. Woods, J. H., and G. Winger. 1997. Abuse liability of flunitrazepam. *J. Clin. Psychopharmacol.* 17:1S–57S.
18. Goodwin, R. D., and D. S. Hasin. 2002. Sedative use and misuse in the United States. *Addiction* 97:555–562. *Data from national*

survey of 8098 community-dwelling adults; those who used illicit sedatives were more likely to have major depression (OR 1.47), agoraphobia (OR 1.59), antisocial personality disorder (OR 5.29), suicidal ideation (OR 1.91), and alcohol dependence (OR 4.32) when compared to nonusers of sedatives.

19. Substance Abuse and Mental Health Services Administration. 2004. *Results from the 2003 National Survey on Drug Use and Health: National Findings* (Office of Applied Studies, NSDUH Series H-25, DHHS Publication No. SMA 04-3964). Rockville, MD.

20. Office of Applied Studies. *Drug Abuse Warning Network, 2003: Interim national estimates of drug-related emergency department visits.* Available at http://www.dawninfo.samhsa.gov

21. Ray, W. A., R. L. Fought, and M. D. Decker. 1992. Psychoactive drugs and the risk of injurious motor vehicle crashes in elderly drivers. *Am. J. Epidemiol.* 136:873–883.

22. Darke, S. 1994. Benzodiazepine use among injecting drug users: Problems and implications. *Addiction* 89:379–382.

23. Darke, S., W. Hall, M. Ross, and A. Wodak. 1992. Benzodiazepine use and HIV risk-taking behaviour among injecting drug users. *Drug Alcohol Depend.* 31:31–36

24. Hajak, G., W. E. Muller, H. U. Wittchen, et al. 2003. Abuse and dependence potential for the non-benzodiazepine hypnotics zolpidem and zopiclone: A review of case reports and epidemiologic data. *Addiction* 98:1371–1378.

25. Bailey, D. N., and J. R. Briggs. 2002. Carisoprodol—An unrecognized drug of abuse. *Am. J. Clin. Pathol.* 117:396–400.

26. Olsen, R. W., J. S. Yang, and R. W. Ransom. 1988. GABA-stimulated 36Cl- flux in brain slices as an assay for modulation by CNS depressant drugs. *Adv. Biochem. Psychopharmacol.* 45:125–133.

27. Bramness, J. G., S. Skurtveit, and J. Morland. 2004. Impairment due to intake of carisoprodol. *Drug Alcohol Depend.* 74:311–318.

28. Siddiqi, M., and C. A. Jennings. 2004. A near-fatal overdose of carisoprodol (soma): A case report. *J. Toxicol. Clin. Toxicol.* 42:239–240.

29. Roberge, R. J., E. Lin, and E. P. Krenzelok. 2000. Flumazenil reversal of carisoprodol (soma) intoxication. *J. Emerg. Med.* 18:61–64.

30. Mason, P. E., and W. P. Kerns. 2002. Gamma hydroxybutyric acid (GHB) intoxication. *Acad. Emerg. Med.* 9:730–739.

31. Chin, R. L., K. A. Sporer, B. Cullison, et al. 1998. Clinical course of gamma-hydroxybutyrate overdose. *Ann. Emerg. Med.* 31:716–722.

32. Li, J., S. A. Stokes, and A. Woeckener. 1998. A tale of novel intoxication: Seven cases of gamma-hydroxybutyric acid overdose. *Ann. Emerg. Med.* 31:723–728.

33. Mycyk, M. B., C. Wilemon, and S. E. Aks. 2001. Two cases of withdrawal from 1,4-butanediol use. *Ann. Emerg. Med.* 38:345–346.

34. Tancredi, D. N., and M. W. Shannon. 2003. Case 30-2003: A 21-year-old man with sudden alteration of mental status. *N. Engl. J. Med.* 349:1267–1275.

35. Noyes, R., P. J. Perry, R. R. Crowe, et al. 1986. Seizures following the withdrawal of alprazolam. *J. Nervous Mental Dis.* 174:50–52.

36. Benzodiazepine dependence, toxicity and abuse. 1990. A Task Force Report of the American Psychiatric Association. Washington, DC: American Psychiatric Association.

37. Shader, R. I., and D. J. Greenblatt. 1993. Use of benzodiazepines in anxiety disorders. *N. Engl. J. Med.* 328:1398–1405.
38. Moller, H. J. 1999. Effectiveness and safety of benzodiazepines. *J. Clin. Psychopharmacol.* 19:2S–11S.
39. Busto, U., E. M. Sellers, C. A. Naranjo, et al. 1986. Withdrawal reaction after long-term therapeutic use of benzodiazepines. *N. Engl. J. Med.* 315:854–859.
40. Olnes, M. J., A. Golding, and P. W. Kaplan. 2003. Nonconvulsive status epilepticus resulting from benzodiazepine withdrawal. *Ann. Intern. Med.* 139:956–958.
41. Raja, M., M. C. Altavista, A. Azzoni, and A. Albanese. 1996. Severe barbiturate withdrawal syndrome in migrainous patients. *Headache* 36:119–121.
42. McDonough, M., N. Kennedy, A. Glasper, and J. Bearn. 2004. Clinical features and management of gamma-hydroxybutyrate (GHB) withdrawal: A review. *Drug Alcohol Depend.* 75:3–9.
43. Reeves, R. R., and J. D. Parker. 2003. Somatic dysfunction during carisoprodol cessation: Evidence for a carisoprodol withdrawal syndrome. *JAOA* 103:75–80.
44. Reeves, R. R., J. J. Beddingfield, and J. E. Mack. 2004. Carisoprodol withdrawal syndrome. *Pharmacotherapy* 12:1804–1806.
45. Ghoneim, M. M., and S. P. Mewaldt. 1990. Benzodiazepines and human memory: A review. *Anesthesiology* 72:926–938.
46. Golombok, S., P. Moodley, and M. Lader. 1988. Cognitive impairment in long-term benzodiazepine users. *Psychol. Med.* 18:365–374.
47. Curran, H. V. 1991. Benzodiazepines, memory and mood: A review. *Psychopharmacology* 105:1–8.
48. Foy, A., D. O'Connell, D. Henry, et al. 1995. Benzodiazepine use as a cause of cognitive impairment in elderly hospital inpatients. *J. Gerontol. Med. Sci.* 50A:M99–M106.
49. Tata, P. R., J. Rollings, M. Collins, et al. 1994. Lack of cognitive recovery following withdrawal from long-term benzodiazepine use. *Psychol. Med.* 24:203–213.
50. Salzman, C., J. Fisher, K. Nobel, et al. 1992. Cognitive improvement following benzodiazepine discontinuation in elderly nursing home residents. *Int. J. Gen. Psychiatry* 7:89–93.
51. Larson, E. B., W. A. Kukull, D. Buchner, and B. V. Reifler. 1987. Adverse drug reactions associated with global cognitive impairment in elderly persons. *Ann. Int. Med.* 107:169–173.
52. Lader, M. H., M. Ron, and H. Petursson. 1984. Computed axial brain tomography in long-term benzodiazepine users. *Psychol. Med.* 14:203–206.
53. Moodley, P., S. Golombok, P. H. Shrine, and M. Lader. 1993. Computed axial brain tomograms in long-term benzodiazepine users. *Psychiatr. Res.* 48:135–144.
54. Perera, K. M. H., T. Powell, and F. A. Jenner. 1987. Computerized axial tomographic studies following long-term use of benzodiazepines. *Psychol. Med.* 17:775–777.
55. Poser, W., S. Poser, D. Roscher, and A. Argyrakis. 1983. Do benzodiazepines cause cerebral atrophy? *Lancet* 8326:715.
56. Oster, G., D. M. Huse, S. F. Adams, et al. 1990. Benzodiazepine tranquilizers and the risk of accidental injury. *Am. J. Pub. Health* 12:1467–1470. *Four thousand five hundred fifty-four persons who had been prescribed a benzodiazepine were compared with 13,662*

who had been prescribed another drug. Accident-related care was twofold more likely for those who had been prescribed benzodiazepines, with the probability of an accident-related medical encounter higher during months in which a prescription for a benzodiazepine had recently been filled. Those who had filled three or more prescriptions for a benzodiazepine in the 6 months following initiation of therapy had a significantly higher risk of an accident-related medical event than those who had filled only one.

57. Ray, W. A., R. L. Fought, and M. D. Decker. 1992. Psychoactive drugs and the risk of injurious motor vehicle crashes in elderly drivers. *Am. J. Epidemiol.* 136:873–883.

58. Cumming, R. G., J. P. Miller, J. L. Kelsey, et al. 1991. Medications and multiple falls in elderly people: The St. Louis study. *Age Aging* 20:455–461.

59. Lichtenstein, M. J., M. R. Griffin, J. E. Cornell, et al. 1994. Risk factors for hip fractures occurring in the hospital. *Am. J. Epidemiol.* 140:830–838.

60. Myers, A. H., S. P. Baker, M. L. Van Natta, et al. 1991. Risk factors associated with falls and injuries among elderly institutionalized persons. *Am. J. Epidemiol.* 133:1179–1190.

61. Sorock, G. S., and E. E. Shimkin. 1988. Benzodiazepine sedatives and the risk of falling in a community-dwelling elderly cohort. *Arch. Int. Med.* 148:2441–2444.

62. Wagner, A. K., F. Zhang, and S. B. Soumerai. 2004. Benzodiazepine use and hip fractures in the elderly. *Arch. Intern. Med.* 164:1567–1572. *Analysis of 125,203 New Jersey Medicaid claims over 42 months in which there were 2312 hip fractures. Hip fracture rate was significantly higher in patients with exposure to any benzodiazepine when compared to those with no benzodiazepine exposure (incidence rate ratio [IRR]: 1.24), for a short half-life, high-potency benzodiazepine (IRR: 1.27), during the first 2 weeks after starting a benzodiazepine (IRR: 2.05), during the second 2 weeks after starting a benzodiazepine (IRR: 1.88), and for continued use (IRR: 1.18).*

63. Cummings, S. R., M. C. Nevitt, W. S. Browner, et al. 1995. Risk factors for hip fracture in white women. *N. Engl. J. Med.* 332:767–773.

64. Herings, R. M. C., B. H. Stricker, A. de Boer, et al. 1995. Benzodiazepines and the risk of falling leading to femur fractures. Dosage more important than elimination halflife. *Arch. Int. Med.* 155:1801–1807.

65. Ray, W. A., M. R. Griffin, and W. Downey. 1989. Benzodiazepines of long and short elimination half-life and the risk of hip fracture. *JAMA* 262:3303–3307.

66. Oster, G., D. M. Huse, S. F. Adams, et al. 1990. Benzodiazepine tranquilizers and the risk of accidental injury. *Am. J. Public Health* 80:1467–1470.

67. Lekka, N. P., C. Paschalis, and S. Beratis. 2002. Suicide attempts in high-dose benzodiazepine users. *Compr. Psychiatry* 43:438–442.

68. Oude Voshaar, R. C., W. J. Gorgels, A. J. Mol, et al. 2003. Tapering off long-term benzodiazepine use with or without group cognitive-behavioural therapy: Three-condition, randomized controlled trial. *Br. J. Psych.* 182:498–504.

69. Sullivan, J. T., and E. M. Sellers. 1992. Detoxification for triazolam physical dependence. *J. Clin. Psychopharmacol.* 12:124–127.
70. Schweizer, E., K. Rickels, W. G. Case, and D. J. Greenblatt. 1990. Long-term therapeutic use of benzodiazepines. II. Effects of gradual taper. *Arch. Gen. Psychiatry* 47:908–915.
71. Loder, E., and D. Biondi. 2003. Oral phenobarbital loading: A safe and effective method of withdrawing patients with headache from butalbital compounds. *Headache* 43:904–909. *Study of 19 patients who stopped butalbital (8–20 tablets/day) and were treated with phenobarbital doses of 120 mg/hour until sedated (range of 8–13 doses). There were no adverse effects and all patients were successfully withdrawn.*
72. Chesaux, M., M. Monnat, and D. F. Zullino. 2003. Topiramate in benzodiazepine withdrawal. *Hum. Psychopharmacol.* 18:375–377.
73. Mercier-Guyon, C., J. P. Chabannes, and P. Saviuc. 2004. The role of captodiamine in the withdrawal from long-term benzodiazepine treatment. *Curr. Med. Res. Opin.* 9:1347–1355.
74. Romach, M. K., H. L. Kaplan, U. E. Busto, et al. 1998. A controlled trial of ondansetron, a 5-HT3 antagonist, in benzodiazepine discontinuation. *J. Clin. Psychopharmacol.* 18:121–131.
75. Zitman, F. G., and J. E. Couvee. 2001. Chronic benzodiazepine use in general practice patients with depression: An evaluation of controlled treatment and taper-off. Report on behalf of the Dutch chronic benzodiazepine working group. *Br. J. Psych.* 178:317–324.
76. Cantopher, T., S. Olivieri, N. Cleave, and J. G. Edwards. 1990. Chronic benzodiazepine dependence—A comparative study of abrupt withdrawal under propranolol cover versus gradual withdrawal. *Br. J. Psychiatry* 156:406–411.
77. Rappa, L. R., M. Larose-Pierre, D. R. Payne, et al. 2004. Detoxification from high-dose zolpidem using diazepam. *Ann. Pharmacother.* 38:590–594.
78. Vorma, H., H. Naukkarinen, S. Sarna, and K. Kuoppasalmi. 2004. Symptom severity and quality of life after benzodiazepine withdrawal treatment in participants with complicated dependence. *Addict. Behav.* 29:1059–1065.
79. Vorma, H., H. Naukkarinen, S. Sarna, and K. Kuoppasalmi. 2002. Treatment of out-patients with complicated benzodiazepine dependence: Comparison of two approaches. *Addiction* 97:851–859.
80. Ashton, H. 1987. Benzodiazepine withdrawal: Outcome in 50 patients. *Br. J. Addict.* 82:665–671. *Fifty consecutive patients who completed detoxification from prescribed benzodiazepines were assessed at 10-month to 3.5-year follow-up; 48% were doing "excellent" off benzodiazepines, 22% were "good," 16% were "better," and 6% were "poor." Three were back on benzodiazepines.*
81. Allgulander, C., S. Borg, and B. Vikander. 1984. A 4–6-year follow-up of 50 patients with primary dependence on sedative and hypnotic drugs. *Am. J. Psychiatry* 141:1580–1582.
82. Rickels, K., W. G. Case, E. Schweizer, et al. 1991. Long-term benzodiazepine users 3 years after participation in a discontinuation program. *Am. J. Psychiatry* 148:757–761.

7

Opioids

BACKGROUND

Opioids have been used for centuries for their analgesic effect and for the control of dysenteries, as well as for their pleasurable effects. However, these beneficial uses have been accompanied by the vexing problem of dependence and addiction. *Opioids* are the family of compounds related to opium; *opiates* are drugs derived from opium itself. Opium is produced from the juice of the opium poppy, and its derivatives include morphine, codeine, and heroin. Morphine, the active ingredient of opium, was first purified in 1805. Diacetylmorphine (heroin) was later synthesized from morphine in 1898 and was initially marketed as a safer, less addicting opioid. Methadone is a synthetic opioid developed in Germany during World War II as an analgesic, and it has subsequently found use as a treatment for opioid dependence. Buprenorphine is a partial opioid agonist and antagonist that was developed in the 1970s and is increasingly used for treatment of opioid dependence.

EPIDEMIOLOGY

According to the *2003 National Survey on Drug Use and Health,* approximately 3.7 million Americans reported using heroin at some time in their lives; 314,000 had used heroin in the past year and 189,000 were classified as experiencing dependence on or abuse of the substance. Over 31 million Americans reported lifetime nonmedical use of prescription pain relievers (mainly opioids); 11.7 million of these had used in the past year, of whom 12.2% (1.4 million) were classified as abusing or being dependent on these medications (1).

The nonmedical use of prescription pain relievers had steadily risen during the 1990s; in 2001, an estimated 2.4 million Americans used these agents for the first time, compared with 628,000 in 1990. Codeine and propoxyphene preparations (including Darvocet, Darvon, and Tylenol with codeine) are the most commonly abused, followed by hydrocodone-containing medications (Vicodin, Lortab, Lorcet), oxycodone-containing preparations (Tylox, Percocet, Percodan), long-acting oxycodone (OxyContin), meperidine (Demerol), and methadone.

The misuse of opioids is an important medical problem. One study estimated that the medical care costs associated with heroin addiction in the United States exceeded 5 billion dollars in 1996 (2). In 2002, it was estimated that almost 100,000 emergency department visits in the United States were related to heroin use; for prescription opiates, the number was close to 120,000 (3).

DRUG EFFECTS

Acute Effects

Opioids exert their effect by mimicking the effect of endorphins (endogenous opioid peptides). They are thought to bind to a number of receptors that are responsible for different effects; the major receptors appear to be the mu (μ), delta (δ), and kappa (κ) receptors (4). Stimulation of all three receptors is thought to have an analgesic effect. Stimulation of the mu receptor is also associated with euphoria, respiratory depression, suppression of cough, decreased gastrointestinal motility, and miosis; it is also thought to be the receptor that is most responsible for dependence. Kappa receptors are also associated with sedation, dysphoria, and miosis. Experienced users develop tolerance to the sedative effects and respiratory depression but not to the constipating and miotic effects of opioids.

Users of opioids administer them through a variety of routes: oral, intranasal, through smoking, and by intravenous, intramuscular, or subcutaneous injection. For heroin users, the drug peaks in the serum within a minute of intravenous use, 3–5 minutes of intranasal or intramuscular use, and 5–10 minutes of subcutaneous use. Drug users prefer heroin (over morphine) because its greater lipid solubility allows for better penetration of the blood-brain barrier. Users experience euphoria, sedation, analgesia, and a sense of well-being. Table 7.1 lists selected opioid analgesics and their relative potency.

Overdose

Overdose is a common and serious complication of opioid abuse. In one study of injection heroin users in San Francisco, 48% had reported having at least one overdose and 33% reported two or more in the past (5). In a cohort of 1075 addicts seeking treatment in the U.K. in the mid-1990s who were followed for 4 years, 68% of the deaths were due to overdose, and the risk of overdose was increased with the concurrent use of other substances, especially alcohol, benzodiazepines, and amphetamines (6). The risk of overdose is also heightened by recent abstinence (7) or detoxification (8), because tolerance to opioid side effects is reduced.

The typical presentation of opioid overdose is the triad of depressed level of consciousness, decreased respiration, and miotic (constricted) pupils. Death does not generally occur immediately after use; most individuals are thought to expire hours after their overdose.

The standard treatment for opioid overdose is naloxone, which can be given intravenously (usually 0.4 mg) or subcutaneously (0.8 mg); both appear to be equally effective (9). A higher dose (1–2 mg) can be tried if the initial dose is not effective. Higher doses may be required to treat overdoses with propoxyphene, pentazocine, and buprenorphine. Naloxone can also be given via endotracheal tube in an intubated patient; however, it is not effective orally, since it is highly metabolized by the liver when given by this route. Intranasal administration of naloxone is also effective, though the response is not as rapid as intramuscular administration (10).

Naloxone is relatively short-acting (45–90 minutes); therefore, the overdose victim might have recurrent toxicity, even after a satisfactory initial response. For this reason, it is standard practice to take overdose victims to a hospital after resuscitation in the field; 2–3 hours of observation after an overdose is usually sufficient (11).

There are a number of clinical signs that may help identify overdose victims who can be discharged an hour after receiving

Table 7.1.   Characteristics and dosing of selected opiod analgesics

Generic Name	Trade Names*	Equianalgesic Parenteral Dose†	Equianalgesic Oral Dose†	Starting Oral Dose†‡
Morphine	MSIR, Avinza,[1] Kadian,[1] Oramorph SR,[1] MSContin[1]	10 mg	30 mg	15–30 mg q 3–4 h
Buprenorphine	Buprenex, Subutex, Suboxone[2]	0.4 mg	4 mg (sublingual)	2–4 mg (sublingual)
Butorphanol	Stadol	2 mg	—	—
Codeine	Tylenol #3*	75 mg	130 mg	30–60 mg q 3–4 h
Diacetylmorphine	Heroin	4 mg	—	—
Fentanyl	Duragesic, Sublimaze	0.1 mg	—	—
Hydrocodone	Anexia,* Lortab,* Lorcet,* Vicodin,* Zydone*	—	30 mg	5–10 mg q 3–4 h
Hydromorphone	Dilaudid	1.5 mg	7.5 mg	4–6 mg q 3–4 h
Levorphanol	Levo-Dromoran	2 mg	4 mg	4 mg q 6–8 h
Meperidine	Demerol	75 mg	300 mg	50–100 mg q 3–4 h
Methadone	Dolophine, Methadose	10 mg	20 mg (acute)	10–20 mg q 6–8 h
Oxycodone	Endocet,* Percodan,* Percocet,* Roxicet,* Tylox,* OxyContin[1]	—	20 mg	5–10 mg q 3–4 h

Table 7.1. *Continued*

Generic Name	Trade Names*	Equianalgesic Parenteral Dose†	Equianalgesic Oral Dose†	Starting Oral Dose‡
Pentazocine	Talwin, Talwin NX,[2] Telacen*	50 mg	50 mg	50 mg q 4–6 h
Propoxyphene	Darvon, Darvocet*	—	100 mg	65–100 mg q 4–6 h
Tramadol	Ultram, Ultracet*	—	100 mg	50–100 mg q 4–6 h

* Some trade names are combinations with aspirin or acetaminophen.
† Doses approximately equivalent to 10 mg of parenteral morphine.
‡ For adults ≥50 kg, frequency is for non-sustained-release formulations.
[1] Sustained-release formulations.
[2] Combined with naloxone.

naloxone. In one study of 573 presumed opioid overdose victims, the presence of the following six clinical factors identified those who could be safely discharged an hour after naloxone: (1) patient can mobilize as usual, (2) room air O2 saturation >92%, (3) respiratory rate between 10 and 20 breaths/min, (4) temperature between 35.0 and 37.5°C, (5) heart rate between 50 and 100 beats/min, and (6) Glasgow Coma Scale of 15 (12). Among heroin users who refuse transport to the hospital, the risk of recurrent toxicity appears to be fairly low (13) but is more of a concern for those who overdose on long-acting opioids (14). Overdose may also be complicated by noncardiogenic pulmonary edema; this is generally clinically apparent within 2 hours after an overdose and should be considered in anyone with a cough or hypoxia after overdose. Overdose victims may also develop rhabdomyolysis or compartment syndrome.

Addiction treatment is probably the most effective way to prevent overdose deaths. Several studies have found that methadone maintenance treatment is associated with a lower risk of overdose (15). Furthermore, the introduction of buprenorphine in France for treatment of opioid addiction has been associated with a reduction in overdose deaths in that country (16).

Some have argued that addicts (or their friends and family members) should be supplied with naloxone to treat overdoses (17). Advocates point out that many overdoses occur in the presence of others and medical help is often not sought until it is too late. Increasing the availability of this effective and fairly safe drug has the potential to save many lives. However, there are a number of concerns about this strategy. It may cause addicts to engage in more risky behavior, or their aversion to naloxone may prevent them from using it; furthermore, there is a risk of blood-borne disease from needlesticks. Another harm reduction strategy that has been proposed is the development of "supervised fixing rooms" where addicts can use and receive timely treatment in the event of an overdose (18).

Withdrawal

The withdrawal syndrome typically begins within 12 hours of discontinuation of regular use of short-acting opioids, such as heroin; this may be delayed in users of longer-acting preparations, such as methadone. The typical symptoms include dysphoria, yawning, perspiration, rhinorrhea, lacrimation, nausea, diarrhea, and piloerection ("goose bumps"). The symptoms can be very unpleasant but are generally not life-threatening; however, patients who have coexisting medical conditions may experience serious complications. Withdrawal symptoms generally resolve within a week of abstinence but may be prolonged to 2 weeks or more in patients withdrawing from longer-acting opioids. Figure 7.1 provides the 11-item Clinical Opiate Withdrawal Scale (COWS), which can be used to assess the severity of withdrawal and response to treatment. Alternatively, the 10-item Short Opiate Withdrawal Scale (SOWS; see Figure 7.2) can be used; this can be completed entirely by the patient and may be easier to use in clinical practice (19). It should be noted that there is also a *Subjective* Opiate Withdrawal Scale that is often referred to by the same acronym (SOWS).

Clinical Opiate Withdrawal Scale (COWS)

Resting pulse rate *after resting for 1 minute* 0 <80 beats/minute 1 81–100 bpm 2 101–120 bpm 4 >120 bpm	**GI upset** *over last 1/2 hour* 0 no GI symptoms 1 stomach cramps 2 nausea or loose stool 3 vomiting or diarrhea 5 multiple episodes of diarrhea or vomiting
Sweating *over past 1/2 hour, not accounted for by room temperature or patient activity* 0 no report of chills or flushing 1 subjective report of chills or flushing 2 flushed or observable moistness on face 3 beads of sweat on brow or face 4 sweat streaming off face	**Tremor** *observation of outstretched hands* 0 no tremor 1 tremor can be felt, but not observed 2 slight tremor observable 4 gross tremor or muscle twitching
Restlessness *observation during assessment* 0 able to sit still 1 reports difficulty sitting still, but able to do so 3 frequent shifting or extraneous movements of legs/arms 5 unable to sit still for more than a few seconds	**Yawning** *observation during assessment* 0 no yawning 1 yawning once or twice during assessment 2 yawning three or more times during assessment 4 yawning several times/minute
Pupil size 0 pupils pinned or normal in size for room light 1 pupils possibly larger than normal for room light 2 pupils moderately dilated 4 pupils are so dilated that only rim of iris is visible	**Anxiety or irritability** 0 none 1 patient reports increasing irritability or anxiousness 2 patient obviously irritable or anxious 4 patient is so irritable or anxious that participation in assessment is difficult
Bone or joint aches *if patient was having pain previously, only additional component attributable to opiate withdrawal* 0 not present 1 mild diffuse discomfort 2 patient reports severe diffuse aching of joints or muscles 4 patient rubbing joints or muscles and is unable to sit still because of discomfort	**Gooseflesh skin** 0 skin is smooth 3 piloerection of skin can be felt or hairs standing up on arms 5 prominent piloerection
Runny nose or tearing *not accounted for by cold symptoms or allergies* 0 not present 1 nasal stuffiness or unusually moist eyes 2 nose rubbing or tearing 4 nose constantly running or tears streaming down cheeks	**Total Score**_____ 5–12 mild 13–24 moderate 25–36 moderately severe > 36 severe withdrawal

Figure 7.1. Clinical Opiate Withdrawal Scale (COWS). Adapted with permission from Wesson, D. R., and W. Ling. 2003. The Clinical Opiate Withdrawal Scale (COWS). *J. Psychoactive Drugs* **35:253–259.**

Short Opiate Withdrawal Scale

	None (0 points)	Mild (1 point)	Moderate (2 points)	Severe (3 points)
1. Feeling Sick				
2. Stomach Cramps				
3. Muscle Spasms/Twitching				
4. Feelings of Coldness (Chills)				
5. Heart Pounding				
6. Muscular Tension				
7. Aches and Pains				
8. Yawning				
9. Runny Eyes				
10. Problems Sleeping				

1–10 points: Mild withdrawal
11–20 points: Moderate withdrawal
21–30 points: Severe withdrawal

Figure 7.2. The Short Opiate Withdrawal Scale. From Gossop, M. 1990. The development of a short opiate withdrawal scale. *Addict. Behav.* 15:487–490, with permission.

DIAGNOSIS

The DSM-IV diagnostic criteria for opioid dependence are the same as those for other substances; these are provided in Appendixes A and B. Anyone who uses opioids on a regular basis for an extended period of time will develop physical dependence; that is, they will develop tolerance to the drug effects and withdrawal symptoms if the substance is abruptly discontinued. This is true for patients who take prescribed opioids for chronic pain; with these patients, it is often difficult to distinguish physical dependence from addiction (meaning a pattern of use that is harmful rather than therapeutic); this topic is covered further in Chapter 13, "Prescription Drug Abuse."

Physical Exam

A number of findings on exam should raise the consideration of opioid dependence; these include constricted pupils, drowsiness, or frequent "nodding." Patients may exhibit signs of withdrawal from opioids (covered earlier in this section). Intranasal users may have nasal septal erosion or perforation (especially those who use cocaine as well). Injection drug users often have needle marks or track marks in the antecubital fossae or forearms; however, some inject in other locations, including veins in the neck, legs, groin, or axilla, or subcutaneously into the upper arm, thigh, or buttock.

Laboratory Testing

Opioid use may be detected through urine toxicology screening, though its utility as a screening test in unselected populations is limited. Urine toxicology immunoassays are most sensitive for opioids that are structurally similar to morphine (such as codeine or heroin) and less sensitive to other opioids (such as oxycodone, meperidine, or buprenorphine) (20). Methadone can be differentiated from other opioids; this is useful for monitoring individuals on methadone maintenance. Toxicology testing is covered further in Chapter 3.

In addition, since many injection drug users are infected with hepatitis C (21), the presence of antibodies to this virus or an elevated serum ALT may also be clues to a history of injection drug use.

MEDICAL COMPLICATIONS

Opioids themselves are associated with remarkably few medical complications, even with long-term use. Most of the medical complications that addicts acquire are due to the use of needles to administer the drug; complications of injection drug use are reviewed in Chapter 15, "Medical Care of the Addicted Patient."

Pulmonary Complications

Pulmonary complications with opioid use are not common. Although respiratory depression can be an acute effect of opioid use, most chronic users develop tolerance to this side effect. However, opioid users have been noted to sometimes develop acute noncardiogenic pulmonary edema, generally in the setting of overdose. In one series, of 1278 heroin overdoses treated at one hospital, 27 (2.1%) developed pulmonary edema as a complication and nine required mechanical ventilation; most recovered within 24 hours (22). There has also been one case report of hypersensitivity pneumonitis associated with intranasal heroin use (23). Furthermore, inhalation of heroin may trigger an attack in asthmatic patients (24).

Cardiovascular Complications

A number of studies have reported that the synthetic opioids methadone and levacetylmethadol (LAAM) are associated with a dose-dependent prolongation of the QT interval (25). This topic is covered further in Chapter 15, in the section titled "Care of Patients on Methadone."

Gastrointestinal Complications

Opioids slow gastrointestinal transit; one of their first therapeutic uses was to treat diarrheal illnesses. Constipation is a common problem for chronic opioid users. Use of bulking (e.g., fiber) and osmotic agents generally helps with this. Oral methylnaltrexone, a quaternary opioid receptor antagonist that does not cross the blood-brain barrier, has been reported to be effective at relieving constipation for patients on methadone maintenance (26).

Renal Complications

Opioids seem to have little, if any, deleterious effect on the kidneys (27). However, in the 1970s and 1980s, an association was observed between injection heroin use and nephrotic syndrome (so-called heroin nephropathy), sometimes leading to end-stage renal disease. These patients were generally African-American men, and pathologic evaluation revealed sclerosing glumerulonephritis (28). The etiology of this condition has never been clearly established and may have been due to impurities or adulterants; hepatitis C may also be responsible for some of the renal disease seen in heroin users (29). It appears that the incidence of "heroin nephropathy" has declined since the 1980s (30), though a case-control study in 1991 found that heroin use was associated with the development of end-stage renal disease and was estimated to account for 5–6% of new cases (**31**).

Endocrine Complications

Experimental and clinical studies have shown that opioids can produce hypogonadotrophic hypogonadism; in practice, this is generally seen in individuals on methadone maintenance or high doses of opioids for chronic pain. This topic is covered further in Chapter 15 in the section titled "Care of Patients on Methadone."

Neuromuscular Complications

Patients receiving meperidine (Demerol), especially those with renal failure, are at risk for neurotoxicity due to accumulation of the drug and its active metabolite, normeperidine (32). Symptoms include agitation, tremor, myoclonus, and even seizures (33).

TREATMENT

Screening and counseling outpatients who use heroin (and cocaine) is effective at reducing subsequent drug use (**34**). Beyond simple counseling, the treatment options for an opioid addict can be roughly categorized as (1) abstinence-based ("drug-free") treatment, aided by detoxification, and (2) maintenance treatment with the use of an opioid agonist, such as methadone or buprenorphine. A number of agents are effective at reducing the symptoms of withdrawal. However, most studies of detoxification focus on short-term outcomes (i.e., completion of detoxification) and there is little evidence supporting their long-tem effectiveness. Aftercare in the form of self-help groups, outpatient treatment, or residential programs may help addicts maintain abstinence. Maintenance treatment with an opioid agonist appears to be more effective at reducing illicit opioid use. See Table 7.2 for a summary of opioid abuse and dependence treatment studies.

Table 7.2. Summary of opioid abuse and dependence treatment studies

Intervention	Studies	Outcomes
Brief advice	RCT	Effective for reducing opioid use (in one RCT)
Self-help groups	Observational	Participation associated with better outcomes
Drug counseling	RCT	Effective (in one study)
Contingency management	RCTs Meta-analysis	Effective (while incentives are offered); no evidence of lasting effect
Residential treatment	Observational RCT	Participation associated with better outcomes; better than outpatient treatment in some measures (in one RCT)
Naltrexone	RCTs Meta-analysis	May be effective for a subset of highly motivated individuals
Detoxification		
Methadone taper	RCTs Meta-analysis	Effective at reducing severity of withdrawal
Clonidine	RCTs Meta-analysis	Effective, but no more than methadone for withdrawal symptoms
Buprenorphine	RCTs Meta-analysis	Effective (more so than clonidine, but not methadone) for symptoms
Maintenance Treatment		
Methadone	RCTs Meta-analysis	Effective, more so than detoxification Higher doses more effective; addition of psychosocial support is beneficial

Table 7.2. *Continued*

Maintenance Treatment

Levomethadyl acetate (LAAM)	RCTs	Effective, comparable to methadone
Buprenorphine	RCTs	Effective, comparable to methadone
	Meta-analysis	Effective in office-based setting

See text for references and more details.
RCT: randomized controlled trial.

Detoxification/Abstinence

Opioid withdrawal is unpleasant but not generally life-threatening. Detoxification is a palliative procedure to help relieve the symptoms and to help the addict begin the first step to recovery and abstinence. Unfortunately, long-term abstinence after detoxification is the exception rather than the rule (35). Most controlled trials of detoxification are limited by a focus on short-term outcomes (completion of detoxification), and the data that we have on longer-term outcomes is primarily from observational studies. A number of these studies suggest a modest reduction in drug use and criminal activity in the months following detoxification (36, 37).

Administration of any opioid will relieve the symptoms of withdrawal but will not necessarily help reduce dependence. A number of agents and protocols have been utilized to help ameliorate the symptoms of withdrawal and have been studied for use in detoxification. Withdrawal scales may be helpful to assess and monitor patients during detoxification, as were discussed earlier in this chapter. Most research on detoxification has been done on heroin users; these procedures may not be as effective for those dependent on long-acting opioids such as methadone or OxyContin. We address this specific issue at the end of this section.

Treatment Setting

One of the first decisions that must be made is the optimal treatment setting. Often, this decision is limited by availability, health insurance, and other practical considerations. Many opioid addicts can be safely detoxified in an ambulatory setting, and this can be coordinated in a primary care office. Other options include intensive outpatient treatment, residential treatment, and inpatient hospitalization. Indications for treatment at a more intensive level of care include concurrent dependence on other substances (particularly alcohol or benzodiazepines), previous unsuccessful attempts at detoxification, unstable social situation, or a concurrent medical or psychiatric condition that requires more intensive care. There is some evidence that addicts in inpatient treatment are more likely to complete detoxification (38), and some have argued that this makes it cost-effective (39); however, evidence supporting the longer-term superiority of inpatient treatment is lacking (40).

Agents Used for Opioid Detoxification

METHADONE. Methadone has been used for decades for treatment of opioid addiction, both for detoxification and as a maintenance treatment. A variety of protocols have been utilized with different doses of methadone and lengths of treatment. Starting doses typically vary from 20 to 60 mg/day and duration of treatment from a week to a month (or longer). One study comparing a 10-day with 21-day inpatient methadone taper reported higher and earlier peak withdrawal symptoms with the 10-day protocol; however, completion rates were similar (41). A recent Cochrane review of methadone taper for opioid withdrawal reported that "programs vary widely with regard to duration, design and treatment objectives, impairing the application of meta-analysis"; nevertheless, they concluded that "slow tapering with temporary substitution of long-acting opioids, accompanied by medical supervision and ancillary medications, can reduce withdrawal severity" (42). As a practical consideration, in the United States, the use of methadone (and other opioids) for addiction treatment on an outpatient basis is limited to licensed treatment programs, so it cannot be used for office-based detoxification.

CLONIDINE. Clonidine is a centrally acting alpha2-adrenergic receptor agonist that was originally developed for treatment of hypertension. In 1978, it was first reported that this drug also helped reduce the symptoms of opioid withdrawal (43). Clonidine seems to be associated with fewer withdrawal symptoms in the later phases of detoxification than methadone (44), but long-term outcomes (i.e., abstinence from opioids on follow-up) are no better (45). A recent Cochrane review of the use of alpha2-adrenergic agonists for opioid withdrawal detected no significant difference in efficacy between these agents and the traditional methadone taper (46). Some addiction treatment programs utilize a combination of methadone taper (or some other long-acting opioid) with clonidine.

For opioid detoxification using clonidine, patients are typically given 0.1 to 0.2 mg every 4–6 hours tapered over 5–12 days, with a maximal daily dosage of 1.0 mg/day. Often, treatment programs supplement this with analgesics, antiemetics, and antidiarrheal/antispasmodic medications to further ameliorate the symptoms of withdrawal.

Side effects of clonidine include dry mouth, sedation, and orthostatic hypotension. Abrupt withdrawal of the medication may be complicated by rebound hyperadrenergic symptoms including hypertension, sweating, agitation, flushing, and headache (47). Clonidine is frequently abused by addicts to potentiate opioid effects (48). There have even been reports of clonidine abuse in the absence of concurrent opioid use (49). Use of the transdermal patch may be less subject to abuse, but we have observed overdoses among addicts associated with chewing the transdermal patch (50).

BUPRENORPHINE. Buprenorphine is a long-acting mixed opioid agonist and antagonist that was first proposed as a treatment for opioid dependence in 1978 (51) and is currently the only FDA-approved medication for the treatment of opioid addiction that is accessible to primary care physicians. The partial opioid-antagonistic properties give buprenorphine some advantages over other opioids: It is associated with less euphoria and withdrawal symptoms; furthermore, the risk of overdose is lower than with other opioids. A number of studies have shown it to be effective for treating withdrawal symptoms and superior to clonidine in this regard (52). A recent Cochrane review concluded that "buprenorphine is more effective than clonidine and of similar effectiveness to methadone for management of opioid withdrawal" (53). Studies have also demonstrated the feasibility and effectiveness of using buprenorphine in primary care settings (54). The Substance Abuse and Mental Health Service Administration (SAMHSA) has issued treatment guidelines for the use of buprenorphine for detoxification and maintenance treatment; these can be obtained via the Internet (www.samhsa.gov) or by calling 800-729-6686 (55).

The optimal buprenorphine regimen for detoxification has not yet been established. A symptom-triggered dose-titration study of buprenorphine for heroin withdrawal found that the median dose was 4 mg on day one, 6 mg on day two, 4 mg on day three, and 2 mg on day four; most (72%) required no further medication on the fifth day (56). A small study comparing a 5-day low-dose buprenorphine regimen (2-4-8-4-2 mg/day) with a high-dose regimen (8-8-8-4-2 mg/day) found that the high-dose regimen was more effective at relieving withdrawal symptoms without any reported adverse effects (57). For our inpatient 3-day detoxification protocol, we have utilized 4 mg on admission and 4 mg at bedtime on day one (8 mg total), 4 mg in morning and 4 mg at night on day two (8 mg total), 4 mg in morning and 2 mg at night on day three (6 mg total), and a 2 mg dose on the morning of discharge. This has been effective for most patients and we have not observed any ill effects.

In the outpatient setting, patients can be titrated up to a target dose of 12 to 16 mg/day over 2–3 days and then gradually tapered over 2–4 weeks (or longer); more gradual tapers appear to be better tolerated (58). The higher initial doses with the extended detoxification are closer to usual maintenance doses of buprenorphine (discussed later in this chapter). Table 7.3 gives suggested protocols for 3- to 10-day inpatient detoxification using buprenorphine in the sublingual formulation.

There have been no studies that compare fixed-dose opioid detoxification regimens with symptom-triggered dosing. Fixed-dose protocols (with "rescue dosing" as needed) are simpler and minimize negotiations (or haggling) over dosing; furthermore, it may be better to treat in anticipation of withdrawal symptoms, rather than wait for symptoms to appear.

Both inpatient and outpatient protocols can be supplemented with symptomatic medication (analgesics, antiemetics, antidiarrheal agents). Providing other treatment modalities, such as behavioral therapy, may offer additional benefits, at least with extended detoxification programs (59). A long-acting depot injection formulation of buprenorphine is a promising treatment option on the horizon (60).

TRAMADOL. Tramadol is a centrally acting synthetic analgesic with opioid activity that has been reported to ameliorate the symptoms of opioid withdrawal. There have been two small observational reports that suggest that this agent may be superior to clonidine (61) and comparable to buprenorphine (62); if further studies confirm this observation, tramadol may be an option for practitioners who do not have access to buprenorphine.

Table 7.3.   Inpatient protocols for opioid detoxification with buprenorphine

Suggested Doses (mg of sublingual buprenorphine)

Day	10-Day (fixed dose)	7-Day (fixed dose)	3-Day (fixed dose)	5-Day (flexible dose)
1	8 mg	8 mg	12 mg	4 mg at onset of withdrawal, & additional 2–4 mg as needed
2	6 mg	8 mg	8 mg	4 mg morning, 2–4 mg evening dose as needed
3	4 mg	4 mg	8 mg	4 mg morning, 2 mg evening dose as needed
4	4 mg	4 mg		2 mg morning, 2 mg evening dose as needed
5	4 mg	2 mg		2 mg as needed
6	2 mg	2 mg		
7	2 mg	0 mg		
8	2 mg			
9	2 mg			
10	0 mg			

Adapted from Johnson, R. E., et al. 2003. *Drug Alcohol Depend.* 70:S59–S77, and Lintzeris, N., et al. 2003. *Drug Alcohol Depend.* 70:287–294.

Special Considerations

   RAPID AND ULTRARAPID DETOXIFICATION. The detoxification process can be accelerated by the addition of an opioid antagonist such as naloxone or naltrexone; some have postulated that combining these with a medication that ameliorates withdrawal symptoms (such as clonidine) may improve success rates ("rapid detoxification"). A (nonrandomized) clinical trial comparing clonidine with clonidine plus naltrexone in the ambulatory setting reported better short-term success rates with the combination (**63**). However, a subsequent randomized controlled trial by the same group found no better treatment retention with the combination, though more were "successfully detoxified" (**64**). The addition of naltrexone to buprenorphine can also help shorten the duration of withdrawal, though it increases the intensity of these symptoms (65).
   Some have tried speeding the process further by heavily sedating or anesthetizing addicts while administering an opioid antagonist ("ultrarapid detoxification"). While there have been reports of favorable success rates and safety with this strategy (**66, 67**), there is no evidence that it is more effective than other

detoxification methods, and there are concerns about its safety (68). A recent Cochrane review of this treatment concluded that this "approach must be regarded as experimental with both risks and benefits remaining uncertain" (69).

DETOXIFICATION FROM LONG-ACTING OPIOIDS. As noted earlier in this section, research on detoxification has generally been done on heroin users and less is known about the optimal strategy for users of long-acting opioids. One study of heroin and methadone users who were detoxified with a 10-day methadone taper found more severe withdrawal symptoms among the methadone users, but no significant difference in onset or duration of withdrawal (70). However, this may not apply to addicts who are being detoxified with other agents. In our experience, the withdrawal syndrome from long-acting opioids is generally delayed and prolonged when compared with the withdrawal syndrome from short-acting opioids. Therefore, detoxification will generally need to start later after the last use and continue for a longer period of time. Furthermore, the antagonistic properties of buprenorphine may predominate when given to someone on high doses of long-acting opioids, so its use may precipitate withdrawal symptoms rather than relieve them. It should be noted that many individuals who abuse long-acting oxycodone (OxyContin) crush the tablets and then ingest, snort, or inject the medication, effectively making it a short-acting drug.

We have found that the shorter detoxification protocols generally do not work as well with users of long-acting opioids, and a better strategy may be to slowly taper the dose of the long-acting opioid rather than attempt detoxification over a few days. If detoxification is attempted, it is probably best to try to begin at 36 to 48 hours after the last dose (especially if you are using buprenorphine) and be prepared to extend treatment beyond what is generally needed (a few weeks of withdrawal symptoms is not unusual). The use of buprenorphine is not recommended for those using 60 mg or more of methadone per day (or its equivalent in other long-acting opioids). Another option may be to switch to a short-acting opioid as a bridge to detoxification with buprenorphine, but federal regulations in the United States may limit this to 3 days.

Relapse Prevention

Detoxification is only the first step on the road to recovery, and it is generally believed that it should be followed by some form of "aftercare." Although there is a paucity of experimental data to support this, some observational studies suggest that aftercare is beneficial. In one study of opioid addicts who participated in a variety of drug treatments, those who received detoxification alone did not do as well as those in therapeutic communities or outpatient drug-free programs; in fact, they fared no better than those who received "intake-only" (i.e., no treatment) (71). Aftercare options include self-help groups, such as Narcotics Anonymous (NA), outpatient treatment, or residential treatment.

Self-Help Groups

Self-help groups are probably the most commonly utilized treatment modality. Many of these groups, such as Narcotics Anonymous (www.na.org), are based on the 12-step philosophy of Alcoholics Anonymous and offer meetings throughout North America. While observational studies indicate that participation in these groups is associated with better outcomes (72), there is little experimental data on their effectiveness.

Outpatient Treatment

Outpatient programs take on a variety of forms and use a wide range of strategies. There is some data to support the effectiveness of certain types of programs. One common approach is counseling combined with self-help groups; a randomized controlled trial of a weekly 3-hour recovery training and self-help group reported significant reduction in opioid use and improvements in employment and (self-reported) criminal activity after 1 year (73).

Another approach is to offer incentives for drug abstinence ("contingency management"); this approach appears to lead to more drug abstinence while the incentives are offered, but this effect dissipates thereafter. One example is a study that reported modestly improved short-term (1 month) outcomes utilizing abstinent-contingent reinforcement in the form of access to financial assistance, in addition to individual counseling, as well as job and social skills training (74). In a follow-up of this study, offering abstinent-contingent incentives for a longer period of time (3 months vs 1 month) was associated with high abstinence rates among a select group of opioid addicts over that period of time (75). A 2004 Cochrane meta-analysis of psychosocial treatments for opioid abuse and dependence concluded that these "are not adequately proved treatment modalities" (76).

Residential Treatment

Residential treatment programs differ widely in approach, setting, and length of treatment. Some halfway houses are little more than a place to stay, while other programs, such as "therapeutic communities," offer more intensive treatment. There is limited data on their effectiveness, most of it in the form of observational studies, which are limited by selection bias and incomplete follow-up of subjects. In one study, heroin addicts who participated in one of three therapeutic communities had better outcomes than those who did not, but this was limited by nonrandom assignment and the likelihood of selection bias (77).

Another study that prospectively studied a select group of individuals with a variety of drug abuse problems and randomly assigned them to a day program or a residential program did report significantly better outcomes with residential treatment in some measures, but the study concluded that the outcomes were not significantly better overall (78). With these limitations in mind, it is clear that some addicts are able to maintain sobriety for extended periods in these programs, but they are in the minority (**79**, **80**).

Naltrexone

Naltrexone, a long-acting orally active opioid antagonist, blocks the effects of opioids and has been an attractive theoretical option for relapse prevention. Unfortunately, the drug does not reduce craving for opioids and its effectiveness is limited by adherence to the drug (81). The use of naltrexone in combination with behavioral treatments, such as contingency management, may be more effective (82). It may also be beneficial in a subset of highly motivated individuals, such as health care professionals (83), business executives (84), or parolees (**85**). A 2003 Cochrane review of the efficacy of naltrexone for opioid dependence concluded that "the available trials do not allow a final evaluation"; however, a "trend in favor of treatment with naltrexone was observed for certain target groups (particularly people who are highly motivated)" (86). Long-acting injectable or implantable forms of opioid antagonists may prove to be more effective (87), but they need to be studied further.

Maintenance Treatment

The principle of opioid maintenance treatment is to reduce the medical and societal harm associated with addiction by substituting illicit drug use with the supervised provision of another opioid. Three agents have been studied for use in this way: methadone, levomethadyl acetate (LAAM), and buprenorphine; some have also proposed harm reduction through the provision of heroin to addicts.

Methadone

Methadone has been used for decades as maintenance treatment for opioid addicts, and studies have shown that this reduces illicit opioid use (**88**); furthermore, it has been found to be more effective than detoxification (**89**). Higher doses of methadone appear to be more effective (**90**), and the incorporation of abstinence reinforcement (such as rewards for drug-clean urine toxicology screens) appears to be effective as well (**91**). A 2003 Cochrane review of methadone maintenance that included six studies and 954 participants concluded that it is effective in reducing illicit opioid abuse and retaining users in treatment (92). Another review concluded that doses of 60 to 100 mg are more effective than lower doses (93).

Methadone programs typically provide widely varying levels of psychosocial services to addicts. There have been a number of studies of outcomes at different levels of services. The provision of methadone alone with limited services has been shown to reduce drug use (94). "Standard" services, which include counseling and reinforcement, lead to better outcomes; the addition of on-site medical/psychiatric care, family counseling, and employment counseling ("enhanced" services) is associated with further improvements, at least in the first 6 months of enrollment (**95**). On the other hand, "standard" services appear to be the most cost-effective (**96**). Intensive treatment in the form of a day treatment program does not appear to offer additional benefits over "enhanced services" (**97**). A 2004 Cochrane meta-analysis concluded that the addition of psychosocial support to methadone maintenance improves some outcomes (mainly heroin use), but evidence for other benefits is lacking (98).

The effectiveness of methadone as a treatment for opioid addiction is limited by its restricted availability. Despite evidence that supports the use of this treatment in the primary care setting (**99**), only licensed programs can dispense methadone for the treatment of opioid dependence in the United States (though physicians can prescribe it for pain treatment).

Levomethadyl Acetate (LAAM)

Levomethadyl acetate (also known as levo-alpha-acetylmethadol or LAAM) is a very long-acting opioid that has the advantage of being able to be dispensed three times a week as opposed to the daily administration of methadone. Studies indicate that it is as effective as methadone (**100**). Unfortunately, reports of prolonged QT syndrome and cardiac arrhythmias associated with it (reviewed further in Chapter 15) have limited its use; furthermore, like methadone, its use for opioid addiction is restricted to licensed treatment programs.

Buprenorphine

Buprenorphine is a long-acting mixed opioid agonist and antagonist that has been shown to be effective at treating opioid withdrawal. It has recently been approved for use as maintenance treatment in the United States and is accessible to physicians who undergo the necessary training and licensing. Studies show buprenorphine to be as effective as methadone when dispensed on a three-times-a-week basis by a treatment program (**100**); it can also be dispensed twice weekly (**101**). When given three times a week, a double dose (two times the daily dose) can be given on Monday and Wednesday, and a triple dose on Friday; for twice-weekly treatment, a quadruple dose can be given on Monday and triple on Friday.

Buprenorphine maintenance also appears to be effective when used in primary care settings. In one study, dispensing buprenorphine in a primary care setting was associated with better outcomes than a traditional methadone program (**102**). Furthermore, the provision of buprenorphine (prescribed) in an office-based setting has also been shown to be safe and effective (**103**). A recent Cochrane review concluded that buprenorphine is "an effective intervention for use in the maintenance treatment of heroin dependence, but it is not more effective than methadone at adequate doses" (104). As noted earlier, SAMHSA has issued treatment recommendations for the use of buprenorphine that can be obtained free of charge via the Internet (www.samhsa.gov) or by telephone (800-729-6686) (55). In addition, the California Society of Addiction Medicine has useful tools for evaluation and treatment that can be accessed at their Web site (www.csam-asam.org).

Buprenorphine has some advantages over methadone. It is less likely to cause overdose, even in individuals who have not built up tolerance to opioids. Withdrawal symptoms from buprenorphine are less severe than withdrawal symptoms from methadone. Moreover, when given in repeated doses over time, buprenorphine appears to have minimal effect on cognitive and psychomotor performance (105). One disadvantage of buprenorphine is its higher cost; however, the prescription cost of buprenorphine is fairly comparable to that of a typical methadone program.

Sublingual buprenorphine is available in two formulations, Subutex and Suboxone. Suboxone is a combination of buprenorphine and naloxone in a 4:1 ratio; the naloxone is added to prevent its parenteral use. Both appear to be equally effective and there is no evidence of ill effect from the naloxone when Suboxone is used as directed. It is recommended that all maintenance patients be given the Suboxone formulation, unless they have a sensitivity to naloxone or are pregnant; buprenorphine has not been adequately studied in pregnant women and should be used only if the benefit outweighs the potential risk. Both formulations are available in 2 mg and 8 mg dosage and must be used sublingually because this route bypasses hepatic metabolism. Table 7-4 gives some general guidelines for treatment induction. Most patients can be maintained on a dose of 12–16 mg/day of the sublingual buprenorphine. Although there is no maximum recommended dose, dosages over 32 mg/day are not generally needed; in our experience, dosages over 24 mg/day are rarely necessary.

Table 7.4. Guidance for buprenorphine maintenance therapy

Induction from Short-Acting Opioids (heroin, morphine, oxycodone, etc.)

Day 1:

- Begin the first dose at least 4 hours after last opioid use.
- Administer 4 mg sublingual tablet of buprenorphine.
- If possible, observe patient for 1–2 hours and give another 4 mg if no ill effects noted; otherwise dispense or prescribe another 4 mg for the patient to take 2–4 hours after the first dose.

Days 2 and 3:

- Assess patient's response to previous day's dosing.
- If the previous day's dose fully suppressed their withdrawal symptoms, then give the same dose; if it did not, increase the dose by 2–4 mg.
- Decrease the dose by 2 mg if the patient experiences intoxification.

Days 4–10:

- Once patient is stable, or after a target dose of 16 mg or greater is reached, continue at that dose for 3–7 days until steady state levels are achieved before increasing the dose further.

continued

Table 7.4. *Continued*

Buprenorphine induction from long-acting opioids (methadone, sustained-release oxycodone/morphine)

Step 1:

- If patient is on an opioid maintenance program or has been prescribed long-acting opioids, treatment should be coordinated with the program or prescriber.
- Patients should be warned that they might experience discomfort or dysphoria for up to 2 weeks with the transition.

Step 2:

- If possible, taper to a dose of 30 mg/day of methadone (or its equivalent). Splitting the dose may help.
- If not possible, transfers can be done with a dose of 30–60 mg/day of methadone (or its equivalent), at the lowest dose that is tolerable to the patient.
- For patients who cannot be tapered below 60 mg of methadone/day, transfer is not generally recommended. There have been reports of patients being transferred to a short-acting opioid followed by transition to buprenorphine. (This may be allowable for only 3 days by federal regulations.)
- Normal transfer (methadone dose ≤ 30 mg/d): At least 24 hours should pass following the last dose of long-acting opioid before giving the first dose of buprenorphine.
- High-dose transfer (methadone dose 30–60 mg/d). The first dose of buprenorphine should be given at least 48–96 hours after the last dose of long-acting opioid, or until the patient experiences maximal withdrawal discomfort. Earlier dosing is highly likely to precipitate withdrawal.
- Recommended dosing schedule is given below:

Long-acting opioid dose (mg of methadone/day)	≤ 10 mg	10–40 mg	40–60 mg
First-day buprenorphine target dose	2–4 mg	4–8 mg	4–8 mg
Optional dose review 2–4 hours after first dose	Dose review not required	Dose review not required	Dose review required: give 2–4 mg additional if needed
Second-day buprenorphine target dose	4 mg	8 mg (4–8 mg)	8 mg (6–10 mg)
Third-day buprenorphine target dose	6 mg (6–8 mg)	12 mg (8–12 mg)	12 mg (10–16 mg)

Adapted from *Dosing Guide for Suboxone & Subutex.*
Distributed by Reckitt Benckiser Pharmaceuticals, Inc.

Patients who are dependent on methadone or other long-acting opioids (including OxyContin) may have a difficult transition, especially if they are taking high doses; it is generally recommended that they be tapered down to the equivalent of 30 mg/day of methadone, and the transfer of patients on doses over 60 mg/day is not recommended.

It is generally recommended that patients be evaluated at least weekly during the initial treatment phase to determine that they are not having any adverse effects and that they are handling the medication responsibly. Having the patient sign an agreement at the onset of treatment can be helpful to clarify and document the responsibilities and expectations; Figure 7.3 provides an example of one such agreement. Once the patient is sta-

---

Buprenorphine Treatment Agreement

Patient Responsibilities

____ **The patient will agree to store the medication properly**. The medication can be harmful to others. The pills should be stored in a safe, secure place, out of reach of children. If anyone other than the patient ingests the medication, the patient must call the poison control center or 911 immediately.

____ **The patient is responsible for the safekeeping of the prescription and medication.** Lost or stolen prescriptions or medications will not be replaced.

____ **The patient will agree to take the medication only as prescribed.** The patient must not change or adjust the dose without prior approval of the treating physician. If the patient wishes to have a dose change, the patient must contact their physician first.

____ **The patient will agree to comply with pill counts or urine tests when requested.** The patient must be prepared to provide a urine sample for testing at each visit and to show their pill bottle for a pill count.

____ **The patient will agree to notify the clinic immediately in case of relapse to drug abuse.** The abuse of opiates or other drugs while on buprenorphine maintenance can be life-threatening and an appropriate treatment plan needs to be developed as soon as possible. The physician should be informed of drug use before a urine test shows it.

____ **The patient will agree to follow clinic procedures and rules.** This includes the hours, phone numbers, procedure for making appointments, fees, and appropriate behavior.

Patient Name _____

Patient Signature _____ **Date** _____

Provider Name _____

Provider Signature _____ **Date** _____

Figure 7.3.   Sample Buprenorphine Treatment Agreement.

bilized and has urine samples that are free of illicit opioids, less frequent visits (biweekly or monthly) may be sufficient. Of note, buprenorphine is not detected in most currently available commercial urine toxicology screens, though there are assays available for its detection. For those who have urine toxicology screens positive for other substances, a variety of strategies can be used. Many opioid addicts also use cocaine; continued use while on buprenorphine is generally not grounds for discontinuing treatment, but physicians should counsel patients on their use and may wish to provide incentives to patients for abstinence (such as increasing the interval between visits). Those who are abusing sedatives or alcohol in combination with buprenorphine should be warned of the risks of combining these and should receive treatment for their other substance use disorders. In some cases, it may be best to discontinue treatment with buprenorphine if the individual continues to abuse alcohol or sedatives and does not comply with treatment.

It is generally recommended that maintenance treatment with buprenorphine be part of a broader treatment plan and that patients participate in other psychosocial treatment modalities. This can be in the form of attending self help groups or receiving office-based counseling; the optimal approach probably depends on the patient's background and his or her stage in treatment. One study comparing brief weekly counseling with more intensive thrice-weekly counseling reported equivalent outcomes (106). Another study using an approach that incorporates friends or family members in treatment ("network therapy") reported lower illicit heroin use among patients on buprenorphine who were able to establish a network (107).

Physicians who wish to prescribe buprenorphine are required to undergo 8 hours of training and obtain a special license from the Drug Enforcement Administration (DEA). Courses are regularly offered throughout the United States and the necessary training can be done on the Internet using Web-based training modules; information on both of these is available on the Substance Abuse and Mental Health Services Administration's Web site (www.samhsa.gov). Current federal law limits each physician to treating 30 individuals at a time.

Heroin

Some have advocated the prescription of diacetylmorphine (heroin) to chronic and treatment-refractory addicts as a harm reduction strategy (108). The rationale is that this will reduce the risk of overdose and medical complications, as well as the societal burden of addiction (crime, etc.). One study of 51 heroin addicts in Switzerland who had failed previous treatments suggested that this is a feasible approach (109). A larger study, conducted in the Netherlands, also found that providing supervised heroin coprescription was safe and effective for heroin addicts who continued to use while on methadone maintenance (110); however, the doses of methadone used were modest and it is possible that increasing the methadone dose would have been just as effective.

REFERENCES

1. Substance Abuse and Mental Health Services Administration. 2004. Results from the 2003 National Survey on Drug Use and Health: National Findings (Office of Applied Studies, NSDUH Series H-25, DHHS Publication No. SMA 04-3964). Rockville, MD.
2. Mark, T. L., G. E. Woody, T. Juday, and H. D. Kleber. 2001. The economic costs of heroin addiction in the United States. *Drug Alcohol Depend.* 61:195–206.
3. Substance Abuse and Mental Health Services Administration, Office of Applied Studies. 2003. Emergency Department Trends from the Drug Abuse Warning Network, Final Estimates 1995–2002, DAWN Series: D-24, DHHS Publication No. (SMA) 03-3780. Rockville, MD.
4. Gutstein, H. B., and H. Akil. 2001. Opioid analgesics. In *The pharmacologic basis of therapeutics.* 10th ed. Edited by J. G. Hardman, L. E. Limbird, and G. A. Goodman, 569–619. New York: McGraw-Hill.
5. Seal, K. H., A. H. Kral, L. Gee, et al. 2001. Predictors and prevention of nonfatal overdose among street-recruited injection heroin users in the San Francisco Bay area, 1998–1999. *Am. J. Pub. Health* 91:1842–1846.
6. Gossop, M., D. Stewart, S. Treacy, and J. Marsden. 2002. A prospective study of mortality among drug misusers during a 4-year period after seeking treatment. *Addiction* 97:39–47.
7. Tagliaro, F., Z. DeBattisti, F. P. Smith, and M. Marigo. 1998. Death from heroin overdose: Findings from hair analysis. *Lancet* 351:1923–1925.
8. Strang, J., J. McCambridge, D. Best, et al. 2003. Loss of tolerance and overdose mortality after inpatient opiate detoxification: Follow up study. *BMJ* 326:959–960.
9. Wanger, K., L. Brough, I. Macmillan, et al. 1998. Intravenous vs subcutaneous naloxone for out-of-hospital management of presumed opioid overdose. *Acad. Emerg. Med.* 5:293–299.
10. Kelly, A. M., D. Kerr, P. Dietze, et al. 2005. Randomised trial of intranasal versus intramuscular naloxone in prehospital treatment for suspected opioid overdose. *Med. J. Aust.* 182:24–27.
11. Sporer, K. A. 1999. Acute heroin overdose. *Ann. Intern. Med.* 130:584–590.
12. Christenson, J., J. Etherington, E. Grafstein, et al. 2000. Early discharge of patients with presumed opioid overdose: Development of a clinical prediction rule. *Acad. Emerg. Med.* 7:1110–1118.
13. Vilke, G. M., C. Sloane, A. M. Smith, and T. C. Chan. 2003. Assessment for deaths in out-of-hospital heroin overdose patients treated with naloxone who refuse treatment. *Acad. Emerg. Med.* 10:893–896.
14. Watson, W. A., M. T. Steele, R. L. Muelleman, and M. D. Rush. 1998. Opioid toxicity recurrence after initial response to naloxone. *J. Toxicol. Clin. Toxicol.* 36:11–17.
15. Caplehorn, J. R., M. S. Dalton, F. Haldar, et al. 1996. Methadone maintenance and addicts' risk of fatal heroin overdose. *Subst. Use Misuse* 31:177–196.

16. Lepere, B., L. Gourarier, M. Sanchez, et al. 2001. Reduction in the number of lethal heroin overdoses in France since 1994. Focus on substitution treatments. *Ann. Med. Interne* (Paris) 152(Suppl. 3):IS5–IS12.

17. Strang, J., S. Darke, W. Hall, et al. 1996. Heroin overdose: The case for take-home naloxone. *BMJ* 312:1435–1436.

18. Strang, J., and R. Fortson. 2004. Commentary: Supervised fixing rooms, supervised injectable maintenance clinics—understanding the difference. *BMJ* 328:102–103.

19. Gossop, M. 1990. The development of a short opiate withdrawal scale (SOWS). *Addict. Behav.* 15:487–490.

20. Testing for Drugs of Abuse. 2002. *The Medical Letter* 44:71–73.

21. Fingerhood, M. I., D. R. Jasinski, and J. T. Sullivan. 1993. Prevalence of hepatitis C in a chemically dependent population. *Arch. Intern. Med.* 153:2025–2030.

22. Sporer, K. A., and E. Dorn. 2001. Heroin-related noncardiogenic pulmonary edema: A case series. *Chest* 120:1628–1632.

23. Karne, S., C. D'Ambrosio, O. Einarsson, and P. G. O'Connor. 1999. Hypersensitivity pneumonitis induced by intranasal heroin use. *Am. J. Med.* 107:392–395.

24. Cygan, J., M. Trunsky, and T. Corbridge. 2000. Inhaled heroin-induced status asthmaticus. Five cases and a review of the literature. *Chest* 117:272–275.

25. Martell, B. A., J. H. Arnsten, B. Ray, and M. N. Gourevitch. 2003. The impact of methadone on cardiac conduction in opiate users. *Ann. Intern. Med.* 139:154–155.

26. Yuan, S. C., and J. F. Foss. 2000. Oral methylnaltrexone for opioid-induced constipation. *JAMA* 284:1383–1384.

27. Arruda, J. A., N. A. Kurtzman, and V. K. Pillay. 1975. Prevalence of renal disease in asymptomatic heroin addicts. *Arch. Intern. Med.* 135:535–537.

28. Cunningham, E. E., J. R. Brentjens, M. A. Zielezny, et al. 1980. Heroin nephropathy. A clinicopathologic and epidemiologic study. *Am. J. Med.* 68:47–53.

29. do Sameiro Faria, M., S. Sampaio, V. Faria, and E. Carvalho. 2003. Nephropathy associated with heroin abuse in Caucasian patients. *Nephrol. Dial. Transplant.* 18:2308–2313.

30. Friedman, E. A., and T. K. Tao. 1995. Disappearance of uremia due to heroin-associated nephropathy. *Am. J. Kidney Dis.* 25.689–693.

31. Perneger, T. V., M. J. Klag, and P. K. Whelton. 2001. Recreational drug use: A neglected risk factor for end-stage renal disease. *Am. J. Kid. Dis.* 38:49–56. *Seven hundred sixteen persons with end-stage renal disease (ESRD) were compared with 361 random controls. After adjusting for age, sex, race, socioeconomic status, hypertension, and diabetes, illicit opiate use (ever) was associated with an increased risk of ESRD (OR: 19). However, other potential risk factors were not taken into account, including HIV, HCV, and smoking.*

32. Szeto, H. H., C. E. Inturrisi, R. Houde, et al. 1977. Accumulation of normeperidine, an active metabolite of meperidine, in patients with renal failure or cancer. *Ann. Intern. Med.* 86:738–741.

33. Hershey, L. A. 1983. Meperidine and central neurotoxicity. *Ann. Intern. Med.* 98:548–549.

34. Bernstein, J., E. Bernstein, K. Tassiopoulos, et al. 2005. Brief motivational intervention at a clinic visit reduces cocaine and heroin use. *Drug Alcohol Depend.* 77:49–59. *Patients at walk-in clinics were screened for heroin or cocaine use and randomized to one of the following: (1) a brief intervention (by a trained counselor) including motivational interview, active referrals, and written handout with a list of treatment resources, followed by a phone call 10 days later, or (2) handout only. Of the 23,669 screened, 1232 (5%) were eligible, 1175 enrolled, and 778 were used in the final analysis. At 6-month follow-up, the intervention group was more likely to be abstinent from heroin alone (40.2% vs. 30.6%), cocaine alone (22.3% vs. 16.9%), and both drugs (17.4% vs. 12.8%).*

35. Gossop, M., L. Green, G. Phillips, and B. Bradley. 1987. What happens to opiate addicts immediately after treatment: A prospective follow up study. *BMJ* 294:1377–1380. *Of 57 consecutively admitted addicts, 50 (88%) completed 21-day inpatient detox and were followed for 6 months. Most (76%) used opiates at some point during this period; at 6 months, 26 were opiate-free and 8 reported using less than daily.*

36. Broers, B., F. Giner, P. Dumont, and A. Mino. 2000. Inpatient opiate detoxification in Geneva: Follow-up at 1 and 6 months. *Drug Alcohol Depend.* 58:85–92. *Seventy-three opiate addicts received inpatient detox (most with methadone, average 15 days); 73% completed detox, and at 6 months, 22 of 60 interviewed were abstinent and 11 had at least one overdose.*

37. Chutuape, M. A., D. R. Jasinski, M. I. Fingerhood, and M. L. Stitzer. 2001. One-, three-, and six-month outcomes after brief inpatient opioid detoxification. *Am. J. Drug Alcohol Abuse* 27:19–44. *One hundred sixteen heroin users who agreed to participate after inpatient 3-day detox were followed for 6 months; compared to baseline, they (1) used less heroin, cocaine, and alcohol, (2) engaged in less criminal activity, (3) were more likely to be employed, and (4) were more likely to have a regular place to live. Approximately a third were not using heroin at 6 months, another third were using regularly, and the rest were using intermittently.*

38. Gossop, M., A. Johns, and L. Green. 1986. Opiate withdrawal: Inpatient versus outpatient programmes and preferred versus random assignment to treatment. *BMJ* 293:103–104. *Sixty opioid addicts were asked if they were willing to accept either inpatient or outpatient detox; those who agreed (20) were randomized to one, and the rest (40) were assigned to their choice. Twenty-five out of thirty-one (81%) completed 3-week inpatient methadone taper vs. 5/29 (17%) assigned to 8-week outpatient taper. Those in their treatment choice tended to do better than those randomly assigned (54% vs. 34%).*

39. Gossop, M., and J. Strang. 2000. Price, cost and value of opiate detoxification. *Br. J. Psych.* 177:262–266.

40. Day, E., J. Ison, and J. Strang. 2005. Inpatient versus other settings for detoxification for opioid dependence. *The Cochrane Database of Systematic Reviews.* Issue 2. Art. No.: CD004580.

41. Gossop, M., P. Griffiths, B. Bradley, and J. Strang. 1989. Opiate withdrawal symptoms in response to 10-day and 21-day methadone withdrawal programmes. *Br. J. Psych.* 154:360–363.

42. Amato, L., M. Davoli, M. Ferri, and R. Ali. 2003. Methadone at tapered doses for the management of opioid withdrawal. *The Cochrane Database of Systemic Reviews.* Issue 4. Art. No.: CD:003409.pub2.

43. Gold, M. S., D. E. Redmond, and H. D. Kleber. 1978. Clonidine in opiate withdrawal. *Lancet* 311:929–930.

44. Washton, A. M., and R. B. Resnick. 1980. Clonidine versus methadone for opiate detoxification. *Lancet* 316:1297. *In this double-blind trial, 26 opioid addicts on 15–30 mg/day of methadone were given either a 1 mg/day methadone taper or an "individualized clonidine regimen." Thirty-one percent on methadone were abstinent for 10 days after detox versus 46% on clonidine; this difference was not statistically significant.*

45. Kleber, H. D., C. E. Riordan, B. Rounsaville, et al. 1985. Clonidine in outpatient detoxification from methadone maintenance. *Arch. Gen. Psychiatry.* 42:391–394. *Forty-nine methadone-maintained addicts whose dose had been lowered to 20 mg/day were randomized to (1) methadone taper at 1 mg/day increments or (2) substitution with clonidine (increasing from 0.3 mg/day to 1.0 mg/day on day 10, then tapered over 10 days). Patients on clonidine were more likely to drop out in the first 10 days but did better in the second half. Overall, 30-day success rates were about the same (~40%).*

46. Gowing, L., M. Farrell, R. Ali, and J. White. 2004. Alpha2 adrenergic agonists for the management of opioid withdrawal. *The Cochrane Database of Systematic Reviews,* Issue 4. Art. No · CD002024.pub2.

47. Reid, J. L., H. J. Dargie, D. S. Davies, et al. 1977. Clonidine withdrawal in hypertension. Changes in blood-pressure and plasma and urinary noradrenaline. *Lancet* 309:1171–1174.

48. Dennison, S. J. 2001. Clonidine abuse among opiate addicts. *Psych. Quart.* 72:191–195.

49. Markowitz, J. S., H. Myrick, and W. Hiott. 1997. Clonidine dependence. *J. Clin. Psychopharmacol.* 17:137–138.

50. Rapko, D. A., and D. A. Rastegar. 2003. Intentional clonidine patch ingestion by 3 adults in a detoxification unit. *Arch. Intern. Med.* 163:367–368.

51. Jasinski, D. R., J. S. Pevnick, and J. D. Griffith. 1978. Human pharmacology and abuse potential of the analgesic buprenorphine: A potential agent for treating narcotic addiction. *Arch. Gen. Psychiatry.* 35:501–516.

52. Lintzeris, N., J. Bell, G. Bammer, et al. 2002. A randomized controlled trial of buprenorphine in the management of short-term ambulatory heroin withdrawal. *Addiction* 97:1395–1404. *One hundred fourteen heroin users were randomized to detox with either 8 days of clonidine or 5 days of buprenorphine. Those on buprenorphine had better treatment retention at day 8 (86% vs. 57%) and 35 (62% vs. 39%); they also had less severe withdrawal symptoms.*

53. Gowing, L., R. Ali, and J. White. 2004. Buprenorphine for the management of opioid withdrawal. *The Cochrane Database of Systematic Reviews.* Issue 4. Art. No.: CD002025.pub2.

54. Gibson, A. E., C. M. Doran, J. R. Bell, et al. 2003. A comparison of buprenorphine treatment in clinic and primary care

settings: A randomised trial. *Med. J. Aust.* 179:38–42. *One hundred fifteen heroin addicts were randomized to 5-day out-patient detox at either a drug treatment center or a general practice. There were no significant differences in detox completion (~75%) or participation in post-detox treatment (~56%). At 3-month follow-up, self-reported heroin use in both arms was about the same but was significantly lower than prior to detox.*

55. Center for Substance Abuse Treatment. 2004. Clinical Guidelines for the Use of Buprenorphine in the Treatment of Opioid Addiction. Treatment improvement protocol (TIP) Series 40. DHHS Publication No. (SMA) 04-3939. Rockville, MD: Substance Abuse and Mental Health Services Administration.

56. Lintzeris, N., G. Bammer, L. Rushworth, et al. 2003. Buprenorphine dosing regimen for inpatient heroin withdrawal: A symptom-triggered dose titration study. *Drug Alcohol Depend.* 70:287–294.

57. Oreskovich, M. R., A. J. Saxon, M. L. K. Ellis, et al. 2005. A double-blind, double-dummy, randomized, prospective pilot study of the partial Mu opiate agonist, buprenorphine, for acute detoxification from heroin. *Drug Alcohol Depend.* 77:71–79. *Thirty heroin-dependent adults with moderate-severe withdrawal symptoms (COWS ≥ 13) were randomized to inpatient detox with (1) low-dose buprenorphine, (2) high-dose buprenorphine, or (3) clonidine. Both buprenorphine regimens were better at suppressing withdrawal than clonidine; high dose was somewhat better than low in some measures.*

58. Amass, L., W. K. Bickel, S. T. Higgins, and J. R. Hughes. 1994. A preliminary investigation of outcome following gradual or rapid buprenorphine detoxification. *J. Addict. Dis.* 13:33–45.

59. Bickel, W. K., L. Amass, S. T. Higgins, et al. 1997. Effects of adding behavioral treatment to opioid detoxification with buprenorphine. *J. Consult. Clin. Psychol.* 65:803–810. *Thirty-nine opioid addicts in a 26-week detox program were randomized to behavioral treatment (vouchers for clean urines, community reinforcement, and individual counseling) or standard treatment (weekly individual counseling). Those assigned to behavioral treatment were more likely to complete the 26-week course (53% vs. 20%) and to have extended opioid abstinence; use of other drugs was not significantly reduced.*

60. Sigmon, S. C., C. J. Wong, A. L. Chausmer, et al. 2004. Evaluation of an injection depot formulation of buprenorphine: Placebo comparison. *Addiction* 99:1439–1449. *Fifteen opioid addicts were randomized to depot-buprenorphine or placebo in a double-blind fashion and monitored for 6 weeks on an inpatient unit. Those on buprenorphine needed less medication for withdrawal and had a blunted response to hydromorphone; there were no ill effects noted.*

61. Sobey, P. W., T. V. Parran, S. F. Grey, et al. 2003. The use of tramadol for acute heroin withdrawal: A comparison to clonidine. *J. Addict. Dis.* 22:13–25.

62. Tamaskar, R., T. V. Parran, A. Heggi, et al. 2003. Tramadol versus buprenorphine for the treatment of opiate withdrawal: A ret-

rospective cohort study. *J. Addict. Dis.* 22:5–12. *Of 64 subjects with mild-moderate opioid withdrawal, 44 were detoxified with tramadol and 20 with buprenorphine. The tramadol group received 100 mg q4 hours day one, 100 mg q6 day two, and then 50 mg q6 and 50 mg q8 days three and four. The buprenorphine protocol was 0.4, 0.3, 0.2, and 0.1 mg SC q4 on four sequential days. Withdrawal symptom severity and completion rates were comparable, but 4 of 44 on tramadol needed supplemental buprenorphine. The paper does not report how subjects were assigned to each treatment.*

63. O'Connor, P. G., M. F. Waugh, and K. M. Carroll, et al. 1995. Primary care-based ambulatory opioid detoxification: The results of a clinical trial. *J. Gen. Intern. Med.* 10:255–260. *One hundred twenty-five opioid addicts were offered detox with clonidine alone (over 12 days) or combined with naltrexone (5 days); 57 chose the first and 68 the latter. Baseline characteristics and withdrawal symptoms were not significantly different, but 94% on the combination completed the program versus 42% on clonidine alone (p < 0.001).*

64. O'Connor, P. G., K. M. Carroll, J. M. Shi, et al. 1997. Three methods of opioid detoxification in a primary care setting: A randomized trial. *Ann. Intern. Med.* 127:526–530. *One hundred sixty-two heroin addicts were randomized to detox with (1) clonidine (7 days), (2) clonidine + naltrexone (3 days), or (3) buprenorphine (5 days). Those in arms 2 and 3 were somewhat more likely to complete detox (80% vs. 65% on clonidine alone; p = 0.07), but 8-day retention was no better (~60% in each arm). Those on buprenorphine had significantly less withdrawal symptoms.*

65. Umbricht, A., I. D. Montoya, D. R. Hoover, et al. 1999. Naltrexone shortened opioid detoxification with buprenorphine. *Drug Alcohol Depend.* 56:181–190.

66. Seoane, A., G. Carrasco, L. Cabré, et al. 1994. Efficacy and safety of two methods of rapid intravenous detoxification in heroin addicts previously treated without success. *Br. J. Psych.* 171:340–345. *Three hundred healthy, motivated volunteers were randomized to ultrarapid (~8 hours duration) detox with light or deep sedation. The complication rate was 4.3%; 6 required intubation and 1 developed nosocomial pneumonia that led to a 5-day hospitalization. After detox, subjects received naltrexone and visits by a physician and psychologist—93% remained abstinent after 1 month.*

67. Hensel, M., and W. J. Kox. 2000. Safety, efficacy, and long-term results of a modified version of rapid opiate detoxification under general anaesthesia: A prospective study in methadone, heroin, codeine and morphine addicts. *Acta Anaesthesiol. Scand.* 44:326–333. *Seventy-two young opioid addicts were detoxified under general anesthesia using naltrexone and clonidine over 6 hours; naltrexone was prescribed after completion and they also received supportive therapy. No significant complications were reported. At 12 months, 49 (67%) were abstinent from opioids; there was no control group for comparison.*

68. Dyer, O. 2001. Doctor struck off after patient dies from detoxification treatment. *BMJ* 323:955.

69. Gowing, L., R. Ali, and J. White. 2002. Opioid antagonists under heavy sedation or anaesthesia for opioid withdrawal. *The Cochrane Database of Systematic Reviews.* Issue 2. Art. No.: CD002022.

70. Gossop, M., and J. Strang. 1991. A comparison of the withdrawal responses of heroin and methadone addicts during detoxification. *Br. J. Psychiatry* 158:697–699.

71. Bracy, S. A., and D. D. Simpson. 1982. Status of opioid addicts 5 years after admission to drug abuse treatment. *Am. J. Drug Alcohol Abuse* 9:115–127.

72. Christo, G., and C. Franey. 1995. Drug users' spiritual beliefs, locus of control and the disease concept in relation to Narcotics Anonymous attendance and six-month outcomes. *Drug Alcohol Depend.* 38:51–56.

73. McAuliffe, W. E. 1990. A randomized controlled trial of recovery training and self-help for opioid addicts in New England and Hong Kong. *J. Psychoactive Drugs* 22:197–209. *One hundred sixty-eight volunteers who completed drug treatment (detox, therapeutic community, halfway house, etc.) were randomized to weekly 3-hour sessions that included recovery training led by a drug counselor and a peer-led self-help group; they also participated in recreational activities and community service. The control arm received no treatment. Among those who had follow-up interviews, opioid abstinence and "rare use" was significantly higher in the treatment arm during the first 6 months (47% vs. 29%) and second 6 months (36% vs. 19%).*

74. Gruber, K., M. A. Chutuape, and M. L. Stitzer. 2000. Reinforcement-based intensive outpatient treatment for inner city opiate abusers: A short-term evaluation. *Drug Alcohol Depend.* 57:211–223. *Twenty-eight of 52 opiate addicts (of 91 initially recruited) who completed inpatient 3-day detox were randomized to a 3-month program that included (during the first month) counseling, social skills training, employment and housing assistance, recreational activities, and abstinent-contingent rewards; during the next 2 months, they had counseling only. Only five completed the program; participants were more likely to be abstinent from heroin/cocaine at 30 days (50% vs. 21%), but not at 3-month follow-up.*

75. Katz, E. C., K. Gruber, M. A. Chutuape, and M. L. Stitzer. 2001. Reinforcement-based outpatient treatment for opiate and cocaine abusers. *J. Subst. Abuse Treat.* 20:93–98. *Thirty-seven recently detoxified opioid addicts in a program like the one in the previous reference were given abstinence-contingent rewards over 3 months instead of over 1 month. Sixteen (43%) completed the program; 92% of their urines were opioid/cocaine-free versus 56% of the dropouts' urines.*

76. Mayet, S., M. Farrell, M. Ferri, et al. 2004. Psychosocial treatment for opiate abuse and dependence. *The Cochrane Database of Systematic Reviews.* Issue 4. Art. No.: CD004330.

77. Bale, R. N., V. P. Zarcone, W. W. Van Stone, et al. 1984. Three therapeutic communities. A prospective controlled study of narcotic addiction treatment: Process and two-year follow-up results. *Arch. Gen. Psychiatry* 41:185–191. *One hundred eighty-one opioid addicts who spent at least a week in one of three therapeutic communities were compared with 166 who completed only detox. After 2 years, those who participated in two of the three programs were more likely to be working or attending school and*

less likely to have been convicted of a crime. Most of the drug and alcohol use outcome measures were not significantly better.

78. Guydish, J., J. L. Sorensen, M. Chan, et al. 1999. A randomized trial comparing day and residential drug abuse treatment: 18-month outcomes. *J. Consult. Clin. Psychol.* 67:428–434. *Five hundred thirty-four drug abusers were randomized to day or residential treatment in a therapeutic community; 261 (49%) completed 2 weeks and 188 (35%) completed all the follow-up interviews over 18 months. Overall, both groups improved. Those assigned residential treatment had better outcomes in terms of psychiatric symptoms and social problem severity but not in terms of other measures, including addiction severity and employment.*

79. Keen, J., P. Oliver, G. Rowse, Mathers. 2001. Residential rehabilitation for drug users: A review of 13 months' intake to a therapeutic community. *Fam. Pract.* 18:545–548. *Of 138 drug users admitted to a residential treatment program in the U.K., 17 (12.5%) completed the 1-year program and remained abstinent.*

80. Gossop, M., J. Marsden, D. Stewart, and T. Kidd. 2003. The national treatment outcome research study (NTORS): 4–5 year follow-up results. *Addiction* 98:291–303. *Four hundred eighteen (of 650 eligible) drug misusers who were treated in a variety of settings, including residential treatment, were followed for 4–5 years. The 142 in residential treatment reported significant declines in criminal activity, and almost half of the heroin users reported being abstinent in the previous 90 days at their follow-up interview.*

81. San, L., G. Pomarol, J. M. Peri, et al. 1991. Follow-up after six month maintenance period on naltrexone versus placebo in heroin addicts. *Br. J. Addict.* 86:983–990.

82. Carroll, K. M., S. A. Ball, C. Nich, et al. 2001. Targeting behavioral therapies to enhance naltrexone treatment of opioid dependence. Efficacy of contingency management and significant other involvement. *Arch. Gen. Psychiatry* 58:755–761.

83. Ling, W., and D. R. Wesson. 1984. Naltrexone treatment for addicted health care professionals: A collaborative private practice experience. *J. Clin. Psych.* 45:46–48.

84. Washton, A. M., M. S. Gold, and A. C. Potash. 1984. Naltrexone in addicted physicians and business executives. *NIDA Res. Monogr.* 55:185–190.

85. Cornish, J. W., D. Metzger, G. E. Woody, et al. 1997. Naltrexone pharmacotherapy for opioid dependent federal probationers. *J. Subst. Abuse Treat.* 14:529–534. *Fifty-one volunteer probationers (of 300 eligible) were randomized to naltrexone or control; all received counseling. Over 6 months, those assigned to naltrexone had better treatment retention (52% vs. 33%); they were less likely to be reincarcerated (26% vs. 56%) or to have opiate-positive urines (8% vs. 30%).*

86. Kirchmayer, U., M. Davoli, and A. D. Verster. 2003. Naltrexone maintenance treatment for opioid dependence. *The Cochrane Database of Systemic Reviews.* Issue 2. Art. No.: CD001333.

87. Foster, J., C. Brewer, and T. Steele. 2003. Naltrexone implants can completely prevent early (1-month) relapse after opiate detoxification: A pilot study of two cohorts totaling 101 patients with a note on naltrexone blood levels. *Addict. Biol.* 8:211–217.

88. Newman, R. G., and W. B. Whitehill. 1979. Double-blind comparison of methadone maintenance treatments of narcotic addicts in Hong Kong. *Lancet* 314:485–488. *One hundred heroin addicts were stabilized on 60 mg of methadone over 2 weeks and then randomized to (1) methadone taper (1 mg/day) followed by placebo or (2) methadone maintenance (30–130 mg/day). Retention rates were better on maintenance, both at 32 weeks (76% vs. 10%) and at 3 years (56% vs. 2%).*

89. Sees, K. L., K. L. Delucchi, C. Masson, et al. 2000. Methadone maintenance vs. 180-day psychosocially enriched detoxification for treatment of opioid dependence. *JAMA* 283:1303–1310. *One hundred seventy-nine opioid addicts were randomized to methadone maintenance or methadone-assisted detox and followed for 12 months. Those on maintenance had better treatment retention, lower rate of drug-related HIV risk behaviors, and fewer legal problems. Heroin use decreased in both arms, more so on maintenance; however, most in both arms still used heroin. There was no difference in employment, family functioning, or alcohol use.*

90. Strain, E. C., G. E. Bigelow, I. A. Liebson, and M. L. Stitzer. 1999. Moderate- vs. high-dose methadone in the treatment of opioid dependence. *JAMA* 281:1000–1005. *One hundred seventy-nine opioid addicts were randomized to low-dose (40–50 mg/day) or high-dose (80–100 mg/day) methadone. At week 30, the high-dose group had lower rates of illicit opioid use (53% vs. 62%) and more completed the 40-week program (33% vs. 20%), but this difference was not statistically significant.*

91. Preston, K. L., A. Umbricht, and D. H. Epstein. 2000. Methadone dose increase and abstinence reinforcement for treatment of continued heroin use during methadone maintenance. *Arch. Gen. Psychiatry* 57:395–404. *One hundred twenty subjects on methadone who had three or more positive urine tox screens (opiates or cocaine) over 5 weeks were randomized to (1) methadone dose increase (from 50 to 70 mg/day), (2) vouchers as a reward for negative tox screens, (3) both dose increase and vouchers, or (4) neither (control). Dose increase and vouchers were equally effective at reducing use over 8 weeks, but the combination was not significantly better.*

92. Mattick, R. P., C. Breen, J. Kimber, and M. Davoli. 2003. Methadone maintenance therapy versus no opioid replacement therapy for opioid dependence. *The Cochrane Database of Systematic Reviews.* Issue 2. Art. No.: CD002209.

93. Faggiano, F., F. Vigna-Taglianti, E. Versino, and P. Lemma. 2003. Methadone maintenance at different dosages for opioid dependence. *The Cochrane Database of Systematic Reviews.* Issue 3. Art. No.: CD002208.

94. Yancovitz, S. R., D. C. DesJarlais, N. P. Peyser, et al. 1991. A randomized trial of an interim methadone maintenance clinic. *Am. J. Pub. Health* 81:1185–1191.

95. McLellan, A. T., I. O. Arndt, D. S. Metzger, et al. 1993. The effects of psychosocial services in substance abuse treatment. *JAMA* 269:1953–1959. *Ninety-two opiate addicts were randomized to (1) "minimum methadone services" (MMS), methadone alone without additional services; (2) "standard methadone services" (SMS), methadone plus counseling and reinforcement; or (3) "enhanced methadone services" (EMS), SMS plus on-site medical/psychiatric*

care, employment counseling, and family therapy. "Treatment failure" was defined as eight consecutive opiate/cocaine-positive urines or three "emergency situations" requiring immediate health care, and was higher over 24 weeks among MMS subjects (69%) than among SMS (41%) or EMS (19%); most were due to cocaine use.

96. Kraft, M. K., A. B. Rothbard, T. R. Hadley, et al. 1997. Are supplementary services provided during methadone maintenance really cost-effective? *Am. J. Psych.* 154:1214–1219. *This study calculated the cost-effectiveness of the three levels of services from the previous reference. The annual cost per abstinent client was $16,485 at the minimum level, $9804 at the standard level, and $11,818 at the enhanced level.*

97. Avants, S. K., A. Margolin, J. L. Sindelar, et al. 1999. Day treatment versus enhanced standard methadone services for opioid-dependent patients: A comparison of clinical efficacy and cost. *Am. J. Psych.* 156:27–33. *Two hundred ninety-one subjects on methadone maintenance were randomized to (1) enhanced treatment (2 hours/week of counseling and other services) or (2) intensive treatment (5 hours/day, 5 days/week of counseling and group therapy). Eighty-one percent in both arms completed the 12-week program; the enhanced treatment had equivalent outcomes (cocaine or opiate use) at less than half the cost of the intensive treatment.*

98. Amato, L., S. Minozzi, M. Davoli, et al. 2004. Psychosocial combined with agonist maintenance treatment versus agonist maintenance treatments alone for the treatment of opioid dependence. *The Cochrane Database of Systematic Reviews.* Issue 4, Art. No.: CD004147.

99. Fiellin, D. A., P. G. O'Connor, M. Chawarski, et al. 2001. Methadone maintenance in primary care. *JAMA* 286:1724–1731. *Forty-seven opioid addicts on methadone for a year without evidence of illicit drug use were randomized to either receive methadone at a primary care office or continue their program. Illicit drug use over 6 months was the same in both groups (40–50%); patients were more satisfied with office-based treatment.*

100. Johnson, R. E., M. A. Chutuape, E. C. Strain, et al. 2000. A comparison of levomethadyl acetate, buprenorphine, and methadone for opioid dependence. *N. Engl. J. Med.* 343:1290–1297. *Fifty-five opioid addicts were randomized to (1) levomethadyl acetate (3X/week), (2) methadone (daily), (3) buprenorphine (3X/week), or (4) low-dose methadone (essentially a control group). The three active treatments were roughly equivalent and were better than low-dose methadone in terms of retention and abstinence (26–36% vs. 8%).*

101. Marsch, L. A., W. K. Bickel, G. J. Badger, and E. A. Jacobs. 2005. Buprenorphine treatment for opioid dependence: The relative efficacy of daily, twice and thrice weekly dosing. *Drug Alcohol Depend.* 77:195–204. *One hundred thirty-four opioid addicts were randomized to daily, thrice-weekly, or twice-weekly buprenorphine (dosage: 4–12 mg/day, mean ~7.5 mg). Sixty-nine percent completed 24 weeks; drug use and addiction severity index improved equally in all three arms.*

102. O'Connor, P. G., A. H. Oliveto, J. M. Shi, et al. 1998. A randomized trial of buprenorphine maintenance for heroin dependence in a primary care clinic versus a methadone clinic.

Am. J. Med. 105:100–105. *Forty-six opioid addicts were randomized to either thrice-weekly buprenorphine dispensed in a primary care clinic or conventional methadone maintenance. Those on buprenorphine had higher 12-week treatment retention (78% vs. 52%), had lower rates of illicit opioid use (63% vs. 85%), and were more likely to have ≥3 consecutive weeks of abstinence (43% vs. 13%). Cocaine use was similar in both arms (~30%).*

103. Fudala, P. J., T. P. Bridge, S. Herbert, et al. 2003. Office-based treatment of opiate addiction with a sublingual-tablet formulation of buprenorphine and naloxone. *N. Engl. J. Med.* 349:949–958. *Three hundred twenty-six opiate addicts were randomized to (1) placebo, (2) buprenorphine, or (3) buprenorphine-naloxone. The trial had two parts: (1) 4-week placebo-controlled trial (16 mg/day), followed by (2) 48–52 open-label efficacy trial. During the first phase, those in either buprenorphine arm had more opiate-negative urine tox screens (~20% vs. 6%) and improved self-rated health and well-being, but cocaine use in all arms was the same (~40%). Buprenorphine appeared to be safe and effective during the efficacy phase.*

104. Mattick, R. P., J. Kimber, C. Breen, and M. Davoli. 2003. Buprenorphine maintenance versus placebo or methadone maintenance for opioid dependence. *The Cochrane Database of Systematic Reviews.* Issue 3. Art. No.: CD002207.

105. Mintzer, M. Z., C. J. Correia, and E. C. Strain. 2004. A dose-effect study of repeated administration of buprenorphine/naloxone on performance in opioid-dependent volunteers. *Drug Alcohol Depend.* 74:205–209.

106. Fiellin, D. A., M. V. Pantalon, M. C. Chawarski, et al. 2005. Counseling and attendance requirements for buprenorphine treatment in primary care [abstract]. *J. Gen. Intern. Med.* 20(Suppl. 1):173–174.

107. Galanter, M., H. Dermatis, L. Glickman, et al. 2004. Network therapy: Decreased secondary opioid use during buprenorphine maintenance. *J. Subst. Abuse Treat.* 26:313–318. *Sixty-six heroin addicts who were willing to bring a drug-free family member or friend were randomized to network therapy (NT) or medication management (MM) and treated for 18 weeks. Seventy percent of those assigned to NT were able to establish a network and had higher rates of opiate-free urines than those in MM (65% vs. 45%).*

108. Drucker, E., and D. Vlahov. 1999. Controlled clinical evaluation of diacetyl morphine for treatment of intractable opiate dependence. *Lancet* 353:1543–1544.

109. Perneger, T. V., F. Giner, M. delRio, and A. Mino. 1998. Randomised trial of heroin maintenance programme for addicts who fail in conventional drug treatments. *BMJ* 317:13–18. *Fifty-one heroin addicts who had failed two or more drug treatments were randomized to supervised heroin maintenance or "conventional treatment" (19/21 on methadone). Over 6 months, those assigned to heroin were less likely to use illicit heroin or to commit property offences but were no better in terms of work, housing, health status, or other drug use.*

110. Van den Brink, W., V. M. Hendricks, P. Blanken, et al. 2003. Medical prescription of heroin to treatment resistant heroin addicts: Two randomised controlled trials. *BMJ* 327:310–312. *Five hundred forty-nine heroin addicts who continued to use despite being on ≥50 mg of methadone/day (mean ~70) were randomized to supervised heroin (in addition to methadone) or methadone alone. "Response" rate, defined as >40% improvement in at least one of three domains (physical/mental/social) after 12 months, was better among those on heroin (55% vs. 29%).*

8

Tobacco

BACKGROUND

Tobacco (*Nicotiana tabacum*) is a broad-leafed plant indigenous to the Americas that was used by natives and introduced to

Europeans when they colonized the Western Hemisphere. Tobacco is now cultivated and used throughout the world. The leaves are most commonly dried and cured and smoked in the form of cigarettes or cigars. The leaves can also be chewed, or sniffed in the powdered form (snuff).

The psychoactive and habit-forming substance in tobacco is nicotine. Nicotine is an organic alkaloid that is found naturally in tobacco and in other plants in the Solanaceae (nightshade) family; this includes eggplant, tomato, potato, paprika, and peppers.

EPIDEMIOLOGY

According to the *2003 National Survey on Drug Use and Health* (NSDUH) (1), 70.8 million Americans (29.8% of the population age 12 or older) reported current (past month) use of a tobacco product; most of them (86%) used cigarettes. Current tobacco use was highest among young adults aged 18–25 (44.8%) and is more prevalent among males (35.9%) than females (24.0%). Cigarette smoking rates decline with increasing level of education and are higher among unemployed when compared with employed individuals.

The number of Americans who smoked for the first time declined from 3.3 million in 1997 to 2.7 million in 2001. However, the number of new smokers each year has been over 2.5 million since 1965; most of these (76%) were under age 18.

In 2003, an estimated 35.7 million Americans were classified as nicotine dependent (15.0% of population aged 12 or older); 4.7% of youths aged 12–17 were dependent, 18.9% of young adults aged 18–25, and 15.8% of adults aged 26 and older.

DRUG EFFECTS

Acute Effects

Nicotine is the psychoactive component of tobacco and is responsible for its habit-forming effects. It can be absorbed through the lungs when smoked and through the oral or nasal mucosa when chewed or sniffed. Nicotine is poorly absorbed from tobacco when ingested. The typical cigarette delivers about 1 mg of nicotine; those who chew may absorb up to 2–3 mg. Nicotine has a half-life of about 2 hours in experienced users and is primarily metabolized by the liver into cotinine, which has a much longer half-life. Nicotine acts on selective acetylcholine receptors that are generally referred to as nicotine receptors, which have a mild stimulating effect and lead to increased alertness, improved attention, and decreased appetite (2). Despite the serious health hazards of tobacco use, nicotine itself seems to have little ill effect and may even have potential therapeutic uses; for example, use of nicotine patches in elderly nonsmokers has been reported to improve short-term verbal memory (3).

Overdose

While smoking is an important cause of morbidity and mortality worldwide, the risk of acute toxicity or overdose is minimal, especially among regular users who have developed tolerance to the side effects. Nevertheless, there are reports of acute toxicity among children who have ingested tobacco or were exposed to nicotine patches. Symptoms of acute toxicity include nausea, vomiting, diarrhea, weakness, and dizziness (4). There is no specific antidote to nicotine poisoning.

Withdrawal

Regular users of tobacco experience a number of signs and symptoms with cessation. During the first few days of abstinence, tobacco users experience craving for tobacco, irritability, anxiety, difficulty concentrating, restlessness, slowing of heart rate, and increased appetite (5). These symptoms are most intense during the first 4 days of abstinence and then decline gradually over a month; however, increased appetite and weight gain seem to persist beyond the first month—for as long as 6 months (or longer) (6).

DIAGNOSIS

The simplest way to assess tobacco use is to ask the patient; this should be a routine part of the assessment of almost any patient. There are a number of biomarkers associated with smoking that are generally used in studies to confirm smoking cessation, but they have limited clinical utility. Smokers have higher exhaled carbon monoxide concentrations when compared with healthy nonsmokers (7); however, exhaled carbon monoxide is also increased with obstructive lung disease (8), passive exposure to cigarette smoke (9), and carbon monoxide poisoning. Serum carboxyhemoglobin levels are also elevated with smoking; in fact, this may falsely elevate smokers' pulse oximetry readings, since these devices cannot distinguish between oxyhemoglobin and carboxyhemoglobin (10). Cotinine is a metabolite of nicotine that can be detected in the serum, saliva, and urine of tobacco users and appears to be the best method to distinguish smokers from nonsmokers (11). Smoking is also associated with higher serum thiocyanate levels due to trace amounts of cyanide in tobacco (12); however, this test has a lower sensitivity than cotinine levels (11).

MEDICAL COMPLICATIONS

Smoking is one of the most significant preventable causes of death and disability. In the year 2000, an estimated 4.83 million premature deaths worldwide were attributable to smoking; the leading smoking-related causes of death were cardiovascular disease (1.69 million deaths), chronic obstructive pulmonary disease (0.97 million), and lung cancer (0.85 million) (13). In the United States, roughly 40% of the deaths attributable to smoking are from cancer, 40% from cardiovascular disease, and 20% from respiratory disease (14). The data on complications of tobacco use comes from observational studies in the form of cohort or case-control studies. This type of data is always limited by the possibility that other factors associated with smoking may account for some of the risk observed. However, adjustment for other demographic and behavioral factors does not substantially affect the observed associations (14).

Smoking cessation has been found to substantially reduce subsequent mortality (15). Furthermore, there is some evidence that smoking interventions are more effective when delivered to those with a serious complication from smoking (16); this reinforces the importance of recognizing these connections and intervening to help smokers quit their habit.

Some illnesses and conditions associated with smoking are summarized in Table 8.1 and are covered briefly in the following section.

Table 8.1.   Medical complications associated with tobacco use

Cutaneous

Premature aging and wrinkling of facial skin
Cutaneous squamous cell carcinoma

Head and Neck

Cataracts
Macular degeneration
Periodontal disease
Squamous cell carcinoma of the head and neck
Oropharyngeal cancer

Pulmonary

Chronic obstructive pulmonary disease (emphysema)
Lung cancer
Respiratory infections (tuberculosis, pneumonia, influenza)

Cardiovascular

Coronary artery disease
Peripheral vascular disease
Thromboangiitis obliterans
Aortic aneurysms

Gastrointestinal

Esophageal cancer
Pancreatic cancer
Stomach cancer
Colorectal cancer
Anal cancer
Peptic ulcer disease
Gastroesophageal reflux

Renal

Renal carcinoma
Renal insufficiency
Renovascular disease

Genitourinary

Bladder cancer
Cervical cancer
Erectile dysfunction

Neuromuscular

Stroke

Cutaneous Complications

Smoking is associated with premature aging of the skin and increased facial wrinkling. These changes are similar to those seen with excessive sun exposure and are greatly increased by the combination of smoking and sun exposure (17). Smoking is also associated with an increased risk of cutaneous squamous cell carcinoma but not of basal cell carcinoma or melanoma (18).

Head and Neck Complications

Individuals who smoke tobacco are at higher risk for periodontal disease and tooth loss; those who chew tobacco can develop gingival recession and tooth abrasion (19). The most serious head and neck complications associated with tobacco use are malignancies. Tobacco smoking is associated with an increased risk of squamous cell carcinoma of the head and neck. In one study, when compared with those who never smoked, those who ever smoked had a fourfold higher risk and active smokers had a 6.5 times higher risk. This is further increased with concomitant alcohol use; heavy drinkers who smoked had a 22-fold higher risk compared with nonsmokers who did not drink or drank moderately (20). Furthermore, among smokers who do develop head and neck cancer, continued smoking is associated with poorer therapeutic outcomes (21).

Some studies have found an association between chewing tobacco and oral and pharyngeal cancers (22). However, in a Swedish study no such association was found; this may be due to differences in the preparation of chewing tobacco used in Sweden (also known as "snus") (20). Smokers also experience higher rates of ocular complications, including cataracts (23) and macular degeneration (24).

Pulmonary Complications

Chronic Obstructive Pulmonary Disease

Smoking is the main risk factor for chronic obstructive pulmonary disease (COPD), and this is one of the most important causes of morbidity and mortality attributable to smoking (25). It is estimated that 50% of smokers will eventually develop COPD, though many of these remain undiagnosed (26). Smoking invariably causes airway inflammation, but those who go on to develop COPD seem to have a more pronounced response, which leads to lung destruction and airway obstruction (27). Quitting smoking will slow the decline in lung function, though this benefit may be partly offset by the deleterious effects of weight gain on lung function (28). Nevertheless, in a cohort study of persons with severe COPD, recent smoking (i.e., smoking after enrollment) was the strongest predictor of mortality, suggesting that smoking cessation will improve survival, even among those with severe disease (29).

For those who have reversible airway obstruction (i.e., asthma), smoking increases the severity of the illness (30) and impairs their response to anti-inflammatory therapy (31).

Lung Cancer

Numerous studies have shown a strong association between smoking and all types of lung cancer; this risk increases with duration and number of cigarettes smoked (32). The risk appears to be highest for users of unfiltered high-tar brands, but there does not seem to be much difference between other types of cigarettes (33). Furthermore, active smoking at the time of diagnosis of lung cancer is associated with shortened survival (34).

Respiratory Infections

Smoking is associated with an increased risk of respiratory infections, including pneumonia and tuberculosis. Moreover, smoking increases the risk of acquiring influenza and the severity of the illness among those who acquire it (35).

The risk of pneumonia among smokers was double that of nonsmokers in a population-based case-control study in Spain; this accounted for an estimated 32% of cases (36). A case-control study in North America found that smoking was the strongest independent risk factor for invasive pneumococcal disease among immunocompetent adults (37).

Pulmonary tuberculosis, in a cohort study in Hong Kong, was found to be associated with smoking in a dose-dependent fashion (38). Similarly, a case-control study conducted in India found that smoking was associated with a fourfold increased risk of mortality from tuberculosis and accounted for 61% of the deaths due to this disease (39). Of note, many Indian men smoke bidis, which contain tobacco but are wrapped in the leaf of another plant, temburni.

Cardiovascular Complications

Coronary Artery Disease

Coronary heart disease is the leading cause of death attributable to smoking. Smoking is one of the major risk factors for heart disease (40); there are a number of physiological effects that probably account for this association, including endothelial impairment (41) and adverse effects on lipid profiles (42). Smokers are also at increased risk of developing aortic aneurysms; in fact, the increased relative risk is even greater than that seen with smoking and coronary artery disease (43). Among smokers who experience a myocardial infarction, continuing to smoke increases their risk for recurrent events; for those who quit, their risk declines to a rate similar to nonsmokers about 3 years after quitting (44).

Peripheral Vascular Disease

Peripheral vascular disease is also strongly associated with smoking in a dose-dependent fashion; in fact, it appears to be the strongest risk factor for this condition (45). There is also a strong association between smoking and thromboangiitis obliterans (Buerger's disease), and the most effective way to prevent limb loss in this devastating disease is to quit smoking (46).

The use of smokeless tobacco, on the other hand, has not been shown to increase cardiovascular risk and is almost certainly less risky than cigarette smoking (47).

Gastrointestinal Complications

Smoking is associated with a number of malignancies of the gastrointestinal tract. The association is the strongest for esophageal carcinoma (squamous [48] and adenocarcinoma [49]) and pancreatic cancer (50). Cigarette smoking has also been associated with colorectal cancers and may account for approximately 12% of colorectal cancer deaths (51). Use of cigarettes and other tobacco products also appears to be associated with stomach cancers (52). Moreover, smoking is associated with a fourfold increased risk of anal carcinoma among men and women (53).

Smokers are also at increased risk for peptic ulcer disease; there appears to be a synergistic effect with concomitant *Helicobacter pylori* infection that greatly increases this risk (54). Smoking is also associated with an increased risk of gastroesophageal reflux disease (55).

Renal Complications

A number of studies suggest that smoking is associated with an accelerated decline in renal function, especially among diabetics (56) and the elderly (57). Given the association between smoking and vascular disease elsewhere in the body, it is not surprising that smoking is also associated with renovascular disease (58). Smokers are also at increased risk for renal cell carcinoma (59).

Genitourinary Complications

Smoking increases the risk of erectile dysfunction among men (60), presumably due to its effects on endothelial function (61). It is also associated with bladder cancer (62).

Furthermore, smoking is associated with an increased risk of cervical cancer among women who are infected with oncogenic human papillomaviruses (63).

Neuromuscular Complications

Smokers are at increased risk for stroke (64) and have poorer outcomes if they require carotid endarterectomy (65). The data on smoking and the risk of dementia is mixed. Earlier (case-control) studies suggested that smoking may actually reduce the risk of Alzheimer's disease (66), while more recent prospective studies have found an increased risk (67) or no significant difference in risk (68).

TREATMENT

Given the tremendous health burden of smoking, efforts to help smokers quit are a public health priority. Moreover, a number of studies have shown that quitting smoking improves health outcomes (**69**). However, there is little evidence that "cutting down" is beneficial or that switching to lower-tar cigarettes makes any difference. Therefore, the goal of treatment should be smoking cessation. Fortunately, a number of treatment modalities have been shown to be effective in well-designed trials, including physician advice, telephone counseling, and group and individual therapy, as well as pharmacological interventions such as nicotine replacement

Table 8.2.   Summary of smoking cessation studies

Intervention	Studies	Outcomes
Self-help educational materials	RCTs Meta-analysis	Small effect, if any
Physician advice	RCTs Meta-analysis	Effective (OR: 1.7); more intensive advice a little more effective
Group counseling	RCTs Meta-analysis	Effective (OR: 2.2)
Individual counseling	RCTs Meta-analysis	Effective (OR: 1.6)
Nicotine replacement	RCTs Meta-analysis	Effective (OR: 1.8)
Bupropion	RCTs Meta-analysis	Effective (OR: 2.1)
Nortriptyline	RCTs Meta-analysis	Effective (OR: 2.9)—not significantly better than bupropion
Clonidine	RCTs Meta analysis	Effective (OR: 1.9), but side effects are common
Hypnosis	RCTs Meta-analysis	Not effective
Acupuncture	RCTs Meta-analysis	Not effective

See text for references and more details.
RCT: randomized controlled trial.
OR: odds ratio of smoking cessation with intervention compared to placebo or
no intervention; figures are from Cochrane meta-analyses.

and antidepressants (bupropion and nortriptyline). Table 8.2 summarizes the data on treatment to date. Unfortunately, no single intervention has yet proven to be effective for the majority of smokers. The US Department of Health and Human Services has issued guidelines on treating tobacco use and dependence that were updated in 2000 and can be accessed at www.guideline.gov (70).

Self-Help

Providing smokers with educational materials to help them quit smoking is a simple intervention and easy to implement, but unfortunately it appears to have minimal (if any) effect (**71**). A 2002 Cochrane review of 51 trials concluded that "self-help materials may increase quit rates compared with no intervention, but the effect is likely to be small" (72).

Counseling and Other Psychosocial Interventions

A number of studies suggest that physician advice can help individuals quit smoking. Guidelines for counseling tobacco users are summarized in Table 8.3. A 2004 Cochrane review of 39 trials concluded that physician advice "has a small effect on smoking cessation" (73). Analysis of pooled data from 17 trials comparing brief advice with no advice found a small increase in

Table 8.3.   Suggested guidelines for counseling tobacco users

1. **ASK—Identify all tobacco users at every visit**
- Expand vital signs to include tobacco use or use an alternative universal identification system.

2. **ADVISE—Strongly urge all tobacco users to quit**

Advice should be:
- *Clear*—"I think it is important for you to quit smoking now and I can help you." "Cutting down while you are ill is not enough."
- *Strong*—"As your clinician, I need you to know that quitting smoking is the most important thing you can do to protect your health now and in the future."
- *Personalized*—Tie tobacco use to:
  - current health or illness
  - social and economic costs
  - motivation level and readiness to quit
  - impact of tobacco use on children and others in household

3. **ASSESS—Determine willingness to make a quit attempt**
- If the patient is willing to make a quit attempt at this time, provide assistance.
- If the patient will participate in an intensive treatment, deliver such treatment or refer to an intensive intervention.
- If the patient clearly states that he or she is unwilling to make a quit attempt, provide motivational intervention.
- If the patient is a member of a special population (e.g., adolescent, pregnant, ethnic minority), consider providing additional information.

4. **ASSIST—Aid the patient in quitting**
- *Set a quit date*—Ideally, this should be within 2 weeks.
- *Tell* family, friends, and coworkers about quitting and request understanding and support.
- *Anticipate* challenges to planned quit attempt, particularly during the critical first few weeks. These include nicotine withdrawal symptoms.
- *Remove* tobacco products from your environment. Prior to quitting, avoid smoking in places where you spend a lot of time (e.g., home, car, work).

Adapted from Fiore, M. C., W. C. Bailey, S. J. Cohen, et al. 2000, October. *Treating tobacco use and dependence.* Quick Reference Guide for Clinicians. Rockville, MD: U.S. Department of Health and Human Services. Public Health Service.

the odds of cessation (odds ratio 1.74; 95% confidence interval (CI): 1.48–2.05); this translates to an absolute increase in cessation rate of 2.5%, or one additional individual for every 40 who were given advice. More intensive advice appeared to be a little better than minimal advice (odds ratio 1.44; 95% CI: 1.24–1.67). Nurse-delivered counseling and education also appears to have a small but significant benefit (**74**). Finally, telephone counseling also seems to have a small effect, but its benefit when used as an adjunct to physician advice (compared to advice alone) is less clear (75).

Group behavioral therapy is a commonly used treatment for smoking and other addictions. The approaches used in these groups vary widely but often include components such as motivational enhancement, advice on relapse prevention, coping skills, relaxation techniques, stress management, and cognitive-behavioral therapy. A recent Cochrane review of this treatment modality concluded that they are "better than self-help and other less intensive interventions." However, they found that there is "not enough evidence to support the use of particular components in a programme beyond the support and skills training normally included" (**76**).

Individual counseling generally utilizes a variety of approaches analogous to group behavioral therapy in a one-on-one setting. A number of studies have shown this approach to be effective, but it has not been shown to be any more effective than group therapy (77). An innovative approach is the use of an Internet-based smoking cessation program using a cognitive behavioral approach; this has recently been studied in a randomized controlled trial and appears to be modestly effective (in conjunction with nicotine replacement) (**78**).

Pharmacological Treatment

Nicotine Replacement

Numerous studies have shown that nicotine replacement therapy is effective for helping individuals to quit smoking (79). Overall, the provision of nicotine replacement increases smoking cessation rates by about 70%; however, since smoking cessation rates with no treatment are about 10%, this translates into an absolute increase of 7%, meaning that, on average, one additional smoker would quit out of 14 treated. Most of these studies measured outcomes 6–12 months after treatment; there is little data on longer-term outcomes.

Nicotine replacement can be given in a variety of forms, including gum, patches, nasal spray, inhaler, or sublingual tablet/lozenge. Table 8.4 gives additional information on available nicotine replacement products. The length of treatment varies in published studies, but 12 weeks is typical; there does not appear to be any additional benefit from using courses of nicotine replacement longer than 8 weeks. Abstinence during the first 2 weeks of treatment (particularly week 2) has been found to be the best predictor of longer-term abstinence (**80**). No form of nicotine replacement therapy has been shown to be more effective than any other. However, use of higher-dose nicotine gum (4 mg) appears to be more effective for highly dependent smokers (defined by number of cigarettes smoked and time to first cigarette in the morning). Likewise,

Table 8-4. Nicotine replacement products*

Type	Brand Names	Dosage Forms	Usual Dosage
Gum	Nicorette	2 mg, 4 mg	<25 cigs/day, use 2 mg >25 cigs/day, use 4 mg Chew every 1–2 hours first 6 weeks, then taper
Lozenge	Commit	2 mg, 4 mg	Begin with 4 mg dose if 1st cigarette is within 30 min of waking; dissolve lozenge in mouth every 1–2 hours for first 6 weeks, then taper
Patch	Nicoderm CQ, Nicotrol patch	7, 14, & 21 mg/24 hr (Nicoderm) 5, 10, & 15 mg/24 hr (Nicotrol)	If smoking >10 cigs/day, apply highest-dose patch daily for 6 weeks, then next lower doses daily for 2 weeks each sequentially
Nasal spray	Nicotrol nasal spray	10 ml bottle (10 mg/ml)	2–4 sprays per hour; up to 80 sprays/day Can taper gradually; do not use for > 3 months
Inhaler	Nicotrol inhaler	10 mg cartridge (4 mg nicotine)	Puff or inhale deeply for up to 20 min, 6–16 cartridges/day for 3–6 weeks, then taper; do not use for > 6 months

* Compiled from manufacturers' instructions.

higher-dose patches may be more effective for heavy smokers; the serum nicotine levels achieved with a 22 mg patch are significantly lower than those found in most smokers, and a 44 mg dose may be closer to what smokers are used to, especially heavy smokers (>31 cigarettes/day) (81). Combining a patch with an as-needed inhaler or nasal spray may modestly improve abstinence rates.

There has been little evidence of serious toxicity from the use of nicotine replacement; this raises the provocative question of whether encouraging ongoing use of alternative nicotine delivery systems would be effective as a harm-reduction strategy (82). Unfortunately, most smokers do not find the available nicotine replacement products to be a satisfying alternative. Some have suggested the use of "snus," an oral moist tobacco product that is commonly used in Sweden and appears to have few detrimental health effects.

Antidepressants

The antidepressants bupropion and nortriptyline have proven to be among the most effective treatments for smoking cessation, while other antidepressants, including selective serotonin reuptake inhibitors and venlafaxine, have not been shown to be effective (83). Bupropion is FDA-approved for smoking cessation and is generally considered the treatment of choice because of the larger number of studies done on it. Antidepressants appear to be more effective than nicotine replacement alone, but it has not been established that the addition of nicotine replacement to antidepressants is more effective than antidepressants alone (84). Longer-term use of antidepressants (a year or longer) may reduce relapse rates.

The dosage of nortriptyline used in the trials ranged from 50 to 150 mg/day (most used 75 mg); the dosage of bupropion used was 150–300 mg/day (most used 300 mg/day in two divided doses). Nortriptyline may cause dry mouth and sedation. Bupropion can cause insomnia and headaches, and there is a small risk of seizures.

Clonidine

Some studies have reported improved smoking cessation rates with clonidine (85), while other studies have found no benefit (86). A 2004 Cochrane review that included six trials concluded that "clonidine is effective in promoting smoking cessation" but did note that "there are potential sources of bias" and that "side-effects limit the usefulness of clonidine for smoking cessation" (87).

Aversion Therapy

One interesting approach to smoking cessation is to pair the pleasurable stimulus of smoking with an unpleasant stimulus; this is referred to as "aversion therapy" or "aversive conditioning." There are a few approaches that have been tried. One is "rapid puffing" where the smoker puffs rapidly but does not inhale deeply, creating an unpleasant sensation. Another is "smoke holding," where the smoker inhales and holds the smoke in his or her lungs for 30 seconds while focusing on the unpleasant sensations caused by the smoke. Yet another type of aversion therapy is "excessive smoking" where the smoker increases his or her smoking before attempting to quit. None of these approaches has been shown to be effective (88).

Silver acetate is used in another form of aversion therapy. This substance can be used in gum, lozenge, or spray form and creates an unpleasant metallic taste when the user smokes. Unfortunately, this does not appear to be effective (89).

Acupuncture

Some studies of auricular acupuncture have reported modestly reduced smoking rates (**90**). However, a recent randomized controlled trial of acupuncture for smoking cessation failed to show a sustained effect (**91**). Furthermore, a 2002 Cochrane review of 22 studies of acupuncture (and related techniques) for smoking cessation concluded that there "is no clear evidence that acupuncture, acupressure, laser therapy or electrostimulation are effective for smoking cessation" (92).

Hypnosis

Some studies have reported impressive smoking cessation results with hypnosis (93). However, a 1998 Cochrane review of nine studies of hypnotherapy concluded that they "have not shown that hypnotherapy has a greater effect on six month quit rates than other interventions or no treatment" (94).

Tobacco and Other Substance Dependence

Persons who are dependent on alcohol and illicit drugs often smoke as well. Traditionally, most treatment programs focus on the alcohol or illicit drug use before addressing smoking. One recent study seems to support this approach. In this study of alcoholics who were also smokers, those who received concurrent alcoholism treatment and smoking cessation were no more likely to quit smoking and had poorer drinking outcomes when compared with those who received smoking cessation 6 months after their alcohol treatment (95).

REFERENCES

1. Substance Abuse and Mental Health Services Administration. 2004. Results from the 2003 National Survey on Drug Use and Health: National Findings (Office of Applied Studies, NSDUH Series H-25, DHHS Publication No. SMA 04-3964). Rockville, MD.
2. Salomon, M. E. 2002. Nicotine and tobacco preparations. In *Goldfrank's Toxicologic Emergencies*. 7th ed. Edited by L. Goldfrank et al., 1075–1084. New York: McGraw-Hill.
3. Min, S. K., I. W. Moon, R. W. Ko, and H. S. Shin. 2001. Effects of transdermal nicotine on attention and memory in healthy elderly non-smokers. *Psychopharmacology* 159:83–88.
4. Woolf, A., K. Burkhart, T. Caraccio, and T. Litovitz. 1997. Childhood poisoning involving transdermal nicotine patches. *Pediatrics* 99:E4.
5. Hughes, J. R., and D. Hatsukami. 1986. Signs and symptoms of tobacco withdrawal. *Arch. Gen. Psychiatry* 43:289–294.
6. Hughes, J. R., S. W. Gust, K. Skoog, et al. 1991. Symptoms of tobacco withdrawal: A replication and extension. *Arch. Gen. Psychiatry* 48:52–59.

7. Middleton, E. T., and A. H. Morice. 2000. Breath carbon monoxide as an indication of smoking habit. *Chest* 117:758–763.

8. Montuschi, P., S. A. Kharitonov, and P. J. Barnes. 2001. Exhaled carbon monoxide and nitric oxide in COPD. *Chest* 120:496–501.

9. Ece, A., F. Gurkan, K. Haspolat, et al. 2000. Passive smoking and expired carbon monoxide concentrations in healthy and asthmatic children. *Allergol. Immunopathol.* 28:255–260.

10. Glass, K. L., T. A. Dillard, Y. Y. Phillips, et al. 1996. Pulse oximetry correction for smoking exposure. *Mil. Med.* 161:273–276.

11. Jarvis, M. J., H. Tunstall-Pedoe, C. Feyerabend, et al. 1987. Comparison of tests used to distinguish smokers from nonsmokers. *Am. J. Pub. Health* 77:1435–1438.

12. Vogt, T. M., S. Selvin, G. Widdowson, and S. B. Hulley. 1977. Expired air carbon monoxide and serum thiocyanate as objective measures of cigarette exposure. *Am. J. Pub. Health* 67:545–549.

13. Ezzati, M., and A. D. Lopez. 2003. Estimates of global mortality attributable to smoking in 2000. *Lancet* 362:847–852.

14. Thun, M. J., L. F. Apicella, and S. J. Henley. 2000. Smoking vs. other risk factors as the cause of smoking-attributable deaths. Confounding in the courtroom. *JAMA* 284:706–712.

15. Anthonisen, N. R., M. A. Skeans, R. A. Wise, et al. 2005. The effects of a smoking cessation intervention on 14.5-year mortality. *Ann. Intern. Med.* 142:233–239. *Five thousand eight hundred eighty-seven smokers with asymptomatic airway obstruction were randomized to a smoking cessation program or usual care. At 5 years, those in the program were more likely to have quit smoking (21.7% vs. 5.4%); after 14.5 years, they had lower overall mortality (11.8% vs. 13.7%).*

16. Ockene, J., J. L. Kristeller, R. Goldberg, et al. 1992. Smoking cessation and severity of disease: The Coronary Artery Smoking Intervention Study. *Health Psychol.* 11:119–126.

17. Kadunce, D. P., R. Burr, R. Gress, et al. 1991. Cigarette smoking: Risk factor for premature facial wrinkling. *Ann. Intern. Med.* 114:840–844.

18. DeHertog, S. A. E., C. A. H. Wensveen, M. T. Bastiaens, et al. 2001. Relation between smoking and skin cancer. *J. Clin. Oncol.* 19:231–238.

19. Taybos, G. 2003. Oral changes associated with tobacco use. *Am. J. Med. Sci.* 4:179–182.

20. Lewin, F., S. E. Norell, H. Johansson, et al. 1998. Smoking tobacco, oral snuff, and alcohol in the etiology of squamous cell carcinoma of the head and neck. A population-based case-referent study in Sweden. *Cancer* 82:1367–1375.

21. Browman, G. P., G. Wong, I. Hodson, et al. 1993. Influence of cigarette smoking on the efficacy of radiation therapy for head and neck cancer. *N. Engl. J. Med.* 328:159–163.

22. Winn, D. M., W. J. Blot, C. M. Shy, et al. 1981. Snuff dipping and oral cancer among women in the Southern United States. *N. Engl. J. Med.* 304:745–749.

23. Klein, B. E. K., R. Klein, K. E. Lee, and S. M. Meuer. 2003. Socioeconomic and lifestyle factors and the 10-year incidence of age-related cataracts. *Am. J. Ophthalmol.* 136:506–512.

24. Age-related eye disease study research group. Risk factors associated with age-related macular degeneration. 2000. *Ophthalmology* 107:2224–2232.

25. Pauwels, R. A., and K. F. Rabe. 2004. Burden and clinical features of chronic obstructive pulmonary disease. *Lancet* 364:613–620.

26. Lundback, B., A. Lindberg, M. Lindstrom, et al. 2003. Not 15 but 50% of smokers develop COPD? Report from the Obstructive Lung Diseases in Northern Sweden Studies. *Respir. Med.* 97:115–122

27. Hogg, J. C. 2004. Pathophysiology of airflow limitation in chronic obstructive pulmonary disease. *Lancet* 364:709–721.

28. Chinn, S., D. Jarvis, R. Melotti, et al. 2005. Smoking cessation, lung function, and weight gain: A follow-up study. *Lancet* 365:1629–1635.

29. Hersh, C. P., D. L. DeMeo, E. Al-Ansari, et al. 2004. Predictors of survival in severe, early onset COPD. *Chest* 126:1443–1451.

30. Althuis, M. D., M. Sexton, and D. Prybylski. 1999. Cigarette smoking and asthma symptom severity among adult asthmatics. *J. Asthma* 36:257–264.

31. Chadhuri, R., E. Livingston, A. D. McMahon, et al. 2003. Cigarette smoking impairs the therapeutic response to oral corticosteroids in chronic asthma. *Am. J. Respir. Crit. Care Med.* 168:1308–1311.

32. Alberg, A. J., and J. M. Samet. 2003. Epidemiology of lung cancer. *Chest* 123(1 Suppl.):21S–49S.

33. Harris, J. E., M. J. Thun, A. M. Mondul, and E. E. Calle. 2004. Cigarette tar yields in relation to mortality from lung cancer in the cancer prevention study II prospective cohort, 1982–8. *BMJ* 328:72.

34. Tammemagi, C. M., C. Neslund-Dudas, M. Simoff, and P. Kvale. 2004. Smoking and lung cancer survival: The role of comorbidity and treatment. *Chest* 125:27–37.

35. Kark, J. D., M. Lebiush, and L. Rannon. 1982. Cigarette smoking as a risk factor for epidemic a(h1n1) influenza in young men. *N. Engl. J. Med.* 307:1042–1046.

36. Almirall, J., C. A. Gonzalez, X. Balanzo, and I. Bolibar. 1999. Proportion of community-acquired pneumonia cases attributable to tobacco smoking. *Chest* 116:375–379.

37. Nuorti, J. P., J. C. Butler, M. M. Farley, et al. 2000. Cigarette smoking and invasive pneumococcal disease. *N. Engl. J. Med.* 342:681–689.

38. Leung, C. C., T. Li, T. H. Lam, et al. 2004. Smoking and tuberculosis among the elderly in Hong Kong. *Am. J. Respir. Crit. Care Med.* 170:1027–1033.

39. Gajalakshmi, V., R. Peto, S. Kanaka, and P. Jha. 2003. Smoking and mortality from tuberculosis and other diseases in India: Retrospective study of 43000 adult male deaths and 35000 controls. *Lancet* 362:507–515.

40. Greenland, P., M. D. Knoll, J. Stamler, et al. 2003. Major risk factors as antecedents of fatal and nonfatal coronary heart disease events. *JAMA* 290:891–897.

41. Zeiher, A. M., V. Schachinger, and J. Minners. 1995. Long-term cigarette smoking impairs endothelium-dependent coronary arterial vasodilator function. *Circulation* 92:1094–1100.

42. Cullen, P., H. Schulte, and G. Assman. 1998. Smoking, lipoproteins and coronary disease risk. *Eur. Heart J.* 19:1632–1641.

43. Lederle, F. A., D. B. Nelson, and A. M. Joseph. 2003. Smokers' relative for aortic aneurysm compared with other smoking-related diseases: A systematic review. *J. Vasc. Surg.* 38:329–334.

44. Rea, T. D., S. R. Heckbert, R. C. Kaplan, et al. 2002. Smoking status and risk for recurrent coronary events after myocardial infarction. *Ann. Intern. Med.* 137:494–500.

45. Meijer, W. T., D. E. Grobbee, M. Hunink, et al. 2000. Determinants of peripheral arterial disease in the elderly. *Arch. Intern. Med.* 160:2934–2938.

46. Olin, J. W., J. R. Young, R. A. Graor, et al. 1990. The changing clinical spectrum of thromboangiitis obliterans (Buerger's disease). *Circulation* 82(5 Suppl.):IV3–IV8.

47. Gupta, R., H. Gurm, and J. R. Bartholomew. 2004. Smokeless tobacco and cardiovascular risk. *Arch. Intern. Med.* 164:1845–1849.

48. Brown, L. M., R. Hoover, D. Silverman, et al. 2001. Excess incidence of squamous cell esophageal cancer among U.S. black men: Role of social class and other risk factors. *Am. J. Epidemiol.* 153:114–122.

49. Wu, A. H., P. Wan, and L. Bernstein. 2001. A multiethnic population-based study of smoking, alcohol and body size and risk of adenocarcinomas of the stomach and esophagus (United States). *Cancer Causes Control* 12:721–732.

50. Coughlin, S. S., E. E. Calle, A. V. Patel, and M. J. Thun. 2000. Predictors of pancreatic cancer mortality among a large cohort of United States adults. *Cancer Causes Control* 11:915–923.

51. Chao, A., J. Thun, E. J. Jacobs, et al. 2000. Cigarette smoking and colorectal cancer mortality in the cancer prevention study II. *J. Natl. Cancer Inst.* 92:1888–1896.

52. Chao, A., M. J. Thun, E. J. Jacobs, et al. 2002. Cigarette smoking, use of other tobacco products and stomach cancer mortality in U.S. adults. *Int. J. Cancer* 101:380–389.

53. Daling, J. R., M. M. Madeleine, L. G. Johnson, et al. 2004. Human papillomavirus, smoking, and sexual practices in the etiology of anal cancer. *Cancer* 101:270–280.

54. Rosenstock, S., T. Jorgensen, O. Bonnevie, and L. Anderson. 2003. Risk factors for peptic ulcer disease: A population-based prospective cohort study comprising 2416 Danish adults. *Gut* 52:186–193.

55. Kulig, M., M. Nocon, M. Vieth, et al. 2004. Risk factors for gastroesophageal reflux disease: Methodology and first epidemiological results of the proGERD study. *J. Clin. Epidemiol.* 57:580–589.

56. Yokoyama, H., O. Tomonaga, M. Hirayama, et al. 1997. Predictors of the progression of diabetic nephropathy and the beneficial effect of angiotensin-converting enzyme inhibitors in NIDDM patients. *Diabetologia* 40:405–411.

57. Bleyer, A. J., L. R. Shemanski, G. L. Burke, et al. 2000. Tobacco, hypertension, and vascular disease: Risk factors for renal function in an older population. *Kidney Int.* 57:2072–2079.

58. Baggio, B., A. Budakovic, D. Casara, et al. 2001. Renal involvement in subjects with peripheral atherosclerosis. *J. Nephrol.* 14:286–292.

59. Yuan, J. M., J. E. Castelao, M. Gago-Dominguez, et al. 1998. Tobacco use in relation to renal cell carcinoma. *Cancer Epidemiol. Biomarkers Prev.* 7:429–433.

60. Bacon, C. G., M. A. Mittleman, I. Kawachi, et al. 2003. Sexual function in men older than 50 years of age: Results from the health professionals follow-up study. *Ann. Intern. Med.* 139:161–168.

61. McVary, K. T., S. Carrier, H. Wessells, et al. 2001. Smoking and erectile dysfunction: Evidence-based analysis. *J. Urol.* 166:1624–1632.

62. D'Avanzo, B., E. Negri, C. LaVecchia, et al. 1990. Cigarette smoking and bladder cancer. *Eur. J. Cancer* 26:714–718.

63. Shields, T. S., L. A. Brinton, R. D. Burk, et al. 2004. A case-control study of risk factors for invasive cervical cancer among U.S. women exposed to oncogenic types of human papillomavirus. *Cancer Epidemiol. Biomarkers Prev.* 13:1574–1582.

64. Shinton, R., and G. Beevers. 1989. Meta-analysis of relation between cigarette smoking and stroke. *BMJ* 298:789–794.

65. Rothwell, P. M., J. Slattery, and C. P. Warlow. 1997. Clinical and angiographic predictors of stroke and death from carotid endarterectomy: Systematic review. *BMJ* 315:1571–1577.

66. Van Duijin, C. M., and A. Hofman. 1991. Relation between nicotine intake and Alzheimer's disease. *BMJ* 302:1491–1494.

67. Ott, A., A. J. Slooter, A. Hofman, et al. 1998. Smoking and risk of dementia and Alzheimer's disease in a population-based cohort study: The Rotterdam Study. *Lancet* 351:1840–1843.

68. Doll, R., R. Peto, J. Boreham, and I. Sutherland. 2000. Smoking and dementia in male British doctors: Prospective study. *BMJ* 320:1097–1102.

69. Critchley, J. A., and S. Capewell. 2003. Mortality risk reduction associated with smoking cessation in patients with coronary heart disease: A systematic review. *JAMA* 290:86–97. *Data from 20 studies indicated that those who quit reduce their risk of mortality from CHD by 36%.*

70. Fiore, M. C., W. C. Bailey, S. J. Cohen, et al. 2000, June. *Treating tobacco use and dependence. Clinical practice guideline.* Rockville, MD: U.S. Department of Health and Human Services. Public Health Service.

71. Moore, L., R. Campbell, A. Whelan, et al. 2002. Self-help smoking cessation in pregnancy: Cluster randomised controlled trial. *BMJ* 325:1383. *One thousand five hundred twenty-seven pregnant smokers were randomly assigned to receive either a series of five self-help booklets or usual care. Cessation rates were ~20% in both arms (at end of second trimester).*

72. Lancaster, T., and F. Stead. 2002. Self-help interventions for smoking cessation. *The Cochrane Database of Systematic Reviews.* Issue 3. Art. No.: CD001118.

73. Lancaster, T., and L. F. Stead. 2004. Physician advice for smoking cessation. *The Cochrane Database of Systematic Reviews.* Issue 4. Art. No.: CD000165.pub2.

74. Rice, V. H., and L. F. Stead. 2004. Nursing interventions for smoking cessation. *The Cochrane Database of Systematic Reviews.* Issue 1. Art. No.: CD001188.pub2. *The pooled odds ratio from 20 studies comparing a nursing intervention with control or usual care was 1.47 (95% CI: 1.29–1.68).*

75. Stead, L. F., T. Lancaster, and R. Perera. 2003. Telephone counselling for smoking cessation. *The Cochrane Database of*

Systematic Reviews. Issue 1. Art. No.: CD002850. *The pooled odds ratio from 13 trials comparing telephone counseling with a minimal intervention was 1.56 (95% CI: 1.38–1.77). However, four other studies failed to find any benefit from the addition of telephone counseling to a face-to-face intervention.*

76. Stead, F., and T. Lancaster. 2002. Group behavioral therapy programmes for smoking cessation. T*he Cochrane Database of Systematic Reviews.* Issue 2. Art. No.: CD001007. *Group programs were found to be better than no intervention (pooled odds ratio: 2.19; 95% CI: 1.47–3.37) and self-help (pooled odds ratio: 1.97; 95% CI: 1.57–2.48).*

77. Lancaster, T., and F. Stead. 2002. Individual behavioral counselling for smoking cessation. *The Cochrane Database of Systematic Reviews.* Issue 3. Art. No.: CD001292. *The pooled odds ratio from 15 trials comparing individual counseling with minimal intervention was 1.62 (95% CI: 1.35–1.94). Four studies comparing different levels of intensity of counseling failed to show a significant effect.*

78. Strecher, V. J., S. Shiffman, and R. West. 2005. Randomized controlled trial of a web-based computer-tailored smoking cessation program as a supplement to nicotine patch therapy. *Addiction* 100:682–688. *Three thousand nine hundred seventy one smokers who purchased a brand of nicotine patch and provided a valid e-mail address were randomized to treatment (including tailored newsletters and behavioral support e-mail messages) or access to Web-based instructions. Twenty-eight-day abstinence at 12-week follow-up was higher with the treatment (23% vs. 18%).*

79. Silagy, C., T. Lancaster, L. Stead, et al. 2004. Nicotine replacement therapy for smoking cessation. *The Cochrane Database of Systematic Reviews.* Issue 3. Art. No.: CD000146.pub2. *The pooled odds ratio from 102 trials comparing all forms of nicotine replacement therapy (NRT) with placebo or a non-NRT group was 1.77 (95% CI: 1.66–1.88).*

80. Kenford, S. L., M. C. Fiore, D. E. Joronby, et al. 1994. Predicting smoking cessation: Who will quit with and without the nicotine patch. *JAMA* 271:589–594. *Among 210 smokers from two clinical trials of nicotine patch for smoking cessation, smoking status during week 2 was the strongest predictor of 6-month outcomes.*

81. Lawson, G. M., R. D. Hurt, L. C. Dale, et al. 1998. Application of serum nicotine and plasma cotinine concentrations to assessment of nicotine replacement in light, moderate, and heavy smokers undergoing transdermal therapy. *J. Clin. Pharmacol.* 38:502–509.

82. McNeill, A. 2004. ABC of smoking cessation: Harm reduction. *BMJ* 328:885–887.

83. Hughes, J. R., F. Stead, and T. Lancaster. 2004. Antidepressants for smoking cessation. *The Cochrane Database of Systematic Reviews.* Issue 4. Art. No.: CD000031. *The pooled odds ratio of quitting smoking from 19 trials of buproprion monotherapy was 2.06 (95% CI: 1.77–2.40) and from four trials of nortriptyline, 2.79 (95% CI: 1.70–4.59)*

84. Jorenby, D. E., S. J. Leischow, M. A. Nides, et al. 1999. A controlled trial of sustained-release bupropion, a nicotine patch or both for smoking cessation. *N. Engl. J. Med.* 340:685–691. *Eight hundred ninety-three smokers were randomized to (1) bupropion SR, (2) nicotine patch, (3) bupropion + nicotine patch, or (4)*

placebo for 9 weeks. Twelve-month abstinence rates were 30.3% (B), 16.4% (N), 35.5% (B+N), and 15.6% (P), respectively.

85. Glassman, A. H., F. Stetner, B. T. Walsh, et al. 1988. Heavy smokers, smoking cessation and clonidine. Results of a double-blind, randomized trial. *JAMA* 259:2863–2866.

86. Prochazka, A. V., T. L. Petty, L. Nett, et al. 1992. Transdermal clonidine reduced some withdrawal symptoms but did not increase smoking cessation. *Arch. Intern. Med.* 152:2065–2069.

87. Gourlay, S. G., L. F. Stead, and N. L. Benowitz. 2004. Clonidine for smoking cessation. *The Cochrane Database of Systematic Reviews.* Issue 3. Art. No.: CD000058.pub2. *The pooled odds ratio of quitting smoking from six trials was 1.89 (95% CI: 1.30–2.74), but the "quality of the trials was poor" and side effects were common.*

88. Hajek, P., and L. F. Stead. 2004. Aversive smoking for smoking cessation. *The Cochrane Database of Systematic Reviews.* Issue 3. Art. No.: CD000546.pub2.

89. Lancaster, T., and L. F. Stead. 1997. Silver acetate for smoking cessation. *The Cochrane Database of Systematic Reviews.* Issue 3. Art. No.: CD000191.

90. He, D., J. I. Melbø, and A. T. Høstmark. 2001. Effect of acupuncture on smoking cessation or reduction: An 8-month and 5-year follow-up study. *Prev. Med.* 33:364–372. *Forty-six smokers were randomized to ear or sham acupuncture twice weekly for 3 weeks. More in the acupuncture group quit smoking at the end of treatment and 8-month follow-up. At 5-year follow-up, quit rates were similar (18%).*

91. Bier, I. D., J. Wilson, P. Studt, and M. Shakleton. 2002. Auricular acupuncture, education and smoking cessation: A randomized, sham-controlled trial. *Am. J. Pub. Health* 92:1642–1647. *One hundred forty-one smokers were randomized to (1) acupuncture + education, (2) sham acupuncture + education, or (3) acupuncture alone. Twenty-three percent dropped out in the first month and 66% by 18 months; dropouts were not counted as treatment failures. Among those who did follow-up, 1-month quit rates were 40% (1), 22% (2), and 10% (3), respectively. The differences were no longer significant at 18 months.*

92. White, A. R., H. Rampes, and E. Ernst. 2002. Acupuncture for smoking cessation. *The Cochrane Database of Systematic Reviews.* Issue 2. Art. No.: CD000009.

93. Elkins, G. R., and M. H. Rajab. 2004. Clinical hypnosis for smoking cessation: Preliminary results of a three-session intervention. *Int. J. Clin. Exp. Hypn.* 52:73–81.

94. Abbot, N. C., L. F. Stead, A. R. White, and J. Barnes. 1998. Hypnotherapy for smoking cessation. *The Cochrane Database of Systematic Reviews.* Issue 2. Art. No.: CD001008.

95. Joseph, A. M., M. L. Willenbring, S. M. Nugent, and D. B. Nelson. 2004. A randomized trial of concurrent versus delayed smoking intervention for patients in alcohol dependence treatment. *J. Stud. Alcohol.* 65:681–691.

9

Cocaine and Other Stimulants

BACKGROUND

The stimulants are a class of drugs that includes cocaine and the amphetamines. Cocaine is an alkaloid derived from the leaves of the coca plant, which is indigenous to South America. The leaves were chewed by natives for centuries as a mild stimulant. In the mid-1800s, cocaine was extracted from the leaves by Europeans and subsequently used as an anesthetic and as an additive to beverages and patent medicines. The nonprescription use of cocaine was banned in the United States by the passage of the Harrison Narcotics Act in 1914.

Amphetamine-like compounds (technically, phenylethylamines) also have a long history dating back to the use of the alkaloid ephedrine derived from *Ephedra mahuang* in China. Medicinal amphetamines were developed in the early 20th century and were originally used for the treatment of rhinitis and asthma; they were subsequently employed as a stimulant for soldiers in combat during World War II and later to treat obesity. Methamphetamine is easily synthesized from readily available precursors, such as ephedrine or pseudoephedrine.

There are a number of so-called designer drugs that are pharmacologically similar to the amphetamines, such as MDA, MDEA, and MDMA ("Ecstasy"); these have stimulant properties, but they are used more for their hallucinogenic effect. These agents are covered in Chapter 10 on hallucinogens.

Khat (or "qat") is a plant that has been traditionally used on the Arabian Peninsula and in East Africa. The leaves of this plant (*Catha edulis*) contain an alkaloid—cathinone—that resembles amphetamines. The leaves are typically chewed and have mild effects similar to other stimulants. A related drug—methcathinone—can be synthesized from ephedrine. The yellowish white powder is injected, snorted, or ingested, with effects similar to methamphetamine. Methcathinone is sometimes referred to as "cat" or "ephedrone" and is one of the most commonly abused stimulants in Russia.

Caffeine is another mild stimulant and the most commonly used psychoactive substance worldwide; this is discussed briefly at the end of this chapter.

Stimulants have a number of therapeutic uses, including the treatment of attention deficit hyperactivity disorder (ADHD), depression, and narcolepsy and the promotion of weight loss. Table 9.1 provides a list of some of the available prescription stimulants and medications with stimulant effects.

EPIDEMIOLOGY

According to the *2003 National Survey on Drug Use and Health* (NSDUH), approximately 34 million Americans reported using cocaine at some time in their lives; 5.9 million Americans had used in the past year, and almost 1.5 million were classified as experiencing

Table 9.1.   Selected prescription stimulants

Generic Name	Trade Names	Usual Daily Dose	Indication/Use
Amphetamine	Adderall	10 mg	ADHD
Dextroamphetamine	Dexedrine	10 mg	ADHD Narcolepsy
Methylphenidate	Methylin, Ritalin, Concerta	15–20 mg 36 mg	ADHD
Pemoline	Cylert	56.25 mg	ADHD
Modafinil	Provigil	200 mg	Narcolepsy
Benzphetamine	Didrex	25–300 mg	Obesity
Diethylpropion	Tenuate	75 mg	Obesity
Phendimetrazine	Bontril	70–210 mg	Obesity
Phentermine	Adipex-P, Ionamin	15–37.5 mg	Obesity
Caffeine	Cafergot, Norgesic, Fioricet/Fiorinal*	40–600 mg	Headache Musculoskeletal pain
Theophylline	Theo-24, Uniphyl	100–600 mg	Chronic obstructive pulmonary disease
Ephedrine	Rynatuss*	10–40 mg	Cough
Pseudoephedrine	Dimetapp, Duratuss, Entex, Robitussin-CF*	30–240 mg	Cough

* Combination medications.

dependence on or abuse of the substance (0.6% of the population 12 or older). Over 20 million Americans reported lifetime nonmedical use of other stimulants (including methamphetamine); 2.7 million of these had used in the past year, of whom 378,000 were classified as being dependent or abusing these medications (1).

There are some demographic variations in stimulant use. According to the 2003 NSDUH, among adults aged 18 or older, recent (past month) cocaine use was higher among men (1.4%) than among women (0.6%), higher among those with less than high school education (1.4%) than among college graduates (0.7%), and higher among unemployed individuals (2.7%) than among full-time employed (1.1%).

According to the Drug Abuse Warning Network (DAWN) (2), in 2002, cocaine was associated with the highest number of illicit-drug-related emergency department (ED) visits in the 21 metropolitan areas that were sampled. Cocaine accounted for 78 ED visits per 100,000 population, while for methamphetamine, the number was 7 per 100,000. There is a great deal of geographic variation in stimulant use in the United States; the top five cities for cocaine-related ED visits were Chicago, Philadelphia, Baltimore, Miami, and Atlanta. On the other hand, the top five cities for methamphetamine-related ED visits were San Francisco, Seattle, San Diego, Los Angeles, and Phoenix.

DRUG EFFECTS

Acute Effects

Cocaine is used in the hydrochloride (crystal), sulfated (powder), or alkaloid (crack) form; the latter has a lower melting point, which makes it conducive for smoking. The effects of cocaine peak after 60–90 minutes with oral use, 30–60 minutes with snorting, and within minutes of intravenous use or smoking, and the effects are generally short-lived. Methamphetamine is used in a powder or crystal form and can also be ingested, snorted, smoked, or injected with similar results, but the effects are longer-lasting than with cocaine.

The stimulants exert their effect by increasing levels of catecholamines through stimulation of release or blockage of reuptake; direct stimulation of receptors may also play a role. Users of cocaine and methamphetamine experience a "high" or "rush" of intense euphoria accompanied by tachycardia and elevated blood pressure and followed by depression, which may lead to repeated use. Cocaine also has a local anesthetic effect when applied to the mucus membranes.

Oral amphetamines promote wakefulness, alertness, concentration, and self-confidence; they can also improve physical performance by athletes. They also suppress appetite. Prolonged use is often followed by depression and fatigue (3).

Overdose

High doses of stimulants produce generalized sympathomimetic effects, including tachycardia or cardiac arrhythmia, severe hypertension, and agitation. The cardiovascular effects may lead to myocardial infarction, aortic dissection, or stroke (as discussed later in this chapter); hyperthermia and rhabdomyolysis can also occur. In one study of 146 cocaine-related deaths over a 10-year period in Australia, most of the fatalities were associated with injection use (86%), and in most cases other substances were also involved (81%) (4).

There is no specific antidote for stimulant overdose. Benzodiazepines are frequently used for agitation and phenothiazines for psychotic symptoms; beta-blockers should be avoided because they may potentiate coronary artery vasoconstriction. One animal study suggests that activated charcoal may reduce methamphetamine toxicity after ingestion of the drug (5).

Withdrawal

Regular users of stimulants seem to experience withdrawal symptoms upon cessation, but they do not have a clear-cut, easily observable syndrome as can be seen with opioid, sedative, or alcohol withdrawal. The typical symptoms include dysphoria, fatigue, insomnia, and psychomotor agitation; these generally peak 2–4 days after cessation but can persist for several weeks (6). Other possible symptoms include drug craving, increased appetite, psychomotor retardation, and vivid, unpleasant dreams. The symptoms of amphetamine withdrawal are similar but may be delayed in onset and are longer lasting than symptoms of cocaine withdrawal due to amphetamines' longer half-life.

DIAGNOSIS

The diagnostic criteria for abuse of and dependence on cocaine and other stimulants are the same as for other substances (see Appendixes A and B). Although physical dependence with stimulants (i.e., tolerance and withdrawal) is generally less severe than with opioids, sedatives, or alcohol, individuals who use cocaine do develop tolerance to its effects (7) and, as noted earlier, can experience withdrawal symptoms after cessation of use.

Physical Exam

Stimulant users may exhibit signs of use such as tachycardia, elevated blood pressure, or agitation. They may present with one of the medical complications discussed in the next section. Intranasal users may have nasoseptal erosions or perforation. Injection drug users may have the stigmata of needle use on their arms, legs, or other sites.

Laboratory Testing

While cocaine has a short half-life, its metabolites (specifically benzoylecgonine) can be detected in the urine for 2–3 days after last use and up to 8 days with heavy use; false-positive results are uncommon. Amphetamines can likewise be detected in the urine for 2–3 days after last use; there are a number of drugs that can cause false-positive amphetamine screen, including ephedrine, pseudoephedrine, trazodone, bupropion, desipramine, amantadine, and ranitidine (8).

MEDICAL COMPLICATIONS

Most of the complications of stimulant use are related to their effect on the vascular system and damage to various organs that occurs as a result. Some of the medical complications are due to the use of needles, not the drug per se; the medical complications of injection drug use are covered in more detail in Chapter 15.

Ear, Nose, and Throat Complications

Intranasal use of cocaine has been associated with a variety of nasopharyngeal complications including nasal septal erosions and perforation, oronasal fistulas (9), perforation of the hard palate (10), and saddle-nose deformity. The clinical presentation may mimic a vasculitis such as Wegner's granulomatosis (11). There are also anecdotal reports of severe dental disease among methamphetamine addicts ("meth mouth"); it is not clear if this is due to a drug effect or simply neglect.

Pulmonary Complications

Smoking the alkaloid ("crack") form of cocaine causes acute bronchoconstriction and may lead to wheezing and asthma attacks (12). It has been found (on bronchoalveolar lavage) to be associated with alveolar hemorrhage and microvascular injury; however, the clinical significance of this finding is unclear (13). Pulmonary hypertension has been reported in association with intravenous cocaine use (14), as well as inhaled methamphetamine use (15). On the other hand, cocaine smoking has not been found to have significant acute or chronic effects on diffusing capacity of the lung (16).

Drug users who inject talc-containing crushed tablets are at risk for pulmonary granulomatosis, which may lead to pulmonary hypertension (17) and chronic obstructive lung disease (18). This complication has been generally (but not exclusively) associated with intravenous methylphenidate (Ritalin) use.

Cardiovascular Complications

Myocardial Infarction

Cocaine users often experience chest pain with use, and cocaine-related chest pain is a frequent reason for emergency department visits. In one study, 17% of all patients presenting to four emergency departments with nontraumatic chest pain had used cocaine; among those 18–30 years old, 29% had used cocaine, and among those 31–40 years old, 48% (**19**). A minority of these patients will suffer a myocardial infarction; in one series, approximately 6% of patients with cocaine-associated chest pain experienced this complication (20).

Cocaine-induced myocardial infarction is thought to be due to vasoconstriction of coronary arteries (due to stimulation of alpha-adrenergic receptors) as well as increased myocardial oxygen demand (due to increased heart rate, arterial pressure, and ventricular contractility) (21). Cocaine-induced vasoconstriction is potentiated by β-blockade (22); therefore, it is generally recommended that β-blockers be avoided when treating patients with cocaine-associated chest pain or myocardial infarction.

Most of those who experience myocardial infarction are male cigarette smokers and many have preexisting coronary artery disease; however, myocardial infarction can occur in those with normal coronary arteries (**23**). Furthermore, one cannot reliably predict which patients will experience myocardial infarction on the basis of clinical presentation or ECG findings (20). Patients with cocaine-associated chest pain should be evaluated with serum troponin measurement; serum creatine kinase is felt to be less reliable, since it can be elevated due to rhabdomyolysis. For those who have normal troponin levels, no new ischemic changes on ECG, and no evidence of cardiovascular complications, a 9- to 12-hour observation period is probably sufficient (**24**).

Less is known about the cardiac effects of methamphetamine, but there have been reports of chest pain and myocardial infarction associated with its use as well (25).

Cardiomyopathy

Cocaine users appear to be at increased risk for the development of cardiomyopathy (**26**); although some of these cases are due to myocardial damage from coronary artery disease and myocardial infarction, others occur in the absence of any evidence of ischemia and may be due to myocarditis (27) or the direct toxic effect of cocaine (28). Similarly, there have been reports of cardiomyopathy with methamphetamine use (29).

Arrhythmia

Cocaine use has also been associated with a variety of arrhythmias, often in the setting of cardiac ischemia or myocardial infarction, or in patients with cardiomyopathy, hypotension, or hypoxemia (21). These may lead to syncope or sudden death.

Aortic Dissection

Cocaine use has been associated with acute aortic dissection. In one series, 37% of cases of acute aortic dissection were associated with cocaine use; many of these patients also had untreated hypertension (30).

Endocarditis

While all injection drug users are at risk for endocarditis, those who use cocaine appear to be at higher risk for this complication (31). Endocarditis is discussed in more detail in Chapter 15.

Peripheral Vascular Disease

Cocaine use has been associated with limb ischemia; this can occur acutely after inadvertent injection into an artery (32) or even after intranasal use (33). There may also be an association between cocaine use and thromboangiitis obliterans (Buerger's disease) (34).

Gastrointestinal Complications

The vasoconstrictive effects of cocaine can affect the gastrointestinal tract and lead to ischemic colitis (35); this has also been observed with methamphetamine (36) and prescription stimulants (37).

Renal Complications

Cocaine use has been associated with declines in kidney function (**38**) and kidney failure (**39**), especially among hypertensive patients. Cocaine-induced rhabdomyolysis may also be complicated by renal failure (40). Renal infarction associated with cocaine use has also been reported (41).

Neuromuscular Complications

Stroke

Cocaine use has been associated with ischemic and hemorrhagic stroke, as well as subarachnoid hemorrhage; in one series of 214 young adults (age 15–44) with stroke, 27 (13%) had used cocaine shortly before the onset (**42**). Methamphetamine use has likewise been associated with hemorrhagic and ischemic stroke (43).

Rhabdomyolysis

Cocaine and methamphetamine users are at risk for rhabdomyolysis, which can be complicated by renal failure or compartment syndrome and can occur with any route of use (44). In one California series of nontraumatic rhabdomyolysis, 43% of the patients had a positive toxicology screen for methamphetamines; those with methamphetamine-associated rhabdomyolysis tended to be younger and were more likely to be agitated on presentation (45).

Hyperthermia / Heat Stroke

Epidemiological studies have noted an association between high ambient temperature (>88°F) and mortality associated with cocaine use (46). This is probably at least partly due to an increased risk of hyperthermia among cocaine users; cocaine has been found to impair heat dissipation by inhibiting sweating and cutaneous vasodilation (47).

Psychiatric Complications

Cocaine users may develop a variety of psychiatric symptoms including anxiety, agitation, paranoia, and psychosis. Cocaine-induced psychosis and paranoia appear to be a relatively common experience for users (48). This phenomenon seems to be partly dose-related (49), but individual predisposition probably also plays a role (50). Amphetamine users can experience similar complications, but they tend to be longer in duration. As with other substances, those who abuse or are dependent on stimulants are at increased risk of a variety of psychiatric illnesses including depression, bipolar disorder, anxiety disorders, personality disorders, and schizophrenia, though a cause-and-effect relationship has not been established (51).

TREATMENT

Most of the research done on the treatment of stimulant addiction has been performed on cocaine addicts. There is less data on the treatment of methamphetamine dependence, but given its similarity to cocaine, it is reasonable to postulate that treatment effects would be comparable (52). The treatment modalities that have been utilized can be roughly divided into two types: (1) psychosocial treatment and (2) pharmacotherapy and other intervention. (See Table 9.2 for a summary of stimulant abuse and dependence treatment intervention studies.) A variety of psy-

Table 9.2.   Summary of stimulant abuse and dependence treatment studies

Intervention	Studies	Outcomes
Psychosocial		
Self-help groups	Observational	Participation is associated with better outcomes
Brief advice	RCT	Effective for reducing cocaine use in one RCT
Group counseling	RCTs	Effective, more intensive (3X/week), no more effective than weekly
Individual counseling	RCTs	Effective, may offer some benefit when added to group counseling
Cognitive-behavioral therapy (CBT)	RCTs	Effective (in some studies)
Contingency management	RCTs	Effective (while incentives are offered)
Analytic psychotherapy	RCTs	No benefit when added to group counseling; outcomes better with CBT
Residential treatment	Observational	> 90 days participation associated with better outcomes
Pharmacotherapy		
Antidepressants	RCTs Meta-analysis	Not effective
Dopamine agonists	RCTs Meta-analysis	Not effective
Dopamine antagonists	RCTs	Not effective
Disulfiram	RCTs	Effective in two 12-week RCTs
Topiramate	RCT	Modestly effective in one 12-week RCT
Stimulants	RCTs	Effective in two RCTs
Acupuncture	RCTs Meta-analysis	Not effective

Most studies were of cocaine users; see text for references and more details.
RCT: randomized controlled trial.

chosocial interventions appear to be effective for selective individuals. As of yet, no medical agent has consistently been shown to be effective, but disulfiram, topiramate, and long-acting amphetamines are agents that may be beneficial. Combinations of psychosocial treatment and pharmacotherapy may prove to be the most effective approach.

Psychosocial Treatment

There are a variety of psychosocial modalities that have been used in treating cocaine dependence. Participation in self-help groups is associated with improved outcomes. Individual and group drug counseling also appear to be helpful. A number of behavioral approaches have been found to be modestly effective (at least during the treatment phase), but psychotherapeutic approaches have not been shown to be helpful.

Self-Help Groups

As with other forms of addiction, self-help (or mutual-help) groups are the most commonly used form of treatment; Narcotics Anonymous (www.na.org) and Cocaine Anonymous (www.ca.org) both sponsor meetings throughout North America and other countries. These groups utilize the 12-step approach developed by Alcoholics Anonymous but may vary quite a bit depending on the makeup of their members. The data on the effectiveness of these groups is limited but suggests a benefit for some individuals. In one observational study of patients in a variety of treatment modalities, those who afterward participated in self-help groups twice weekly or greater for more than 6 months had better outcomes in terms of drug use and illegal activity; this effect was sustained even when correcting for measures of motivation and demographic factors (53). Another observational study similarly found that participation at least weekly in 12-step groups was associated with lower drug and alcohol use, even when motivational measures were taken into account; on the other hand, less-than-weekly participation was no better than no participation at all (54). A recent study suggests that cocaine-dependent individuals who actively participate in the self-help process—in the form of speaking or performing duties at meetings, talking with a sponsor, reading 12-step literature, or working on a step—have better outcomes than those who simply attend meetings (**55**). An important factor to keep in mind is that these studies generally looked at individuals who had gone through another form of drug treatment before (or while) attending these groups.

Drug Counseling

Drug counseling is another commonly used therapeutic modality and can be offered in a group or individual setting. Simple screening and counseling of outpatients who use cocaine (and heroin) has been found to be modestly effective at reducing subsequent drug use (**56**). A study of intensive group counseling (three 3-hour sessions/week for 12 weeks) found no better outcomes when compared with weekly individual counseling alone or with a weekly group session (**57**). Individual drug counseling may offer some benefit over traditional group therapy. In one study of cocaine-dependent adults, this type of treatment (when combined with group drug counseling) was associated with (modestly) better outcomes than cognitive therapy, supportive-expressive therapy, or group drug counseling alone (**58**).

Behavioral Therapy

A variety of behavioral approaches appear to provide modest benefits, though the data on their effectiveness is mixed. Coping skills therapy was associated with reduced cocaine use in a short-term study (59), but this effect appeared to dissipate after a year (60). A subsequent study failed to find any benefit associated with coping skills therapy but did find that motivational enhancement therapy appeared to benefit individuals with lower initial motivation (61). In another study (mentioned earlier), the addition of cognitive therapy to group drug counseling did not appear to offer any additional benefit and performed worse than individual drug counseling (**58**). On the other hand, a study of amphetamine users reported that 2–4 sessions of cognitive behavioral therapy was effective at reducing amphetamine use (**62**). Finally, in a study of the treatment of methamphetamine dependence, an approach that combines cognitive-behavioral therapy with family education, social support, and individual counseling (the "Matrix Model") was found to perform better than "treatment as usual" in the short term, but not beyond the treatment phase (**63**).

The application of incentives contingent on abstinence—"contingency management"—appears to be a useful approach, though the long-term effectiveness (i.e., beyond the period of incentives) has not been established. For example, in one 24-week trial, contingency management with vouchers (in combination with behavioral treatment and community reinforcement) was found to reduce cocaine use (**64**). The use of community reinforcement with vouchers (compared to vouchers alone) appears to reduce cocaine use further, at least during the treatment phase (**65**). On the other hand, in a study of individuals on methadone maintenance therapy, cognitive-behavioral therapy performed as well as contingency management, and the combination of the two was no better than either alone (**66**). Nevertheless, a recent systematic review of community reinforcement concluded that this approach is effective, especially when combined with abstinence-contingent incentives (such as vouchers) (**67**).

Analytic Psychotherapy

For those who are addicted to stimulants, there is little evidence that analytic psychotherapeutic approaches are effective. In one study, once-weekly psychotherapy was not shown to be effective; this was true for once-weekly family therapy and group therapy as well (**68**). Another study (mentioned earlier) found no benefit associated with the addition of supportive-expressive therapy to group drug counseling for cocaine-dependent individuals (**58**). Furthermore, another study found that outcomes with interpersonal therapy were poorer than with cognitive behavior therapy (**69**).

Residential Treatment

The most intensive form of treatment for cocaine dependence is residential treatment; this is generally in the form of a therapeutic community, but a variety of approaches are used. A large observational study of treatment outcomes reported that long-term residential treatment, when compared with short-term outpatient and outpatient drug-free programs, was associated with lower cocaine use for a subset of individuals with a high level of addiction severity, provided they stayed 90 days or longer in treatment (70).

Pharmacotherapy (and Acupuncture)

There have been studies of numerous agents in search of one that would help reduce cocaine use; unfortunately, to date there is little evidence that any of these interventions is effective. Recent studies suggest that disulfiram, topiramate, modafinil, and long-acting amphetamines may be effective, but more research needs to be done to confirm initial observations and assess their long-term impact. The development of vaccines against cocaine or methamphetamine is another intriguing therapeutic option that is being explored (71).

Antidepressants

Studies on the use of antidepressants for cocaine dependence have generally failed to show a benefit (72). A 2003 Cochrane review of the use of antidepressants for the treatment of cocaine dependence that included 18 studies with 1177 participants concluded that there is "no current evidence supporting the clinical use of antidepressants in the treatment of cocaine dependence" (73).

Dopamine Agonists

Some early trials suggested that dopamine agonists, such as amantadine and bromocriptine, were effective for treatment of cocaine withdrawal symptoms (74). However, subsequent studies of their chronic administration did not find any reduction in cocaine use (75, 76). A 2003 Cochrane review of 17 studies with 1224 participants on the use of dopamine agonists for cocaine dependence concluded that "current evidence does not support the clinical use of dopamine agonists in the treatment of cocaine dependence" (77).

Dopamine Antagonists

Dopamine may be responsible for the reinforcing effects of cocaine. As a result, it has been postulated that dopamine antagonists, such as the antipsychotics olanzapine and risperidone, may reduce cocaine craving and use; unfortunately, clinical trials have shown no benefit (**78, 79**).

Carbamazepine

One study of carbamazepine reported a reduction in cocaine use over a 12-week period (80). However, other studies did not find any benefit, and a 2003 Cochrane review of five studies on the use of carbamazepine for cocaine dependence concluded that there is "no current evidence supporting the clinical use of carbamazepine in the treatment of cocaine dependence" (81).

Disulfiram

Many cocaine-dependent individuals also abuse alcohol. It was noted in studies of disulfiram treatment of individuals with concurrent alcohol and cocaine dependence that use of this medication was associated with reduced cocaine use (82). It was subsequently reported that disulfiram reduced cocaine use in individuals (on methadone maintenance) who were not alcohol dependent (83). A recent 12-week trial found significantly greater reduction in cocaine use with disulfiram, especially when combined with cognitive-behavioral therapy (69). It remains to be seen whether this treatment effect can be replicated in other settings and maintained over longer periods of time.

Topiramate

The gamma aminobutyric acid (GABA) system is thought to play a role in mediating the reinforcing effects of cocaine. Thus, it has been postulated that the GABAergic anticonvulsant topiramate may reduce cocaine craving. A recent 13-week pilot study on a cohort with mild cocaine dependence found that its use was associated with significant reduction in cocaine-positive urine toxicology screens, but not other measures of cocaine use (84).

Modafinil

Modafinil is a glutamate-enhancing agent that promotes wakefulness and is approved for treatment of narcolepsy. Since cocaine depletes extracellular glutamate, it has been postulated that this agent may help reduce craving and use. Moreover, modafinil appears to have low abuse potential. An 8-week pilot study reported that its use was associated with a reduction in cocaine use, without serious side effects (85). However, its effectiveness and long-term safety need to be studied further.

Amphetamines

Some have proposed the use of long-acting agonists for individuals dependent on stimulants, analogous to the use of methadone to treat opioid addicts. A pilot study of dexamphetamine reported favorable results in 30 cocaine-dependent adults over 14 weeks (86); a subsequent larger randomized controlled trial (utilizing sustained-release D-amphetamine) supported this initial evaluation (79). However, further research on the long-term effects and safety needs to be done before the use of these agents can be recommended.

Acupuncture

An initial study of 82 cocaine-dependent subjects on methadone maintenance reported a reduction in cocaine use among subjects who received auricular acupuncture (87). However, a subsequent larger trial involving 620 cocaine addicts found that it was no more effective than sham needle insertion or relaxation controls (88). A recent meta-analysis of nine studies concluded that the evidence "does not support the use of acupuncture for the treatment of cocaine dependence" (89).

CAFFEINE

Caffeine is a naturally occurring methylxanthine similar to the drug theophylline. It blocks adenosine receptors, leading to release of noradrenaline. Caffeine is found in coffee, tea, and chocolate and as an additive in a variety of beverages. It is also an ingredient in a variety of over-the-counter and prescription medications, including headache preparations and drugs to promote wakefulness. A cup (8 ounces) of coffee can contain 25–135 mg of caffeine, tea 15–80 mg, and soft drinks 20–60 mg (12 ounces); over-the-counter preparations may have as much as 200 mg in each dose. The toxic effects of caffeine include nausea, vomiting, tremulousness, and agitation. Caffeine appears to promote cardiac arrhythmias but probably not at the doses usually consumed (90). Caffeine overdose generally occurs only with consumption of caffeine-containing medications and can be fatal in some cases (91). Many regular caffeine users do experience mild withdrawal symptoms with cessation of use, including headaches, fatigue, and drowsiness (92). Some believe that caffeine use can lead to dependence; it appears that some users exhibit signs of dependence, including unsuccessful attempts to cut down and continued use despite harmful effects (93). However, there is little evidence that caffeine causes significant harm to individuals or society at large.

REFERENCES

1. Substance Abuse and Mental Health Services Administration. 2004. Results from the 2003 National Survey on Drug Use and Health: National Findings (Office of Applied Studies, NSDUH Series H-25, DHHS Publication No. SMA 04-3964). Rockville, MD.

2. Substance Abuse and Mental Health Services Administration, Office of Applied Studies. 2004, May. Major drugs of abuse in ED visits, 2002 update. *The DAWN Report.*

3. Hoffman, B. B. 2001. Catecholamines, sympathomimetic drugs and adrenergic receptor antagonists. In *Goodman and Gilman's The pharmacologic basis of therapeutics.* Edited by J. G. Hardman and L. E. Limbird, 215–268. New York: McGraw-Hill.

4. Darke, S., S. Kaye, and J. Duflou. 2005. Cocaine-related fatalities in New South Wales, Australia 1993–2002. *Drug Alcohol Depend.* 77:107–114.

5. McKinney, P. E., C. Tomaszewski, S. Phillips, et al. 1994. Methamphetamine toxicity prevented by activated charcoal in a mouse model. *Ann. Emerg. Med.* 24:220–223.

6. Lago, J. A., and T. R. Kosten. 1994. Stimulant withdrawal. *Addiction* 89:1477–1481.

7. Mendelson, J. H., M. Sholar, N. K. Mello, et al. 1998. Cocaine tolerance: Behavioral, cardiovascular, and neurodendocrine function in men. *Neuropsychopharmacology* 18:263–271.

8. Testing for drugs of abuse. 2002. *The Medical Letter* 44:71–73.

9. Vilela, R. J., C. Langford, L. McCullagh, and E. S. Kass. 2002. Cocaine-induced oronasal fistulas with external nasal erosion but without palate involvement. *Ear Nose Throat* 81:562–563.

10. Mattson-Gates, G., A. D. Jabs, and N. E. Hugo. 1991. Perforation of the hard palate associated with cocaine use. *Ann. Plast. Surg.* 26:466–468.

11. Friedman, D. R., and S. D. Wolfsthal. 2005. Cocaine-induced pseudovasculitis. *Mayo Clin. Proc.* 80:671–673.

12. Tashkin, D. P., E. C. Kleerup, S. N. Koyal, et al. 1996. Acute effects of inhaled and IV cocaine on airway dynamics. *Chest* 110:904–910.

13. Baldwin, G. C., R. Choi, M. D. Roth, et al. 2002. Evidence of chronic damage to the pulmonary microcirculation in habitual users of alkaloidal ("crack") cocaine. *Chest* 121:1231–1238.

14. Yakel, D. L., and M. J. Eisenberg. 1995. Pulmonary artery hypertension in chronic intravenous cocaine users. *Am. Heart J.* 130:398–399.

15. Schaiberger, P. H., T. C. Kennedy, F. C. Miller, et al. 1993. Pulmonary hypertension associated with long-term inhalation of "crank" methamphetamine. *Chest* 104:614–616.

16. Kleerup, E. C., S. N. Koyal, J. A. Marques-Magallanes, et al. 2002. Chronic and acute effects of "crack" cocaine on diffusing capacity, membrane diffusion, and pulmonary capillary blood volume in the lung. *Chest* 122:629–638.

17. Arnett, E. N., W. E. Battle, J. V. Russo, and W. C. Roberts. 1976. Intravenous injection of talc-containing drugs intended for oral use. A cause of pulmonary granulomatosis and pulmonary hypertension. *Am. J. Med.* 60:711–718.

18. Sherman, C. B., L. D. Hudson, and D. J. Pierson. 1987. Severe precocious emphysema in intravenous methylphenidate (Ritalin) abusers. *Chest* 92:1085–1087.

19. Hollander, J. E., K. H. Todd, G. Green, et al. 1995. Chest pain associated with cocaine: An assessment of prevalence in suburban and urban emergency departments. *Ann. Emerg. Med.* 26:671–676. *Among 359 patients with chest pain (8% had a myocardial infarction), 29% of those age 18–30 had a positive urine for cocaine, 18% age 31–40, 18% age 41–50, 3% age 51–60, and 0% age 61 or older.*

20. Hollander, J. E., R. S. Hoffman, P. Gennis, et al. 1994. Prospective multicenter evaluation of cocaine-associated chest pain. *Acad. Emerg. Med.* 1:330–339.

21. Lange, R. A., and L. D. Hillis. 2001. Cardiovascular complications of cocaine use. *N. Engl. J. Med.* 345:351–358.

22. Lange, R. A., R. G. Cigarroa, E. D. Flores, et al. 1990. Potentiation of cocaine-induced coronary vasoconstriction by beta-adrenergic blockade. *Ann. Intern. Med.* 112:897–903.

23. Minor, R. L., B. D. Scott, D. D. Brown, and M. D. Winniford. 1991. Cocaine-induced myocardial infarction in patients with normal coronary arteries. *Ann. Intern. Med.* 115:797–806. *Of 114 cases of cocaine-associated myocardial infarction, 92 had angiography or autopsy and 38% of these had normal coronary arteries.*

24. Weber, J. E., F. S. Shofer, G. L. Larkin, et al. 2003. Validation of a brief observation period for patients with cocaine-associated chest pain. *N. Engl. J. Med.* 348:510–517. *Three hundred forty-four consecutive patients with cocaine-associated chest pain were evaluated; 42 (12%) were admitted. Those with normal troponin-I levels, no new ischemic ECG changes, and no cardiovascular*

complications during 9- to 12-hour observational period (302 patients) were discharged. At 30-day follow-up, none had died of a cardiovascular event; 4 of 256 (1.6%) had a nonfatal myocardial infarction—all 4 had continued to use cocaine.

25. Turnipseed, S. D., J. R. Richards, J. D. Kirk, et al. 2003. Frequency of acute coronary syndrome in patients presenting to the emergency department with chest pain after methamphetamine use. *J. Emerg. Med.* 24:369–373.

26. Roldan, C. A., D. Aliabadi, and M. H. Crawford. 2001. Prevalence of heart disease in asymptomatic chronic cocaine users. *Cardiology* 95:25–30. *In comparison with 32 age-matched controls, 35 cocaine users were more likely to have a positive stress test (34% vs. 9%) and decreased LV function (14% vs. 0%, p = 0.055); they were also more likely to smoke (47% vs. 19%).*

27. Turnicky, R. P., J. Goodin, J. E. Smialek, et al. 1992. Incidental myocarditis with intravenous drug use: The pathology, immunopathology, and potential implications for human immunodeficiency virus-associated myocarditis. *Hum. Pathol.* 23:138–143.

28. Peng, S. K., W. J. French, and P. C. Pelikan. 1989. Direct cocaine cardiotoxicity demonstrated by endomyocardial biopsy. *Arch. Pathol. Lab. Med.* 113:842–845.

29. Hong, R., E. Matsuyama, and K. Nur. 1991. Cardiomyopathy associated with the smoking of crystal methamphetamine. *JAMA* 265:1152–1154.

30. Hsue, P. Y., C. L. Salinas, A. F. Bolger, et al. 2002. Acute aortic dissection related to crack cocaine. *Circulation* 105:1592–1595.

31. Chambers, H. F., D. L. Morris, M. G. Täuber, and G. Modin. 1987. Cocaine use and the risk for endocarditis in intravenous drug users. *Ann. Intern. Med.* 106:833–836.

32. Silverman, S. H., and W. W. Turner. 1991. Intraarterial drug abuse: New treatment options. *J. Vasc. Surg.* 14:111–116.

33. Mizrayan, R., S. E. Hanks, and F. A. Weaver. 1998. Cocaine-induced thrombosis of common iliac and popliteal arteries. *Ann. Vasc. Surg.* 12:476–481.

34. Marder, V. J., and I. K. Mellinghoff. 2000. Cocaine and Buerger disease: Is there a pathogenic association? *Arch. Intern. Med.* 160:2057–2060.

35. Linder, J. D., K. E. Monkemuller, I. Raijman, et al. 2000. Cocaine-associated ischemic colitis. *South. Med. J.* 93:909–913.

36. Johnson, T. D., and M. M. Berenson. 1991. Methamphetamine-induced ischemic colitis. *J. Clin. Gastroenterol.* 13:687–689.

37. Comay, D., J. Ramsay, and E. J. Irvine. 2003. Ischemic colitis after weight-loss medication. *Can. J. Gastroenterol.* 17:719–721.

38. Vupputuri, S., V. Batuman, P. Munter, et al. 2004. The risk for mild kidney function decline associated with illicit drug use among hypertensive men. *Am. J. Kidney Dis.* 43:629–635. *Among 647 hypertensive veterans followed for a median of 7 years, cocaine use was associated with mild kidney function decline (adjusted relative risk 3.0).*

39. Norris, K. C., M. Thornhill-Joynes, C. Robinson, et al. 2001. Cocaine use, hypertension, and end-stage renal disease. *Am. J. Kidney Dis.* 38:523–528. *Among 201 subjects at two urban dial-*

ysis units, cocaine use was associated with a diagnosis of hyper-tension-related renal failure (odds ratio of 9.4).

40. Singhal, P., B. Horowitz, M. C. Quinones, et al. 1989. Acute renal failure following cocaine abuse. *Nephron* 52:76–78.

41. Sharff, J. A. 1984. Renal infarction associated with intravenous cocaine use. *Ann. Emerg. Med.* 13:1145–1147.

42. Kaku, D. A., and D. H. Lowenstein. 1990. Emergence of recreational drug abuse as a major risk factor for stroke in young adults. *Ann. Intern. Med.* 113:821–827. *In this case-control study, drug abuse was associated with an increased risk of stroke (relative risk: 6.5); 74% had used cocaine or methamphetamines.*

43. Perez, J. A., E. L. Arsura, and S. Strategos. 1999. Methamphetamine-related stroke: Four cases. *J. Emerg. Med.* 17:469–471.

44. Horowitz, B. Z., E. A. Panacek, and N. J. Jouriles. 1997. Severe rhabdomyolysis with renal failure after intranasal cocaine use. *J. Emerg. Med.* 15:833–837.

45. Richards, J. R., E. B. Johnson, R. W. Stark, and R. W. Derlet. 1999. Methamphetamine abuse and rhabdomyolysis in the ED: A 5-year study. *Am. J. Emerg. Med.* 17:681–685.

46. Marzuk, P. M., K. Tardiff, A. C. Leon, et al. 1998. Ambient temperature and mortality from unintentional cocaine overdose. *JAMA* 279:1795–1800.

47. Crandall, C. G., W. Vongpatanasin, and R. G. Victor. 2002. Mechanism of cocaine induced hyperthermia in humans. *Ann. Intern. Med.* 136:785–791.

48. Brady, K. T., R. B. Lydiard, R. Malcom, and J. C. Ballenger. 1991. Cocaine-induced psychosis. *J. Clin. Psychiatry* 52:509–512.

49. Batki, S. L., and D. S. Harris. 2004. Quantitative drug levels in stimulant psychosis: Relationship to symptom severity, catecholamines and hyperkinesia. *Am. J. Addict.* 13:461–470.

50. Satel, S. L., and W. S. Edell. 1991. Cocaine-induced paranoia and psychosis proneness. *Am. J. Psychiatry* 148:1708–1711.

51. Regier, D. A., M. E. Farmer, D. S. Rae, et al. 1990. Comorbidity of mental disorders with alcohol and other drug abuse. Results from the Epidemiologic Catchment Area study. *JAMA* 264:2511–2518.

52. Cretzmeyer, M., M. V. Sarrazin, D. L. Huber, et al. 2003. Treatment of methamphetamine abuse: Research findings and clinical directions. *J. Subst. Abuse Treat.* 24:267–277.

53. Etheridge, R. M., S. G. Craddock, R. L. Hubbard, and J. L. Rounds-Bryant. 1999. The relationship of counseling and self-help participation to patient outcomes in DATOS. *Drug Alcohol Depend.* 57:99–112.

54. Fiorentine, R. 1999. After drug treatment: Are 12-step programs effective in maintaining abstinence? *Am. J. Drug Alcohol Abuse* 25:93–116.

55. Weiss, R. D., M. L. Griffin, R. J. Gallop, et al. 2005. The effect of 12-step self-help group attendance and participation on drug use outcomes among cocaine-dependent patients. *Drug Alcohol Depend.* 77:177–184. *This observational study included 336 cocaine addicts from a randomized controlled trial of different treatment modalities (ref. #56). Active participation in 12-step activities was associated with reduced subsequent drug use, while attendance at the groups was not.*

56. Bernstein, J., E. Bernstein, K. Tassiopoulos, et al. 2005. Brief motivational intervention at a clinic visit reduces cocaine and heroin use. *Drug Alcohol Depend.* 77:49–59. *Patients attending walk-in clinics were screened for heroin and cocaine use and were randomized to (1) brief intervention by a trained counselor consisting of a motivational interview, active referrals, and a written handout with a list of treatment resources, followed by a phone call 10 days later, or (2) handout only. Of 23,669 screened, 1232 (5%) were eligible, 1175 enrolled, and 778 used in the final analysis. At 6-month follow-up, those in the intervention group were more likely to be abstinent from cocaine alone (22.3% vs. 16.9%), heroin alone (40.2% vs. 30.6%), and both drugs (17.4% vs. 12.8%).*

57. Gottheil, E., S. P. Weinstein, R. C. Sterling, et al. 1998. A randomized controlled study of the effectiveness of intensive outpatient treatment for cocaine dependence. *Psychiatr. Serv.* 49:782–787. *Four hundred forty-seven cocaine addicts (of 862 offered treatment) were randomized to (1) weekly individual counseling, (2) individual counseling plus a weekly group session, or (3) intensive group treatment (three 3-hour sessions / week). There was no difference after 12 weeks of treatment and at 9-month follow-up; the 24% who completed treatment did better, regardless of type.*

58. Crits-Christoph, P., L. Siqueland, J. Blaine, et al. 1999. Psychosocial treatments for cocaine dependence. *Arch. Gen. Psychiatry* 56:493–502. *Four hundred eighty-seven cocaine addicts (of 2197 screened) were randomized to (1) individual drug counseling + group drug counseling (GDC), (2) cognitive therapy + GDC, (3) supportive-expressive therapy + GDC, or (4) GDC alone; 28% of the total completed the 6-month treatment. Over 12 months, the mean addiction severity index (ASI) scores and cocaine use in all four arms decreased, but more so in the first arm.*

59. Monti, P. M., D. J. Rohsenow, E. Michalec, et al. 1997. Brief coping skills treatment for cocaine abuse: Substance use outcomes at three months. *Addiction* 92:1717–1728.

60. Rohsenow, D. J., P. M. Monti, R. A. Martin, et al. 2000. Brief coping skills treatment for cocaine abuse: 12-month substance use outcomes. *J. Consult. Clin. Psychol.* 68:515–520.

61. Rohsenow, D. J., P. M. Monti, R. A. Martin, et al. 2004. Motivational enhancement and coping skills training for cocaine abusers: Effects on substance use outcomes. *Addiction* 99:862–874.

62. Baker, A., N. K. Lee, M. Claire, et al. 2005. Brief behavioural interventions for regular amphetamine users: A step in the right direction. *Addiction* 100:367–378. *Two hundred fourteen amphetamine users were randomized to (1) two sessions of cognitive-behavioral therapy (CBT), (2) four sessions of CBT, or (3) self-help booklet; at 6-month follow-up, abstinence rates were 34%, 38%, and 18%, respectively.*

63. Rawson, R. A., P. Marinelli-Casey, M. D. Anglin, et al. 2004. A multi-site comparison of psychosocial approaches for the treatment of methamphetamine dependence. *Addiction* 99:708–717. *Nine hundred seventy-eight methamphetamine addicts were randomized to (1) Matrix Model (MM) or (2)*

treatment as usual—a variety of community treatment programs. Overall, those assigned to MM were more likely to complete their program (41% vs. 34%), had longer periods of abstinence, and were more likely to give methamphetamine-negative urine over 16 weeks. The 86% who completed 6-month follow-up (in both groups) reported reduced use and 69% had negative urines, but there was no significant difference between the groups.

64. Higgins, S. T., A. J. Budney, W. K. Bickel, et al. 1994. Incentives improve outcome in outpatient behavioral treatment of cocaine dependence. *Arch. Gen. Psychiatry* 51:568–576. *Forty cocaine addicts were randomized to behavioral treatment and community reinforcement with or without voucher incentives over 12 weeks. Both received the same treatment for the second 12 weeks. The voucher group had higher 12-week retention (90% vs. 65%) and 24-week retention (75% vs. 40%); they were also more likely to be cocaine-abstinent during both 12-week periods (but this declined in both groups).*

65. Higgins, S. T., S. C. Sigmon, C. J. Wong, et al. 2003. Community reinforcement therapy for cocaine-dependent outpatients. *Arch. Gen. Psychiatry* 60.1043–1052. *One hundred cocaine addicts were randomized to (1) community reinforcement + vouchers (CR) or (2) vouchers alone. All received 24 weeks of treatment followed by 6 months aftercare and were assessed at 12, 15, and 24 months. Those assigned to CR had better treatment retention (84% vs. 51%) and were more likely to give cocaine-negative urine at 12 weeks (78% vs. 51%), but not subsequently. CR subjects had more paid employment days during treatment and at 9 to 12 month follow-up, but not at 15- to 24-month follow-up. Legal, medical, psychiatric, and family problems were about the same.*

66. Rawson, R. A., A. Huber, M. McCann, et al. 2002. A comparison of contingency management and cognitive-behavioral approaches during methadone maintenance treatment for cocaine dependence. *Arch. Gen. Psychiatry* 59:817–824. *One hundred twenty cocaine addicts on methadone maintenance were randomized to (1) cognitive behavioral therapy (CBT), (2) contingency management (i.e., vouchers for cocaine-negative urines) (CM), (3) CBT + CM, or (4) usual care. During 16 weeks of treatment, the two CM arms had the highest rate of cocaine-negative urines (54% vs. 40% with CBT and 23% with usual care). At 52-week follow-up, the CBT-only group had the highest rate (60%) followed by CM-only (53%), CBT + CM (40%), and usual care (27%).*

67. Roozen, H. G., J. J. Boulogne, M. W. Tulder, et al. 2004. A systematic review of the effectiveness of the community reinforcement approach in alcohol, cocaine and opioid addiction. *Drug Alcohol Depend.* 74:1–13.

68. Kang, S. Y., P. H. Kleinman, G. E. Woody, et al. 1991. Outcomes for cocaine abusers after once-a-week psychosocial therapy. *Am. J. Psychiatry* 148:630–635. *One hundred sixty-eight cocaine abusers were randomized weekly: (1) individual supportive-expressive psychotherapy, (2) family therapy, or (3) group therapy. Of the 122 who had 6-month and 1-year follow-up, 23 (19%) re-*

ported at least 3 months of abstinence, but there was no differ-ence between the three arms.

69. Carroll, K. M., L. R. Fenton, S. A. Ball, et al. 2004. Efficacy of disulfiram and cognitive behavior therapy in cocaine-dependent outpatients. *Arch. Gen. Psychiatry* 61:264–272. *One hundred twenty-one cocaine addicts were randomized in a 2X2 factorial trial to (1) disulfiram or placebo, and (2) cognitive behavior therapy (CBT) or interpersonal psychotherapy (IPT) for 12 weeks. About half were alcohol dependent or abusers. There was greater reduction in cocaine use among those assigned to disulfiram versus placebo and those assigned CBT versus IPT.*

70. Simpson, D. D., G. W. Joe, B. W. Fletcher, et al. 1999. A national evaluation of treatment outcomes for cocaine dependence. *Arch. Gen. Psychiatry* 56:507–514.

71. Haney, M., and T. R. Kosten. 2004. Therapeutic vaccines for substance dependence. *Expert Rev. Vaccines* 3:11–18.

72. Oliveto, A. H., A. Feingold, R. Schottenfeld, et al. 1999. Desipramine in opioid-dependent cocaine abusers maintained on buprenorphine vs. methadone. *Arch. Gen. Psychiatry* 56:812–820.

73. Lima, M. S., A. A. P. Reisser Lima, B. G. O. Soares, and M. Farrell. 2003. Antidepressants for cocaine dependence. *The Cochrane Database of Systemic Reviews.* Issue 2. Art. No.: CD002950.

74. Tennant, F. S., Jr., and A. A. Sagherian. 1987. Double-blind comparison of amantadine and bromocriptine for ambulatory withdrawal from cocaine dependence. *Arch. Intern. Med.* 147:109–112.

75. Handelsman, L., L. Limpitlaw, D. Williams, et al. 1995. Amantadine does not reduce cocaine use or craving in cocaine-dependent methadone maintenance patients. *Drug Alcohol Depend.* 39:173–180.

76. Handelsman, L., A. Rosenblum, M. Palij, et al. 1997. Bromocriptine for cocaine dependence. A controlled clinical trial. *Am. J. Addict.* 6:54–64.

77. Soares, B. G. O., M. S. Lima, A. Lima Reisser, and M. Farrell. 2003. Dopamine agonists for cocaine dependence. *The Cochrane Database of Systemic Reviews.* Issue 2. Art. No.: CD003352.

78. Kampman, K. M., H. Pettinati, K. G. Lynch, et al. 2003. A pilot trial of olanzapine for the treatment of cocaine dependence. *Drug Alcohol Depend.* 70:265–273. *Thirty cocaine addicts were randomized to 10 mg of olanzapine or placebo for 12 weeks; those given placebo were more likely to be abstinent.*

79. Grabowski, J., H. Rhoades, A. Stotts, et al. 2004. Agonist-like and antagonist-like treatment for cocaine dependence with methadone for heroin dependence: Two double-blind randomized clinical trials. *Neuropsychopharmacology* 29:969–981. *Cocaine and heroin-dependent adults were recruited for two parallel trials; all received methadone maintenance and cognitive behavior therapy. Trial I: 94 were randomized to placebo or one of two doses of sustained release D-amphetamine (15–30 mg vs. 30–60 mg); 34 completed the 6-month trial. Those on the higher D-amphetamine dose had fewer cocaine (and opiate)*

positive tox screens. Trial II: 96 were randomized to placebo or one of two doses of risperidone (2 or 4 mg); after 6 months, there was no difference in cocaine (or opiate) positive drug screens.

80. Halikas, J. A., R. D. Crosby, V. L. Pearson, and N. M. Graves. 1997. A randomized double-blind study of carbamazepine in the treatment of cocaine abuse. *Clin. Pharmacol. Ther.* 62:89–105.

81. Lima Reisser, A., M. S. Lima, B. G. O. Soares, and M. Farrell. 2002. Carbamazepine for cocaine dependence. *The Cochrane Database of Systemic Reviews.* Issue 2. Art. No.: CD002023.

82. Carroll, K. M., C. Nich, S. A. Ball, et al. 1998. Treatment of cocaine and alcohol dependence with psychotherapy and disulfiram. *Addiction* 93:713–728.

83. Petrakis, I. L., K. M. Carroll, C. Nich, et al. 2000. Disulfiram treatment for cocaine dependence in methadone-maintained opioid addicts. *Addiction* 95:219–228. *Sixty-seven cocaine addicts on methadone were randomized to disulfiram or placebo with their methadone; 78% completed the 12 weeks of treatment. Both arms reported decreased cocaine and alcohol use; those on disulfiram had a greater reduction in cocaine (but not alcohol) use. The absolute difference was modest (~5 vs. 7 days of use in the previous 30 days at the end of treatment).*

84. Kampman, K. M., H. Pettinati, K. G. Lynch, et al. 2004. A pilot trial of topiramate for the treatment of cocaine dependence. *Drug Alcohol Depend.* 75:233–240. *Forty cocaine addicts with 3 days abstinence and low cocaine withdrawal symptom severity were randomized to topiramate (8-week titration to 200 mg/day) or placebo. All received cognitive behavioral therapy. Those on topiramate were more likely to have cocaine-negative tox screens at week 8; however, they did not report fewer days of cocaine use, fewer dollars spent on drugs, or less drug craving.*

85. Dackis, C. A., K. M. Kampman, K. G. Lynch, et al. 2005. A double blind placebo-controlled trial of modafinil for cocaine dependence. *Neuropsychopharmacology* 30:205–211. *Sixty-two cocaine addicts were randomized to 400 mg/day of modafinil or placebo. Sixty-four percent completed the 8-week study; those on modafinil had more cocaine-negative urines (mean 42% vs. 24%) but did not report less use or craving.*

86. Shearer, J., A. Wodak, I. van Beek, et al. 2003. Pilot randomized double blind placebo-controlled study of dexamphetamine for cocaine dependence. *Addiction* 98:1137–1141.

87. Avants, S. K., A. Margolin, T. R. Holford, and T. R. Kosten. 2000. A randomized controlled trial of auricular acupuncture for cocaine dependence. *Arch. Intern. Med.* 160:2305–2312.

88. Margolin, A., H. D. Kleger, S. K. Avants, et al. 2002. Acupuncture for the treatment of cocaine addiction. A randomized controlled trial. *JAMA* 287:55–63.

89. Mills, E. J., P. Wu, J. Gagnier, and J. O. Ebbert. 2005. Efficacy of acupuncture for cocaine dependence: A systematic review and meta-analysis. *Harm Reduct. J.* 17:4.

90. Myers, M. G. 1991. Caffeine and cardiac arrhythmias. *Ann. Intern. Med.* 114:147–150.

91. Holmgren, P., L. Nordén-Pettersson, and J. Ahlner. 2004. Caffeine fatalities—four case reports. *Forensic Sci. Int.* 139:71–73.

92. Hughes, J. R., S. T. Higgins, W. K. Bickel, et al. 1991. Caffeine self-administration, withdrawal, and adverse effects among coffee drinkers. *Arch. Gen. Psychiatry* 48:611–617.

93. Strain, E. C., G. K. Mumford, K. Silverman, and R. R. Griffiths. 1994. Caffeine dependence syndrome. Evidence from case histories and experimental evaluations. *JAMA* 272:1043–1048.

10

Phencyclidine and Hallucinogens

BACKGROUND

Hallucinogens are a broad spectrum of substances that alter an individual's perception of reality; they are sometimes referred to as "psychedelics." There are a number of synthetic and naturally

Table 10.1.   Selected agents with hallucinogenic effects

Technical Names	Plant or Animal Sources (if any)*	Street/Popular Names
Piperidines		
Phencyclidine (PCP)		Angel dust
Ketamine		Special K, Ket
Tiletamine		
Phenylethylamines		
3,4-Methylenedioxymethamphetamine (MDMA)		Ecstasy, Adam, STP
3,4-Methylenedioxyamphetamine (MDA)		Eve
4-Bromo-2,5-dimethoxyamphetamine (DOB)		Bromo, Nexus
4-Methylthioamphetamine (4-MTA)		Flatliners
Paramethoxyamphetamine (PMA)		Death
Mescaline	Peyote (*Lophophora williamsii*)	Buttons, Cactus, Mesc
	San Pedro (*Trichocereus pachanoi*)	Cimora
Macromerine	Doña ana (*Coryphantha macromeris*)	Doñana, false peyote
Myristicin	Nutmeg (*Myristica fragrans*)	
Ergot alkaloids		
D-Lysergic acid diethylamide (LSD)		Acid
Lysergic acid amide (LSA, Ergine)	Morning glory (*Ipomoea violacea, Rivea corymbosa*)	Ololiuqui, Tlitliltzin
	Hawaiian Baby Woodrose (*Argyreia nervosa*)	

Table 10.1. *Continued*

Technical Names	Plant or Animal Sources (if any)*	Street/Popular Names
Tryptamines		
Psilocybin/psilocin	*Psilocybe cubensis* & other spp.	Magic Mushrooms
Dimethyltryptamine (DMT)	*Anadenanthera peregrina, Virola* spp.	Ayahuasca, Caapi, Yage
5-HO-DMT (Bufotenine)	Colorado River toad (*Bufo alvarius*)	Bufo
5-MeO-DIPT		Foxy, Foxy methoxy
Ibogaine	*Tabernanthe iboga*	Iboga
Piperazines		
Benzylpiperazine (BZP)		Legal E, Legal X, Rapture
Trifluoromethylphenylpiperazine (TFMPP)		Legal E, Legal X, Rapture
Anticholinergics		
Belladonna alkaloids	Jimsonweed (*Datura stramonium*)	
	Angel's trumpet (*Datura suaveolens*)	
	Mandrake (*Mandragora officinarum*)	
	Henbane (*Hyoscyamus niger*)	
	Deadly nightshade (*Atropa belladonna*)	

continued

Table 10.1. *Continued*

Technical Names	Plant or Animal Sources (if any)*	Street/Popular Names
Terpenoids		
Tetrahydrocannabinol (THC)	Marijuana (*Cannabis sativa*)	Grass, Pot, Reefer, Blunt
Thujone	Wormwood (*Artemisia absinthium*)	Absinthe
Salvinorin-A	Diviner's Sage (*Salvia divinorum*)	Salvia, Yerba de la Pastora
		Sweet Flag
Asarone	Calamus (*Acorus calamus*)	
Humulene	Hops (*Humulus lupulus*)	
Coleon	Coleus (*Coleus blumei & pumila*)	
Others		
Muscimol	Fly agaric (*Amanita muscaria*)	Toadstool
Dextromethorphan (DXM)		Robo, Rojo, DM

* Not all sources are listed.

occurring agents that are used for their hallucinogenic effect. Phencyclidine (PCP) and related agents—such as ketamine—are technically "dissociative anesthetics" but share many characteristics with hallucinogens and will be covered in this chapter. The hallucinogens include MDMA (Ecstasy) and lysergic acid diethylamide (LSD); Table 10.1 lists some hallucinogenic agents. Marijuana and its active ingredient, tetrahydrocannabinol (THC), also have hallucinogenic effects, but these will be covered in a separate chapter.

Piperidines

Phencyclidine (PCP or "angel dust") was initially developed in the 1920s and used as an anesthetic; however, its use declined after it was found to often cause psychosis and dysphoria, and it is no longer used therapeutically. PCP is sold in the form of powder, pills, or rocks that can be smoked. It can be ingested, snorted, smoked, or injected. The powder is often added to marijuana; cigarettes are sometimes dipped into formaldehyde with dissolved PCP. Two related agents, ketamine and tiletamine, are used as veterinary anesthetics and also used illicitly.

Phenylethylamines

Methylenedioxymethamphetamine (MDMA or "Ecstasy") and similar "designer drugs" (MDA, DOB, 4-MTA, PMA, and others) are related to amphetamines and have many similar effects, but they are used primarily for their hallucinogenic effect. They are sometimes referred to as "enactogens" or "empathogens" because of their reported ability to induce feelings of empathy; the latter term has fallen out of favor because of the negative (and perhaps inadvertently accurate) connotations of "pathogen." MDMA is generally taken in a pill form; the MDMA content of these pills varies substantially and many pills contain other substances, including caffeine, ephedrine, methamphetamine, or ketamine (1). Furthermore, many of the related phenylethylamines are sold as "Ecstasy" on the street. There are also a number of phenylethylamines in the "2C" family that have been identified and synthesized that have similar effects, including 2C-B, 2C-T-2, 2C-T-7, and 2C-I.

Mescaline is the active hallucinogenic alkaloid that is found in peyote, a small cactus that grows in the Southwestern United States and northern Mexico; growths on the cactus—called "buttons"   are removed and dried, then chewed and ingested. Native Americans have used these for religious ceremonies and as treatment for a variety of ailments. Mescaline can be extracted from peyote or synthesized and used in a variety of forms; it can also be found in other cacti. Peyote is a schedule I substance, but members of the Native American Church are permitted to use it legally. Mescaline can also be found in lower concentrations in a South American cactus called San Pedro (*Trichocereus pachanoi*); in Peru, the skin is used to produce a drink called *cimora*.

Nutmeg (*Myristica fragrans*) is a popular spice that can be hallucinogenic if consumed in large quantities. Myristicin is the primary hallucinogenic substance in the seeds and is me-

tabolized to 3-methoxy-4,5-methylene-dioxyamphetamine
(MMDA)—a phenylethylamine. Whole nuts or powder may be
ingested or dissolved in water or alcohol before consumption;
the psychogenic effect can be obtained with 1–3 whole nut-
megs or 5–30 grams of the powder (2).

Ergot Alkaloids

Lysergic acid diethylamide (LSD) was developed in the 1940s
and is a colorless, odorless powder that is often sold in impreg-
nated blotting paper. A closely related ergot alkaloid is produced
by a fungus that infects rye and is the cause of ergotism, or "St.
Anthony's Fire." There are a number of other naturally occurring
botanicals that contain lysergamides, including the seeds of the
Hawaiian baby woodrose and a few species of morning glory. The
seeds can be crushed or eaten whole; they are sometimes soaked
in water and then the extract is drunk. The Aztecs used Mexican
morning glory seeds ("ololiuqui") in their religious ceremonies.
Commercially available seeds are often coated with an emetic
toxin to discourage ingestion.

Tryptamines

There are a number of other naturally occurring hallucinogenic tryptamines (these are sometimes referred to as "indoles"
or "indolealkylamines"). Psilocybin (4-phosphoryloxy-*N,N*-di-
methyltryptamine) and psilocin (4-hydroxy-*N,N*-dimethyltrypta-
mine) are hallucinogenic tryptamines found in a variety of
Psilocybe mushrooms that can be found in the Southern and
Western United States, as well as other regions of the world. The
dried mushrooms are typically ingested.

N,N-Dimethyltryptamine (DMT) is found in a number of
natural sources, including the bark of the Amazonian *Virola*
species, referred to locally as "Yakee" or "Parica"; it can also
be found in many other botanical sources worldwide. DMT
can be inhaled, smoked, or injected; tribes in South America
have traditionally used the ground bark of the *Virola* trees as
a snuff. DMT is orally active only when combined with a MAO
inhibitor; a brewed tea called "ayahuasca" is consumed in
South America that contains a natural MAO inhibitor, as well
as DMT.

Bufotenine (5-hydroxydimethyltryptamine, or 5-OH-DMT) is
found in the secretions and skin of "Bufo toads," including the
Colorado river toad (*Bufo alvarius*), and has produced the
strange (and dangerous) practice of "toad-licking"; some smoke
the dried secretions, which are milked from the toad's secretory
glands. A synthetic tryptamine, 5-methoxy-*N,N*-diisopropyl-
tryptamine (5-MeO-DIPT), is reportedly sold under the name
"Foxy" (or "Foxy methoxy") and can be purchased on the Internet
(3).

Ibogaine is derived from a West African shrub (*Tabernanthe
iboga*); an extract of the root has been used by indigenous people
in that region. Ibogaine is unique among hallucinogens because
of its long duration of effect (18–24 hours); some claim that it is
an effective treatment for drug addiction (4).

Anticholinergics

There are a number of plants that contain the anticholinergics atropine and scopolamine that have been used for their hallucinogenic effect throughout the world; however, their toxicity has limited their use. These plants include Jimsonweed (*Datura stramonium*), Angel's trumpet (*Datura suaveolens*), mandrake (*Mandragora officinarum*), henbane (*Hyoscyamus niger*), and deadly nightshade (*Atropa belladonna*). Typically, the leaves are ingested or smoked.

Terpenoids

There are a number of psychoactive terpene-like or terpenoid substances that are found in a variety of plants. The best known (and most used) of these is tetrahydrocannabinol (THC), which is found in marijuana and hashish.

Artemisia absinthium is a shrub in the wormwood family that has been used to flavor the liqueur absinthe. The active ingredient, thujone, has hallucinogenic properties. Thujone is not soluble in water but can be dissolved in alcohol and has a distinctive menthol odor.

Salvinorin-A is a hallucinogenic diterpene that is found in the leaves of *Salvia divinorum*, a plant in the mint family. Natives in Mexico have traditionally used it by chewing the leaves or ingesting the juice of the leaves; the dried leaves can also be smoked. This substance has not been scheduled by the DEA, but it is being monitored as a possible emerging drug of abuse. Hops (*Humulus lupulus*), which are used as a flavoring agent in the production of beer, contain the terpenoid humulene and can have mild marijuana-like effects when smoked or ingested.

Others

Fly agaric (*Amanita muscaria*) is another mushroom that has hallucinogenic properties. A number of substances in the mushroom are thought to produce this effect; the most important is probably muscimol. These mushrooms are typically dried and ingested. Misidentification is risky and potentially lethal, since there are other poisonous *Amanita* varieties that often grow in close proximity (5).

Dextromethorphan (DXM) is an over-the-counter cough suppressant that is sometimes used for its hallucinogenic effects, which are similar to the effects of phencyclidine (PCP) and related compounds. Users must consume large quantities of cough syrup (at least 4 oz) to achieve the desired effect; some use a powdered form of the drug. Many pills sold as "Ecstasy" have been found to contain DXM (6).

EPIDEMIOLOGY

According to the *2003 National Survey on Drug Use and Health,* an estimated 34 million Americans have used hallucinogens (this category includes PCP) at some point in their lives; this is 14.5% of the population aged 12 or older (7). An estimated 3.9 million used hallucinogens in the past year (1.7%) and 1.0 million had used them in the past month (0.4%). Lifetime use was highest for LSD (24 million), followed by psilocybin ("mushrooms"; 19.5 million), MDMA (10.9 million), mescaline (9.4 million), PCP (7.1 million), and peyote (5.7 million). Although lifetime use of LSD was the highest, MDMA was the most commonly used hallucinogen in 2003; 2.1 million Americans were estimated to have used MDMA in the past year, 0.6 million LSD, and 0.2 million PCP. Furthermore, there were an estimated 1.8 million new users of MDMA in 2001, in contrast to 0.6 million new users of LSD. Hallucinogen use was highest in the age 18–25 group; an estimated 6.7% had used a hallucinogen in the past year (3.7% had used MDMA). This percentage declines to 0.6% for those age 26 or older.

DRUG EFFECTS

Acute Effects

Hallucinogens in general alter sensory perception and change the qualities of thought or emotion. Users sometimes describe a slowing or speeding of their perception of time. An individual's experience can vary quite widely depending on the substance used, the person's mind-set, and environmental factors. The experience may be intensely pleasurable or extremely frightening ("a bad trip"). Some may have a sense of profound insight or spirituality with use.

PCP and related compounds typically cause "dissociative" symptoms: feelings of depersonalization, derealization, and analgesia. Users may manifest slurred speech and ataxia. Some users may quietly stare for extended periods, while others may become psychotic, paranoid, and even violent.

MDMA ("Ecstasy") and related phenylethylamines are said to bring on feelings of energy, euphoria, openness, and heightened sensation. Users may also experience restlessness, loss of appetite, and difficulty concentrating.

The belladonna alkaloids, in addition to their hallucinogenic effect, have significant anticholinergic effects that make them quite toxic. These include dilated pupils, blurred vision, nausea, tachycardia, ataxia, and delirium.

Overdose and Acute Toxicity

Overall, serious complications or death from hallucinogen use is a rare event, especially when compared with alcohol, opioids, or stimulants. Nevertheless, these substances can be quite dangerous. The perceptual and cognitive changes can result in impaired judgment and risky or violent behavior. The best treatment for most of these individuals is providing a calm and supportive environment; a benzodiazepine may be helpful for some.

Phencyclidine (PCP) overdose can lead to seizures, stupor, catatonia, and even coma; cardiac or respiratory arrest may occur (8).

The growing use of MDMA ("Ecstasy") has been accompanied by increasing reports of fatalities associated with its use; however, these numbers are still small in comparison with alcohol or other drugs (9). Large doses of MDMA (and other phenylethylamines) can produce amphetamine-like effects, including hypertension, hyperthermia, rhabdomyolysis, and cardiac arrhythmias; some users may develop liver or renal failure. The combination of MDMA with MAO inhibitors appears to be particularly dangerous (10). Some of the fatalities associated with MDMA use are due to hyponatremia complicated by cerebral edema. This is due to a combination of excessive fluid intake and inappropriate antidiuretic hormone (ADH) secretion (11). On the other hand, there have been reports of users surviving ingestion of a large number of pills (40–50), without long-term sequelae (12).

Withdrawal

Cessation of hallucinogen use is not associated with a physical withdrawal syndrome. Some regular users of MDMA report tolerance to the drug's effect and after cessation experience fatigue and low mood (13); these are similar to the symptoms that some stimulant users report with cessation.

DIAGNOSIS

Hallucinogen use should be suspected in individuals who present with acute psychosis, confusion, or obtundation, especially if they are an adolescent or young adult. The specific medical complications discussed in the next section may be a clue to use.

Phencyclidine can be detected in urine toxicology testing, and many commercially available assays test for its presence; ketamine and dextromethorphan may cause a false-positive test result. MDMA and LSD can also be detected in the urine but are not generally included in the commonly used commercial screens for drugs of abuse.

MEDICAL COMPLICATIONS

Most of the reports of complications of hallucinogen use are associated with Ecstasy. This is not surprising, given that this is by far the most commonly used of these substances. Most of these complications are probably due to the stimulant effect of this drug; however, given the varied content of pills sold, some of these complications may be due to substances other than MDMA. Furthermore, one must always keep in mind that case reports do not establish cause and effect, especially when the substance is commonly used.

Cardiovascular Complications

MDMA acutely increases heart rate, blood pressure, and myocardial oxygen consumption (14). There have been case reports of myocardial infarction associated with Ecstasy use, presumably due to these sympathomimetic effects (15).

Gastrointestinal Complications

There are reports of severe hepatotoxicity associated with Ecstasy use; in one series in Spain, of 62 patients admitted with acute liver failure, 5 (8%) were thought to be due to Ecstasy use (16). Severe liver damage has also been reported as a complication of phencyclidine-associated malignant hyperthermia (17).

Renal and Electrolyte Complications

There have been a number of reports of serious hyponatremia, some complicated by cerebral edema (18) and even death (19), associated with Ecstasy use. These have generally occurred in the setting of "rave" dance parties, and ironically advice given to these partygoers to ingest large quantities of fluids to avoid dehydration may be partly to blame; inappropriate secretion of antidiuretic hormone also appears to contribute to this (11). There is also one report of severe (and fatal) hyperkalemia associated with Ecstasy use in the absence of renal failure (20).

Neuromuscular Complications

Hyperthermia

Like other stimulants, Ecstasy use can be complicated by hyperthermia, which may in turn lead to rhabdomyolysis and renal failure (21). Phencyclidine (PCP) has also been associated with severe hyperthermia (17).

Stroke

Ecstasy use has been implicated in cerebral infarction (22) and hemorrhage; many of the hemorrhages occur in individuals with underlying vascular malformations (23). PCP use has likewise been associated with intracranial hemorrhage (24) and stroke; in one case series in Baltimore, 11 of 116 cases of stroke were associated with drug use and two of these were associated with PCP (25).

Movement Disorders

There have been a few reports of Parkinsonism among Ecstasy users, but given the numbers of individuals who have used Ecstasy, the association may be entirely coincidental (26). Furthermore, studies on nonhumans have failed to demonstrate dopaminergic neurotoxicity associated with MDMA (27).

Cognitive Impairment

There is some concern about the long-term effects of MDMA use on cognitive function. A number of studies suggest that Ecstasy users have poorer short- and long-term memory, as well as impaired attention and processing speed on tests of cognitive function (28). However, a number of possible confounding factors may contribute to the observed differences; one such factor is the use of other drugs. For example, one recent study found that Ecstasy users tended to perform poorer on tests of memory; however, this difference disappeared when cannabis (marijuana) and amphetamine use was taken into account (29). On the other hand, a study that recruited individuals with minimal exposure to other drugs reported a tendency toward poorer performance on tests of cognitive function (most were not statistically significant); a post hoc analysis of "heavy" users (60–450 lifetime doses) found significant impairment in a number of measures, when compared with nonusers or moderate users (30).

Another possible confounding factor is that Ecstasy users (or heavier users) may have lower baseline cognitive function;

that is, those with poorer cognitive function may be more likely to use Ecstasy, rather than Ecstasy use itself causing poorer cognitive function. A recent study of memory performance among MDMA users who stopped using compared with those who continued found that those who stopped had no improvement and those who continued had no deterioration in memory (31).

Psychiatric Complications

Hallucinogens have numerous acute psychiatric effects, which have already been discussed. For many years, there have been concerns that they may also have psychiatric effects that persist long after use has subsided. Unfortunately, there is little good data on the psychiatric complications of hallucinogens. A 1999 review of this topic that utilized the results of nine studies of mostly LSD users concluded that the "general impression to emerge from these studies is that such [neuropsychological] effects, if present, are modest" and that "the dire predictions...appear unjustified" (32).

As Ecstasy use has grown, so have concerns about its long-term psychiatric effects. There have been many reports of chronic psychiatric symptoms associated with Ecstasy use, including depression, anxiety, delusions, somatization, and even psychosis (33). MDMA acutely promotes the release of serotonin (5-HT) and it also appears to stimulate dopamine receptors; however, in the long term, MDMA causes depletion of serotonin and this may lead to chronic psychiatric complications. One study of 150 MDMA users presenting for addiction treatment reported that 53% had one or more psychiatric problems, including depression, psychotic disorders, panic disorders, and others (34). This was a select group of users (those requesting drug treatment) and most had used other substances as well. As with the studies on the effect of MDMA on cognitive function, it is difficult to establish causality with these types of retrospective descriptive analyses.

Some hallucinogen users may transiently reexperience perceptual disturbances that were associated with previous hallucinogen use ("flashbacks"). This uncommon phenomenon, technically known as "hallucinogen persisting perception disorder" (HPPD), is most associated with LSD use and may occur months to years after last use. Little is known about the etiology, risk factors, or effective treatment of this disorder (35).

TREATMENT

There is little data on treatment for hallucinogen use. Counseling users on the (realistic) health risks associated with these substances would be prudent, and research with other substances indicates that brief advice is effective. As with other substances, treatment outcomes will likely be influenced by an individual's desire to stop and other motivating factors. In one published study of outpatient treatment (group therapy) for 37 phencyclidine users, only 4 (11%) achieved a year of abstinence; 16 (48%) dropped out of treatment and 10 (30%) transferred to residential treatment or a recovery home (36).

For MDMA users, it is thought that regular use depletes serotonin; therefore serotonin reuptake inhibitors (SSRIs) may function as a kind of replacement therapy. Furthermore, in animal models, SSRIs have been found to attenuate the effect of MDMA (37). At this time, it is not known whether SSRIs are clinically useful for reducing MDMA use or toxicity.

REFERENCES

1. Cole, J. C., M. Bailey, H. R. Sumnall, et al. 2002. The content of ecstasy tablets: Implications for the study of their long-term effects. *Addiction* 97:1531–1536.
2. Stein, U., H. Greyer, and H. Hentschel. 2001. Nutmeg (myristicin) poisoning—report on a fatal case and a series of cases recorded by a poison information centre. *Forensic Sci. Int.* 118:87–90.
3. Meatherall, R., and P. Sharma. 2003. Foxy, a designer tryptamine hallucinogen. *J. Anal. Toxicol.* 27:313–317.
4. Vastag, B. 2005. Addiction research. Ibogaine therapy: A "vast, uncontrolled experiment." *Science* 308:345–346.
5. Halpern, J. H. 2004. Hallucinogens and dissociative agents naturally growing in the United States. *Pharmacol. Ther.* 102:131–138.
6. Baggot, M., B. Heifets, R. T. Jones, et al. 2000. Chemical analysis of ecstasy pills. *JAMA* 284:2190.
7. Substance Abuse and Mental Health Services Administration. 2004. Results from the 2003 National Survey on Drug Use and Health: National Findings (Office of Applied Studies, NSDUH Series H-25, DHHS Publication No. SMA 04-3964). Rockville, MD.
8. McCarron, M. M., B. W. Schulze, G. A. Thompson, et al. 1981. Acute phencyclidine intoxication: Incidence of clinical findings in 1,000 cases. *Ann. Emerg. Med.* 10:237–242.
9. McKenna, C. 2002. Ecstasy is in low league table of major causes of death. *BMJ* 325:296.
10. Vuori, E., J. A. Henry, I. Ojanperä, et al. 2002. Death following ingestion of MDMA (ecstasy) and moclobemide. *Addiction* 98:365–368.
11. Hartung, T. K., E. Schofield, A. I. Short, et al. 2002. Hyponatremic states following 3,4-methylenedioxymethamphetamine (MDMA, "ecstasy") ingestion. *Q. J. Med.* 95:431–437.
12. Regenthal, R., M. Krüger, K. Rudolph, et al. 1999. Survival after massive "ecstasy" (MDMA) ingestion. *Intensive Care Med.* 25:640–641.
13. Jansen, K. L. R. 1999. Ecstasy (MDMA) dependence. *Drug Alcohol Depend.* 53:121–124.
14. Lester, S. J., M. Baggott, S. Welm, et al. 2000. Cardiovascular effects of 3,4-methylenedioxymethamphetamine. A double-blind placebo-controlled trial. *Ann. Intern. Med.* 133:969–973.
15. Qasim, A., J. Townsend, and M. K. Davies. 2001. Ecstasy induced acute myocardial infarction. *Heart* 85:e10.
16. Andreu, V., A. Mas, M. Bruguera, et al. 1998. Ecstasy: A common cause of severe hepatotoxicity. *J. Hepatol.* 29:394–397.

17. Armen, R., G. Kanel, and T. Reynolds. 1984. Phencyclidine-induced malignant hyperthermia causing submassive liver necrosis. *Am. J. Med.* 77:167–172.

18. Traub, S. J., R. S. Hoffman, and L. S. Nelson. 2002. The "ecstasy" hangover: Hyponatremia due to 3,4-methylenedioxymethamphetamine. *J. Urban Health* 79:549–555.

19. Parr, M. J., H. M. Low, and P. Botterill. 1997. Hyponatremia and death after "ecstasy" ingestion. *Med. J. Aust.* 166:136–137.

20. Raviña, P., J. M. Quiroga, and T. Raviña. 2004. Hyperkalemia in fatal MDMA ("ecstasy") toxicity. *Int. J. Cardiol.* 93:307–308.

21. Dar, K. J., and M. E. McBrien. 1996. MDMA induced hyperthermia: Report of a fatality and review of current therapy. *Intensive Care Med.* 22:995–996.

22. Manchanda, S., and M. J. Connolly. 1993. Cerebral infarction in association with Ecstasy abuse. *Postgrad. Med. J.* 69:874–875.

23. McEvoy, A. W., N. D. Kitchen, and D. G. Thomas. 2000. Intracerebral haemorrhage and drug abuse in young adults. *Br. J. Neurosurg.* 14:449–454.

24. Bessen, H. A. 1982. Intracranial hemorrhage associated with phencyclidine abuse. *JAMA* 248:585–586.

25. Sloan, M. A., S. J. Kittner, D. Rigamonti, and T. R. Price. 1991. Occurrence of stroke associated with use/abuse of drugs. *Neurology* 41:1358–1364.

26. Kish, S. J. 2003. What is the evidence that ecstasy (MDMA) can cause Parkinson's disease? *Mov. Disorders* 18:1219–1223.

27. Ricaurte, G. A., J. Yuan, G. Hatzidimitriou, et al. 2003. Retraction: Severe dopaminergic neurotoxicity in primates after a common recreational dose of methylenedioxymethamphetamine (MDMA). *Science* 301:1479.

28. Verbaten, M. N. 2003. Specific memory deficits in ecstasy users? The results of a meta-analysis. *Hum. Psychopharmacol.* 10.201–290.

29. Simon, N. G., and R. P. Mattick. 2002. The impact of regular ecstasy use on memory function. *Addiction* 97:1523–1529.

30. Halpern, J. H., H. G. Pope, A. R. Sherwood, et al. 2004. Residual neuropsychological effects of illicit 3,4-methylenedioxymethamphetamine (MDMA) in individuals with minimal exposure to other drugs. *Drug Alcohol Depend.* 75:135–147.

31. Gouzoulis-Mayfrank, E., T. Fischermann, M. Rezk, et al. 2005. Memory performance in polyvalent MDMA (ecstasy) users who continue or discontinue use. *Drug Alcohol Depend.* 78:317–323.

32. Halpern, J. H., and H. G. Pope. 1999. Do hallucinogens cause residual neuropsychological toxicity? *Drug Alcohol Depend.* 53:247–256.

33. Montoya, A. G., R. Sorrentino, S. E. Lukas, and B. H. Price. 2002. Long-term neuropsychiatric consequences of "ecstasy" (MDMA): A review. *Harvard Rev. Psychiatry* 10:212–220.

34. Schifano, F., L. DiFuria, G. Forza, et al. 1998. MDMA ("ecstasy") consumption in the context of polydrug abuse: A report on 150 patients. *Drug Alcohol Depend.* 52:85–90.

35. Halpern, J. H., and H. G. Opoe. 2003. Hallucinogen persisting perception disorder: What do we know after 50 years? *Drug Alcohol Depend.* 69:109–119.

36. Gorelick, D. A., J. N. Wilkins, and C. Wong. 1989. Outpatient treatment of PCP abusers. *Am. J. Drug Alcohol Abuse* 15:367–374.
37. Lingford-Hughes, A., and D. Nutt. 2003. Neurobiology of addiction and implications for treatment. *Br. J. Psychiatry* 182:97–100.

11

Marijuana

BACKGROUND

Marijuana comes from plants in the genus *Cannabis* that are found worldwide. Humans have used the leaves for thousands of years. The leaves are typically smoked but can be ingested. A concentrated preparation of the resin, known as hashish, can also be used. The psychoactive ingredient of marijuana and hashish is tetrahydrocannabinol (THC). THC is part of a broad class of agents known as terpenoids. A number of other terpenoids are found in plants and are used for their psychoactive effects. These plants include wormwood (used in absinthe), salvia, calamus, coleus, and hops; they are covered further in the chapter on hallucinogens.

EPIDEMIOLOGY

According to the *2003 National Survey on Drug Use and Health,* marijuana is the most commonly used illicit drug in the United States; 75% of "illicit drug users" use marijuana and 55% use only marijuana (1). An estimated 3.1 million Americans use marijuana on a daily or almost daily basis; 2.6 million (1.1% of the population aged 12 or older) were judged to be dependent. Among those aged 18 or older, 40.6% have used marijuana at some time, 10.6% in the past year, and 6.2% in the past month. Almost 20% of youth aged 12 to 17 have used marijuana at some time; this rises to 54% among those aged 18 to 25.

This survey also found some variation in recent (past month) marijuana use among different demographic groups. Of those aged 12–17, 7.9% reported recent use; this rises to 17.0% of those aged 18–25 and declines to 4.0% among those aged 26 or older. Among those aged 18 or older, recent marijuana use is twice as high among males (8.0%) than females (4.0%) and higher among unemployed individuals (13.8%) when compared with full-time employed (6.3%).

DRUG EFFECTS

Acute Effects

THC appears to exert its effects through the stimulation of endogenous cannabinoid receptors. These receptors are thought to have analgesic effect and to inhibit nociceptive responses in the central nervous system. Users may feel a sense of relaxation and euphoria, while others may experience anxiety, nausea, and dizziness. Marijuana or hashish may also produce hallucinogenic effects such as depersonalization, visual distortions, and perceptual changes. Users typically report an increased sense of hunger; a prescription form of THC (dronabinol) is used as an appetite stimulant and antiemetic.

Overdose and Acute Toxicity

Serious toxicity with marijuana use is rare, even with consumption of large amounts. Nevertheless, users can experience significant side effects including drowsiness, ataxia, nausea, and vomiting, as well as cardiovascular complications including tachycardia and other arrhythmias, hypotension, and even syncope. There is also a report of coma in two young children who had eaten cookies containing marijuana (2).

Withdrawal

Abstinence from regular marijuana use does not cause an observable physical withdrawal syndrome, as is seen with alcohol and opioids. Nevertheless, regular users often experience unpleasant symptoms with abstinence, including drug craving, insomnia, anorexia, irritability, and restlessness (3).

DIAGNOSIS

A metabolite of THC can be detected in urine for 1–7 days after use; for heavy users, it may be detected up to a month after last use. A number of other drugs may cause false-positive results including dronabinol, efavirenz, ibuprofen, and naproxen (4). Hemp seed oil, which is found in some foods, may cause a false-positive screen, but this is unlikely at the levels usually consumed (5).

MEDICAL COMPLICATIONS

Head and Neck Complications

Marijuana smoke may, like tobacco, contain a number of carcinogens. A case-control study published in 1999 reported that marijuana use was associated with an increased risk of head and neck cancers (6).

Pulmonary Complications

Studies suggest that smoking marijuana is associated with an increased frequency of respiratory symptoms such as wheezing, cough, and sputum production, similar to that seen in tobacco smokers (7, 8). However, it does not appear that marijuana smoking leads to an irreversible decline in lung function in the way that tobacco smoking does (9).

Cardiovascular Complications

Marijuana use acutely stimulates sympathetic activity with increased heart rate and blood pressure; at higher doses, parasympathetic effects may predominate resulting in bradycardia and orthostatic hypotension (10). Chronic users develop tolerance to these effects. These effects do not generally lead to serious complications for young, healthy users, but there are reports of acute, sometimes fatal, cardiovascular events in association with marijuana use (11) and it may be a (rare) trigger for myocardial infarction for individuals with other risk factors (12.)

Gastrointestinal Complications

Marijuana, specifically THC, has a number of effects on the gastrointestinal system that are mediated by cannabinoid receptors in the gut and have generated interest in its therapeutic use (13). Cannabinoids have been shown to be effective antiemetics (14). They also reduce gastrointestinal motility and may be beneficial for irritable bowel syndrome, Crohn's disease, and secretory diarrhea.

Neuromuscular Complications

Heavy marijuana use (generally defined as daily use or more) impairs neurocognitive function (15), and these effects may persist for a day or longer after last use (16). Whether marijuana leads to residual or irreversible cognitive deficits is controversial. Some studies have found cognitive deficits among heavy users after 28 days of abstinence (17), particularly among those with early onset of use (before age 17) (18). However, it is possible that this may be due to innate differences in heavy users—that is, that those with poorer cognitive function are more likely to become heavy users (19). A 2003 meta-analysis of studies on the residual neurocognitive effects of marijuana "failed to reveal a substantial, systematic effect of long-term, regular cannabis consumption on the neurocognitive functioning of users who were not acutely intoxicated." However, this review did concede that there might be a "very small" negative effect on learning and memory (20).

Psychiatric Complications

A number of studies have found an association between marijuana use and psychiatric illness, including depression (21), anxiety (22), and psychosis (23,24). There are a few possible explanations for these observations: (1) those at higher risk for psychiatric illness are more likely to use marijuana (use is a consequence, not a cause), (2) marijuana exacerbates or unmasks mental illness among those with preexisting illness or a predisposition, or (3) marijuana use causes mental illness. Some believe that the evidence supports a causal relationship (25). However, a recent review of this issue concluded that the "[a]vailable evidence does not strongly support an important causal relation between cannabis use by young people and psychosocial harm, but cannot exclude the possibility that such a relation exists" (26).

Other Drug Use

There is a great deal of debate about whether marijuana use leads to the use of other "hard" drugs; this is a prominent argument against the legalization (or decriminalization) of marijuana. An association between marijuana use and subsequent use of "hard drugs" has been demonstrated (27). The argument for a cause-and-effect relationship is strengthened by the association of "hard" drug use with marijuana use among twins who are discordant for marijuana use (i.e., one uses, the other does not); this suggests that shared environmental and genetic factors do not account for the connection (28). However, it is difficult (if not impossible) to establish a causal relationship with these types of observational studies. Furthermore, a recent analysis concluded that the so-called gateway effect could be entirely explained by a "common-factor model," a model in which individuals have a random propensity to use drugs (both marijuana and "hard" drugs) and one does not necessarily lead to the other (29).

TREATMENT

Overall, there has been comparatively little research done on the treatment of persons who abuse or are dependent on marijuana. This may be partly due to a perception that marijuana use is not as much of a problem as other substances. Almost all of the available research is on psychosocial approaches.

Self-Help Groups

As with other substances, there are self-help groups for individuals who want help with marijuana use. These groups are typically modeled on Alcoholics Anonymous and use the 12-step approach. "Marijuana Anonymous" (www.marijuana-anonymous.org) is one such group and holds meetings in many states, as well as Australia and some European countries, and online. We were unable to find any data on its effectiveness.

Psychosocial Treatment

There have been a number of studies on psychosocial treatments for individuals who want treatment for their marijuana use. These studies have generally reported short-term reduction in use with a variety of strategies that have been utilized previously for alcoholism and other substance use problems. These approaches include motivational enhancement, cognitive-behavioral therapy, and contingency management (voucher-based incentives). However, these studies were performed on volunteers who wanted treatment and excluded individuals who had alcohol or other drug problems. Furthermore, most of these studies are limited by the use of a "best-case scenario"; those who did not complete follow-up were not counted as treatment failures.

A randomized controlled trial of treatment for marijuana users "who wanted help quitting" (this study excluded those with signs of marijuana dependence) compared cognitive-behavioral sessions with a therapist-led social support group. Individuals in both groups who completed the follow-up (79% of original cohort) reported significantly reduced marijuana use over 12 months; however, the treatment effect seemed to dissipate over time and neither treatment modality was superior to the other (30). A subsequent trial reported that a brief two-session individual motivational enhancement intervention performed as well as a 14-session group cognitive-behavioral treatment; abstinence rates with either treatment were better than with no treatment (31). Another trial comparing a brief (one-session) cognitive-behavioral intervention with a six-session treatment reported improved outcomes among those who completed follow-up (74% of the original cohort); outcomes with the six-session treatment were marginally better than outcomes with the one-session treatment by some measures (32). Similarly, a study found that five sessions of motivational enhancement and cognitive-behavioral therapy performed as well as 12 sessions; the addition of family education and therapy did not improve outcomes further (33).

In contrast to earlier studies that indicated that brief interventions were as effective as longer treatment, a recent study suggests that a longer and more intensive course of treatment may be more effective. This multicenter randomized controlled trial compared two sessions of motivational enhancement with a nine-session treatment that included motivational enhancement, cognitive-behavioral therapy, and case management. Among those who completed follow-up (only 59% of the original cohort), the nine-session intervention performed better (at least in the short term) (34).

The addition of abstinence-contingent rewards (sometimes referred to as "contingency management") also appears to improve abstinence rates. A small randomized controlled trial reported higher short-term abstinence rates among individuals given vouchers for cannabinoid-negative urines, when compared with others who received motivational enhancement or cognitive-behavioral treatment (35). It is not clear whether this approach has any lasting effect beyond the period when these rewards are provided; research on this approach with other substances suggests that the effects diminish with time.

There is very little data on pharmacotherapy for marijuana dependence. One small study of divalproex sodium failed to show a benefit after 12 weeks of treatment (36). A cannabinoid receptor antagonist has been recently developed and shown to block the effects of smoked marijuana (37). However, the use of cannabinoid antagonists in the treatment of marijuana abuse or dependence has not been established, and the experience with drug antagonists in the treatment of other substance use disorders has not been very promising to date.

REFERENCES

1. Substance Abuse and Mental Health Services Administration. 2004. Results from the 2003 National Survey on Drug Use and Health: National Findings (Office of Applied Studies, NSDUH Series H-25, DHHS Publication No. SMA 04-3964). Rockville, MD.
2. Boros, C. A., D. W. Parsons, G. D. Zoanetti, et al. 1996. Cannabis cookies: A cause of coma. *J. Paediatr. Child Health* 32:194–195.
3. Budney, A. J., J. R. Hughes, B. A. Moore, and P. L. Novy. 2001. Marijuana abstinence effects in marijuana smokers maintained in their home environment. *Arch. Gen. Psychiatry* 58:917–924.
4. Tests for drugs of abuse. 2002. *The Medical Letter*. 44:71–73.
5. Leson, G., P. Pless, F. Grotenhermen, et al. 2001. Evaluating the impact of hemp food consumption on workplace drug tests. *J. Anal. Toxicol.* 25:691–698.
6. Zheng, Z. F., H. Morgenstern, M. R. Spitz, et al. 1999. Marijuana use and increased risk of squamous cell carcinoma of the head and neck. *Cancer Epidemiol. Biomarkers Prev.* 8:1071–1078.
7. Tashkin, D. P., A. H. Coulson, V. A. Clark, et al. 1987. Respiratory symptoms and lung function in habitual heavy smokers of marijuana alone, smokers of marijuana and tobacco, smokers of tobacco alone, and nonsmokers. *Am. Rev. Respir. Dis.* 135:209–216.
8. Taylor, D. R., R. Poulton, T. E. Moffitt, et al. 2000. The respiratory effects of cannabis dependence in young adults. *Addiction* 95:1669–1677.
9. Tashkin, D. P., M. S. Simmons, D. L. Sherrill, and A. H. Coulson. 1997. Heavy habitual marijuana smoking does not cause accelerated decline in FEV1 with age. *Am. J. Respir. Crit. Care Med.* 155:141–148.
10. Jones, R. T. 2002. Cardiovascular system effects of marijuana. *J. Clin. Pharmacol.* 42:58S–63S.
11. Bachs, L., and H. Mørland. 2001. Acute cardiovascular fatalities following cannabis use. *Forensic Sci. Int.* 124:200–203.
12. Mittleman, M. A., R. A. Lewis, M. Maclure, et al. 2001. Triggering myocardial infarction by marijuana. *Circulation* 103:2805–2809.
13. DiCarlo, G., and A. A. Izzo. 2003. Cannabinoids for gastrointestinal diseases: Potential therapeutic applications. *Expert Opin. Investig. Drugs* 12:39–49.
14. Tramèr, M. R., D. Carroll, F. A. Campbell, et al. 2001. Cannabinoids for control of chemotherapy induced nausea and vomiting: Quantitative systematic review. *BMJ* 323:1–8.
15. Block, R. I., and M. M. Ghoneim. 1993. Effects of chronic marijuana use on human cognition. *Psychopharmacology* 110:219–228.
16. Pope, H. G., Jr., and D. Yurgelun-Todd. 1996. The residual cognitive effects of heavy marijuana use in college students. *JAMA* 275:521–527.
17. Bolla, K. I., K. Brown, B. A. Eldreth, et al. 2002. Dose-related neurocognitive effects of marijuana use. *Neurology* 59:1337–1343.
18. Pope, H. G., A. J. Gruber, J. I. Hudson, et al. 2003. Early-onset cannabis use and cognitive deficits: What is the nature of the association? *Drug Alcohol Depend.* 69:303–310.

19. Pope, H. G., Jr. 2002. Cannabis, cognition, and residual confounding. *JAMA* 287:1172–1174.
20. Grant, I., R. Gonzalez, C. L. Carey, et al. 2003. Non-acute (residual) neurocognitive effects on cannabis use: A meta-analytic study. *J. Int. Neuropsychol. Soc.* 9:679–689.
21. Bovasso, G. B. 2001. Cannabis abuse as a risk factor for depressive symptoms. *Am. J. Psychiatry* 158:2033–2037.
22. Patton, G. C., C. Coffey, J. B. Carlin, et al. 2002. Cannabis use and mental health in young people: Cohort study. *BMJ* 325:1195–1198.
23. Zammit, S., P. Allebeck, S. Andreasson, et al. 2002. Self-reported cannabis use as a risk factor for schizophrenia in Swedish conscripts of 1969: Historical cohort study. *BMJ* 325:1199–1203.
24. Arseneault, L., M. Cannon, R. Poulton, et al. 2002. Cannabis use in adolescence and risk for adult psychosis: Longitudinal prospective study. *BMJ* 325:1212–1213.
25. Rey, J. M., and C. C. Tennant. 2002. Cannabis and mental health. *BMJ* 325:1183–1184.
26. Macleod, J., R. Oakes, A. Copello, et al. 2004. Psychological and social sequelae of cannabis and other illicit drug use by young people: A systematic review of longitudinal, general population studies. *Lancet* 363:1579–1588.
27. Degenhardt, L., W. Hall, and M. Lynskey. 2001. The relationship between cannabis use and other substance use in the general population. *Drug Alcohol Depend.* 64:319–327.
28. Lynskey, M. T., A. C. Heath, K. K. Bucholz, et al. 2003. Escalation of drug use in early-onset cannabis users vs. co-twin controls. *JAMA* 289:427–433.
29. Morral, A. R., D. F. McCaffrey, and S. M. Paddock. 2002. Reassessing the marijuana gateway effect. *Addiction* 97:1493–1504.
30. Stephens, R. S., R. A. Roffman, and E. E. Simpson. 1994. Treating adult marijuana dependence: A test of the relapse prevention model. *J. Consult. Clin. Psychol.* 62:92–99. *Two hundred and twelve adults who wanted help quitting marijuana were randomized to (1) a cognitive behavioral group or (2) a therapist led support group. Both were 10 sessions over 12 weeks followed by booster sessions 3 and 6 months later. There were no significant differences in attendance, completion, or abstinence rates. Of the 167 (79%) who completed all the assessments, 63% reported abstinence during the last 2 weeks of treatment; this fell to 49% at 3-month follow-up and 20% at 12 months.*
31. Stephens, R. S., R. A. Roffman, and L. Curtin. 2000. Comparison of extended versus brief treatments for marijuana use. *J. Consult. Clin. Psychol.* 68:898–908. *Two hundred ninety-one treatment-seeking marijuana users were randomized to (1) 14 cognitive-behavioral group treatments over 18 weeks, (2) two 90-minute individual motivational interviewing sessions 1 month apart, or (3) delayed treatment (control). Of the 85% who completed 4-month follow-up, there was no difference between the active treatments, but both had higher abstinence rates than the control arm. There was no comparison between active and delayed treatment after 4 months, when the delayed arm could enter treatment. At 7-, 13-, and 16-month follow-up, the abstinence rates in the active treatment arms were about 34%, 27%, and 28%, respectively.*

32. Copeland, J., W. Swift, R. Roffman, and R. Stephens. 2001. A randomized controlled trial of brief cognitive-behavioral interventions for cannabis use disorder. *J. Subst. Abuse Treat.* 21:55–64. *Two hundred and twenty-nine treatment-seeking marijuana users were randomized to (1) six weekly individual sessions incorporating motivational interview with cognitive-behavioral therapy, (2) one 90-minute version of the same with a self-help booklet, or (3) 24-week delayed treatment (control). Of the 74% with complete follow-up, those in active treatment were more likely to report continuous abstinence, but there was no difference between the two active treatments. Those in active treatment also had lower "dependence severity scores," and these were significantly lower with six-session treatment compared to one-session.*

33. Dennis, M., S. H. Godley, G. Diamond, et al. 2004. The Cannabis Youth Treatment (CYT) Study: Main findings from two randomized trials. *J. Subst. Abuse Treat.* 27:197–213. *Six hundred adolescent marijuana users were assigned to one of five treatments at four sites: (1) five sessions of motivational enhancement/cognitive behavioral therapy, (2) 12 sessions of same, (3) #2 plus family education and therapy, (4) community reinforcement, (5) multidimensional family therapy. Self-reported marijuana use declined significantly in all groups in the 12 months after assignment (~24% reported no past-month drug use); no group was significantly better than any other and there was no control group.*

34. Marijuana treatment research group. 2004. Brief treatments for cannabis dependence: Findings from a randomized multisite trial. *J. Consult. Clin. Psychol.* 72:455–466. *Four hundred and fifty marijuana-dependent adults were randomized to (1) two sessions of motivational enhancement, 5 weeks apart, (2) nine sessions over 3 months including motivational enhancement, case management, and cognitive-behavioral therapy, or (3) delayed treatment (control). The outcomes included only those who completed 4 months (59%) and 9 months (55%) of follow-up, respectively. At 4-month follow-up, subjects in both active arms did better than the control arm; the nine-session group had higher 90-day abstinence rates compared to the two-session group (22.6% vs. 8.6%), but this difference was no longer significant at 9 months (15.6% vs. 9.5%).*

35. Budney, A. J., S. T. Higgins, K. J. Radonovich, and P. L. Novy. 2000. Adding voucher-based incentives to coping skills and motivational enhancement improves outcomes during treatment for marijuana dependence. *J. Consult. Clin. Psychol.* 68:1051–1061. *Sixty marijuana-dependent adults were randomized to (1) four individual motivational enhancement sessions, (2) 14 weekly individual cognitive-behavioral sessions, or (3) cognitive-behavioral sessions (same as #2) plus financial vouchers for cannabinoid-negative urine tox screens. After 14 weeks, subjects in the third arm had higher rates of abstinence; 40% achieved at least 7 weeks of abstinence compared with 5% in the first two arms.*

36. Levin, F. R., D. McDowell, S. M. Evans, et al. 2004. Pharmacotherapy for marijuana dependence: A double-blind placebo-controlled pilot study of divalproex sodium. *Am. J. Addict.* 13:21–32. *Twenty-five marijuana-dependent adults were randomized to divalproex sodium or placebo for 6 weeks, then crossed over for another 6 weeks; all re-*

ceived weekly relapse prevention therapy. About half completed treatment; there was no difference between the arms in retention or marijuana use.

37. Huestis, M. A., D. A. Gorelick, S. J. Heishman, et al. 2001. Blockade of effects of smoked marijuana by the CB1-selective cannabinoid receptor antagonist SR141716. *Arch. Gen. Psychiatry* 58:322–328.

12

Inhalants: Volatile Organic Compounds, Nitrites, and Anesthetics

BACKGROUND

Inhalants are a pharmacologically heterogeneous group of substances that have been traditionally grouped together because of their predominant route of use. There is no technical definition for this group of agents, which are sometimes referred to as "volatile substances," but it generally includes three classes of chemicals: volatile organic compounds, volatile anesthetics, and nitrites. Table 12.1 lists some of these chemicals and their sources.

The volatile organic compounds are a diverse group of chemicals that can be found in fuels (gasoline, butane, and propane), solvents (nail polish remover, paint thinner, correction fluid), cleaning agents, adhesives, aerosols (spray paint, hair spray), and refrigerants. Table 12.2 lists some of the organic compounds that are found in each of these substances. These organic compounds can be roughly divided into aromatic hydrocarbons, alkanes, chlorinated hydrocarbons, ketones, and fluorocarbons.

Abused volatile anesthetics include nitrous oxide (also known as "laughing gas"), which is also used as a propellant in whipped cream. Other volatile anesthetics can be abused, including ether, halothane, and enflurane.

The nitrites include amyl, butyl, cyclohexyl, and isobutyl nitrite. These chemicals are volatile liquids with a yellowish color and "fruity" odor. Amyl nitrite was originally developed as a treatment for angina and was produced in glass capsules that were popped open to release the liquid and thus referred to as "poppers." Amyl, butyl, and isobutyl nitrite are sold (legally) in small bottles that are sometimes referred to as "poppers" as well. These agents can be purchased on the Internet or at stores (typically adult bookstores or "head shops") and are sometimes labeled as "room deodorizers" or "video head cleaners." Cyclohexyl nitrite is found in room deodorizers. Nitrites are often used in bars and nightclubs and for this reason are referred to as a "club drug" along with Ecstasy, ketamine, gamma-hydroxybutyric acid (GHB), and others.

EPIDEMIOLOGY

According to the *2003 National Survey on Drug Use and Health* (NSDUH), almost 23 million Americans have used inhalants at some time in their lives (9.7% of the population age 12 or older); 2.1 million had used in the past year (0.9%) and 570,000 had used in the past month (0.2%) (1). An estimated 169,000 Americans abused or were dependent on inhalants. Among the inhalants, lifetime use of nitrous oxide was the highest (11.6 million Americans), followed by amyl nitrite (9.0 million), glue, shoe polish or toluene (4.3 million), and gasoline or lighter fluid (3.9 million).

Recent (past month) use was highest among individuals aged 12–17 (1.3%) and declined to 0.4% among those aged 18–25 and to 0.1% among those aged 26 or older. An analysis of data from the 2000 and 2001 NHDSA (now called the NSDUH) found that adolescent inhalant abuse or dependence was associated with participation in mental health treatment, delinquency, history of incarceration, history of foster care placement, and use of alcohol and other drugs, but not with gender, race/ethnicity, or family income (2). Although inhalant use declines with age, it appears that many adolescent inhalant users switch to other substances as they grow older (3, 4). Moreover, the risk of drug use and binge or frequent drinking among college students has been found to be strongly associated with early inhalant use, more so than early marijuana use (5).

Table 12.1.   Chemical agents found in abused inhalants

Substance	Source	Other Names
Volatile Organic Compounds*		
Aromatic Hydrocarbons		
Toluene	Airplane glue, rubber cement,	
Benzene	nail polish & nail polish remover;	
Xylene	paint thinner, gasoline	
Naphthalene	Mothballs	
Alkanes		
Butane	Fuel for lighters, portable stoves, barbecues,	
Propane	& recreational vehicles	
Isopropane	Spray paint, hair spray, deodorants,	
Hexane	room fresheners, gasoline	
Chlorinated hydrocarbons		
Monochloroethane	Dry cleaning agents, video head cleaner,	Ethyl chloride
Trichloroethane	spot removers, degreasers, correction	Methyl chloroform
Trichloroethene	fluid, gasoline	Trichloroethylene
Tetrachloroethylene		Perchloroethylene (PCE)
Dichloromethane		Methylene chloride

Table 12.1. *Continued*

Substance	Source	Other Names
Ketones		
Acetone	Nail polish remover, rubber cement, varnish, lacquers, paint remover	
Methyl ethyl ketone		2-butanone
Methyl butyl ketone		2-hexanone
Fluorocarbons		
	Asthma inhalers, air fresheners, hair spray, spray paint, fire extinguishers, refrigerants	Chlorofluorocarbons CFCs, Freon
Anesthetics		
Nitrous oxide	Whipping cream canisters	Whippets
Ether		
Halothane		
Enflurane		
Nitrites		
Amyl nitrite		Poppers, snappers
Butyl nitrite		Poppers, rush, bolt, video head cleaner
Isobutyl nitrite		Poppers
Cyclohexyl nitrite	Room deodorizers	

Organic compounds are found in multiple sources; many of the sources listed may contain more than one of the compounds listed.

Table 12.2.   Organic compounds found in abused inhalants*

Source	Compounds
Fuels	
Gasoline	Aromatic hydrocarbons (benzene, xylene), alkanes (butane, hexane, octane, paraffins), alkenes, chlorinated hydrocarbons
Bottled fuel gas	Butane, isobutane, propane, isopropane
Lighter fluid	Butane, isopropane
Solvents	
Paint thinner	Toluene, xylene, methylene chloride, methanol
Nail polish remover	Acetone, toluene
Correction fluid	Trichloroethane, trichloroethylene
Cleaning agents	
Dry cleaning	Tetrachloroethylene, trichloroethylene
Spot removers	Tetrachloroethylene, trichloroethylene
Degreasers	Dichloromethane, trichloroethylene
Paint remover	Dichloromethane, toluene
Adhesives	
Airplane glue	Toluene, hexane, acetone
Rubber cement	Toluene, hexane, acetone, methyl ethyl ketone
Aerosols	
Spray paint	Methylene chloride, toluene, butane, propane, fluorocarbons
Hair spray	Butane, propane, fluorocarbons
Deodorants	Butane, propane, fluorocarbons
Room fresheners	Butane, propane, fluorocarbons
Others	
Varnish	Xylene, methyl ethyl ketone
Lacquers	Toluene, methyl ethyl ketone
Fingernail polish	Toluene
Mothballs	Naphthalene, paradichlorobenzene (para-DCB)

*Note: Ingredients vary by manufacturer and brand.

The epidemiology of nitrite use appears to be different from that of other inhalants. Some studies have found comparatively high rates of nitrite use among cohorts of homosexual men (6) and an association between nitrite use and high-risk sexual behavior (7).

The drug effects and complications of each of the three classes of inhalants will be covered separately. There will be a brief discussion of treatment issues at the end of the chapter.

VOLATILE ORGANIC COMPOUNDS: FUELS, SOLVENTS, ADHESIVES, CLEANING AGENTS, AND AEROSOLS

Drug Effects

Acute Effects

The exact mechanism of the neuropsychological effects of abused organic compounds is not well understood. These substances are typically "sniffed" from their original containers or "huffed" from a cloth that is soaked in the chemical; some users may place the substance in a plastic bag and inhale the fumes ("bagging"). The acute effects of these substances are often likened to those of alcohol. Users typically experience a sense of euphoria followed by CNS depression. They may also have visual or auditory hallucinations. Users may become hyperactive or agitated and do impulsive, even dangerous acts that lead to injuries. They may also exhibit slurred speech, psychomotor retardation, ataxia, and disorientation.

Overdose and Acute Toxicity

While deaths due to inhalant abuse are relatively uncommon, it is clear that fatalities do occur. A 1970 article reported on a series of 110 sudden deaths in the 1960s among adolescents and young adults after inhaling organic compounds (toluene, benzene, gasoline, trichloroethane, and fluorocarbons); this phenomenon was dubbed "sudden sniffing death" and was postulated to be due to cardiac arrhythmia (8). A later series in Virginia reported 39 deaths associated with inhalant abuse from 1987 to 1996; the majority of these were male (95%) and age 22 or younger (70%). Thirty-six (92%) of these fatalities were from abuse of organic compounds: butane, 13 fatalities; propane, 5; fluorocarbons, 10; trichloroethane, 4; dichloromethane, 1; toluene, 2; gasoline, 1 (9). Another series from Texas reported 144 deaths related to inhalant abuse from 1988 to 1998; the mean age was 25.6, most were males (92%), and many were in occupations that employed these compounds. As in Virginia, most of these fatalities were associated with abuse of organic compounds: fluorocarbons (35%), chlorinated hydrocarbons (25%), toluene (17%), alkanes (3%), and gasoline (2%) (10).

The exact mechanism of death in these fatalities is often unclear; autopsies, when performed, generally show no anatomical abnormalities that can explain the deaths. Many of these deaths appear to be due to fatal arrhythmias; others may be due to respiratory arrest (11) or aspiration (12). Some cases are due to inadvertent asphyxiation, such as when a user places a plastic bag with the substance over his or her head and then loses consciousness.

Treatment of the intoxicated individual is generally supportive; there are no specific antidotes to these chemicals. Gastric lavage may be helpful in cases of ingestion.

Withdrawal

It appears that regular users of organic compounds develop tolerance to their effects over time. Some may experience unpleasant symptoms with abstinence, including insomnia, irritability, nausea, sweating, and tremulousness (13).

Diagnosis

Organic compound abuse should be considered in anyone who presents with signs of intoxication, particularly among adolescents or individuals who work with these substances. Regular users may have a characteristic perioral rash. Other clues may include paint or solvent stains on clothing, "chemical" odor on breath, and stained fingernails.

Solvents can be detected by gas chromatography in the serum, but this test is not widely available for clinical use. Organic compounds are not detected in routine urine drug tests but some of their metabolites can be detected in the urine, including phenol (metabolite of benzene), hippuric acid (toluene), methylhippuric acid (xylene), and trichloroacetic acid (trichloroethylene) (14).

Medical Complications

Cutaneous Complications

As mentioned earlier, an inhalant abuser may have perioral dermatitis from exposure to these substances. This is typically described as red spots or sores around the mouth and nose. Volatile inhalant abusers are also at risk for burns from accidental fires (15) and hypothermic injuries from aerosols or propellants (16).

Pulmonary Complications

Exposure to volatile organic compounds has been associated with (modestly) diminished lung function among asthmatics (17). Furthermore, a number of studies on occupational exposure to solvents suggest that they are associated with respiratory complaints including wheezing (18) and asthma-related symptoms (19). There is also a report of acute eosinophilic pneumonia after intentional inhalation of trichloroethane (in the commercial product "Scotchguard") (20).

Cardiovascular Complications

Inhalation of organic compounds may lead to ventricular arrhythmias and sudden death. In some of these cases, death occurred in the setting of inhalant use followed by physical exertion, suggesting that endogenous catecholamines may play a role. Ventricular fibrillation has been observed after abuse of lighter fluid (butane) (21), abuse of air freshener (butane and isobutane) (22), and glue sniffing (23). There is also a report of ventricular tachycardia in a child after accidental exposure to non-fluorocarbon propellants (isobutane, butane, and propane) in a deodorant (24). In addition, there is a report of a dilated cardiomyopathy in an adolescent glue-sniffer (25).

Gastrointestinal Complications

One case series of adults hospitalized with "problems related to paint sniffing" reported that six of the 25 individuals presented with gastrointestinal complaints, including abdominal pain, nausea, and vomiting (26). There are also reports of hepatotoxicity associated with occupational exposure to chlorinated hydrocarbons (27) and hydrochlorofluorocarbons (28).

Renal and Electrolyte Complications

Toluene exposure (typically among paint- or glue-sniffers) has been associated with Fanconi's syndrome and distal renal tubular acidosis, resulting in hypokalemia, hypocalcemia, hypophosphatemia, and hyperchloremic metabolic acidosis (29, 30). These individuals can present with profound generalized weakness.

There are also reports of acute renal failure associated with toluene abuse (31–33); however, one study of workers found no evidence of renal toxicity at a moderate level of exposure to toluene (34).

Hematologic Complications

Occupational exposure to benzene (especially at high levels) has been associated with aplastic anemia (35), and there is a case report of aplastic anemia associated with glue sniffing (36). Benzene exposure has also been linked with a number of hematologic malignancies including leukemia, lymphoma, and myelodysplastic syndrome (37).

Neuromuscular Complications

The most serious long-term complications of exposure to organic compounds are the neurologic sequelae. Acutely, users may exhibit a variety of neurological and cognitive deficits, including ataxia, tremor, chorea, myoclonus, nystagmus, delirium, and encephalopathy (38, 39). Many of these problems resolve with elimination of the substance from the body; however, some regular users may develop irreversible residual deficits. These include cognitive deficits (apathy, attention and memory impairment), peripheral neuropathy (40), and cerebellar ataxia. Among gasoline-sniffers, some of these complications may be due to the toxicity of lead in the gasoline (41). However, users of other organic compounds (especially toluene) can have acute and chronic deficits; for example, a 1966 report described a 33-year-old man who inhaled toluene daily for 14 years and had ataxia, tremulousness, and emotional lability (42). A case series in 1981 described 19 children aged 8–14 who were hospitalized with encephalopathy; presentations included coma, ataxia, convulsions, behavior disturbance, and diplopia—one developed persistent cerebellar ataxia (43). Some of these chronic neurological deficits appear to correlate with white matter changes on MRI (**44**).

VOLATILE ANESTHETICS: NITROUS OXIDE AND OTHERS

Drug Effects

Acute Effects

The acute effects of volatile anesthetics include euphoria, dizziness, drowsiness, ataxia, and blurred vision. Some users may experience visual illusions or hallucinations. Higher levels of exposure lead to loss of consciousness and respiratory depression.

Overdose and Acute Toxicity

The main hazard of volatile anesthetic abuse is hypoxia and asphyxiation due to inhalation of high concentrations of the anesthetic. There have been a number of reports of fatalities due to abuse of these substances (45), some among workers who handle nitrous oxide (such as "food-serving establishments") (46) or other volatile anesthetics (hospital employees) (47). While use of nitrous oxide alone does not generally produce deep anesthesia, abuse of other volatile anesthetics can lead to profound respiratory depression and death; the therapeutic window between anesthesia and death is fairly narrow. Nevertheless, the reports of deaths associated with volatile anesthetic abuse tend to be smaller in number than those associated with volatile organic compounds (9, 10).

Withdrawal

It appears that regular users of volatile anesthetics develop tolerance to their effects. There does not appear to be a well-defined withdrawal syndrome, but some users do experience drug craving.

Diagnosis

Abuse of volatile anesthetics should be considered in individuals who present with an acute change in level of consciousness, especially those with occupational access to these agents (food preparation and health care workers). There are no specific physical findings or laboratory tests for detection of illicit use.

Medical Complications

Pulmonary Complications

Volatile anesthetics do not appear to have any pulmonary toxicity, but abuse may result in hypoxia due to inhalation of the anesthetic with insufficient quantities of oxygen.

Cardiovascular Complications

Nitrous oxide and other anesthetics can depress myocardial function (48), and there has been a case report of cardiovascular collapse associated with its therapeutic use (49). There have also been reports of acute myocardial infarction associated with general anesthesia (enflurane and isoflurane) (50). It is possible that illicit users have also had these complications and that some of the fatalities associated with anesthetic use are due to these cardiovascular complications.

Gastrointestinal Complications

There are case reports of hepatotoxicity (fatal in one case) associated with halothane abuse among hospital personnel (51).

Hematologic Complications

Nitrous oxide irreversibly oxidizes the cobalt ion in cyanocobalamin (vitamin B12), thus inactivating cobalamin-dependent enzymes and leading to symptoms typical of vitamin B12 deficiency, including megaloblastic anemia (52).

Neuromuscular Complications

When nitrous oxide causes clinical vitamin B12 deficiency, users may present with peripheral neuropathy, ataxia, and even cognitive changes (53, 54). There have been a number of reports of seizures associated with (therapeutic) use of enflurane (55).

NITRITES

Drug Effects

Acute Effects

Nitrites are potent vasodilators and smooth muscle relaxers. Users describe a "rush" with a feeling of warmth and giddiness. This is often accompanied by removal of inhibitions, heightened sensation, and pleasure, especially when used during sexual intercourse. Some users may experience headaches and visual disturbances.

Overdose and Acute Toxicity

Nitrites may cause hypotension and even syncope. However, the most serious complication of nitrite abuse appears to be methemoglobinemia (56), which can be fatal in some cases (57). Methemoglobinemia presents with cyanosis and the diagnosis can be established by the use of co-oximetry with arterial blood analysis. It can be reversed with intravenous methylene blue (58).

Withdrawal

It is clear that, as with nitrates, frequent exposure to nitrites leads to tolerance to their effects within a few days. There does not appear to be a withdrawal syndrome associated with cessation of use.

Diagnosis

Nitrite abuse should be considered in individuals who present with complications such as hypotension or syncope and especially among those with unexplained methemoglobinemia. There are no specific physical findings or laboratory tests for nitrite abuse.

Medical Complications

Cutaneous Complications

There are reports of acrocyanosis associated with butyl nitrite use; this can present with painless, gray-bluish discoloration of the nose, ears, and distal extremities (59).

Pulmonary Complications

Nitrite users can develop cyanosis due to methemoglobinemia (discussed earlier). There is one case report of severe tracheobronchitis associated with nitrite use (60).

Cardiovascular Complications

As mentioned earlier, the vasodilatory effects of nitrites may lead to hypotension and even syncope. This effect may be potentiated by concurrent use of phosphodiesterase (PDE) inhibitors, such as sildenafil (Viagra) (61).

Hematologic Complications

As noted earlier, nitrites can cause methemoglobinemia. The use of nitrites has also been associated with acute hemolytic anemia (62), especially among individuals who have G6PD deficiency (63).

Infectious Complications

A number of epidemiological studies have found that nitrite use among homosexual and bisexual men is associated with high-risk sexual behavior and sexually transmitted diseases, including HIV (64). In fact, this association was noted before the discovery of the HIV virus, leading some to postulate that AIDS was caused by amyl nitrite (65).

TREATMENT

There is very little data on the treatment of inhalant abusers. Brief counseling has been shown to be effective for alcohol (and other substance) misuse and may be effective for periodic inhalant abusers as well. It would be prudent to advise users of the health hazards of these substances and recommend that they stop using. However, the available data suggests poor response to conventional treatment. For example, one case series of 10 adults admitted for treatment of chronic solvent abuse reported that one-half did not complete inpatient rehabilitation and all had relapsed by 6 months (66). Another study reported on 14 adolescent chronic solvent abusers who were offered outpatient treatment (individual or family therapy); 11 kept appointments, and there was "no change" in 6 and "improvement" in 5 of these (67). The poor outcomes observed may be partly due to selection of severe cases; the high prevalence of antisocial personality disorder among regular users may also be a factor (68).

There is no data on treatment of nitrite abusers. However, given the association between nitrite use and unsafe sexual practices, users should be carefully evaluated for HIV infection and other sexually transmitted diseases and counseled on safe sexual practices.

REFERENCES

1. Substance Abuse and Mental Health Services Administration. 2004. Results from the 2003 National Survey on Drug Use and Health: National Findings (Office of Applied Studies, NSDUH Series H-25, DHHS Publication No. SMA 04-3964). Rockville, MD.
2. Wu, L. T., D. J. Pilowsky, and W. E. Schlenger. 2004. Inhalant abuse and dependence among adolescents in the United States. *J. Am. Acad. Child Adolesc. Psychiatry* 43:1206–1214.
3. Dinwiddie, S. H., T. Reich, and C. R. Cloninger. 1991. Solvent use as a precursor to intravenous drug abuse. *Compr. Psychiatry.* 32:133–140.
4. Schultz, C. G., H. D. Chilcoat, and J. C. Anthony. 1994. The association between sniffing inhalants and injecting drugs. *Compr. Psychiatry* 35:99–105.

5. Bennett, M. E., S. T. Walters, J. H. Miller, and W. G. Woodall. 2000. Relationship of early inhalant use to substance use in college students. *J. Subst. Abuse* 12:227–240.

6. Woody, G. E., M. L. VanEtten-Lee, D. McKirnan, et al. 2001. Substance use among men who have sex with men: Comparison with a national household survey. *J. Acquir. Immune Defic. Syndr.* 27:86–90.

7. Ostrow, D. G., E. D. Beltran, J. G. Joseph, et al. 1993. Recreational drugs and sexual behavior in the Chicago MACS/CCS cohort of homosexually active men. *J. Subst. Abuse* 5:311–325.

8. Bass, M. 1970. Sudden sniffing death. *JAMA* 212:2075–2079.

9. Bowen, S. E., J. Daniel, and R. L. Balster. 1999 *Br. J. Psychiatry* 150:769–773.

10. Maxwell, J. C. 2001. Deaths related to the inhalation of volitile substances in Texas: 1988–1998. *Am J. Drug Alcohol Abuse* 27:689–697

11. Cronk, S.J., D. E. H. Barlley, and M. F. Farrell. 1985. Respiritory arrest after solvent abuse. *BMJ* 290: 897–898

12. Shepard, R. T. 1989. Mechanism of sudden ndeath associated with volatile substance abuse. *Hum. Toxicol.* 8:287–291

13. Evans, A. C., and D. Raistrick. 1987. Phenomenology of intoxication with toluene-based adhesives and butane gas. *Br. J. Psychiatry* 150:769–773.

14. Broussard, L. A. 2000. The role of the laboratory in detecting inhalant abuse. Clin. Lab. Sci. 13:205–209.

15. Janežič, T. F. 1997. Burns following petrol sniffing. Burns 23:78–80.

16. Kurbat, R. S., and C. V. Pollack. 1998. Facial injury and airway threat from inhalant abuse: A case report. *J. Emerg. Med.* 16:167–169.

17. Harving, H., R. Dahl, and L. Molhave. 1991. Lung function and bronchial reactivity in asthmatics during exposure to volatile organic compounds. *Am. Rev. Respir. Dis.* 143:751–754.

18. Hoppin, J. A., D. M. Umbach, S. J. London, et al. 2004. Diesel exhaust, solvents, and other occupational exposures as risk factors for wheeze among farmers. *Am. J. Respir. Crit. Care Med.* 169:1308–1313.

19. Cakmak, A., A. Ekici, M. Ekici, et al. 2004. Respiratory findings in gun factory workers exposed to solvents. *Respir. Med.* 98:52–56.

20. Kelly, K. J., and R. Ruffing. 1993. Acute eosinophilic pneumonia following intentional inhalation of Scotchguard. *Ann. Allergy* 71:358–361.

21. Gunn, J., J. Wilson, and A. F. Mackintosh. 1989. Butane sniffing causing ventricular fibrillation. *Lancet* 333:617.

22. LoVecchio, F., and S. E. Fulton. 2001. Ventricular fibrillation following inhalation of Glade Air Freshener. *Eur. J. Emerg. Med.* 8:153–155.

23. Cunninghan, S. R., G. W. Dalzell, P. McGirr, and M. M. Khan. 1987. Myocardial infarction and primary ventricular fibrillation after glue sniffing. *BMJ* 294:739–740.

24. Wason, S., W. B. Gibler, and M. Hassan. 1986. Ventricular tachycardia associated with non-freon aerosol propellants. *JAMA* 256:78–80.

25. Wiseman, M. N., and S. Banim. 1987. "Glue-sniffer's" heart? *BMJ* 294:739.

26. Streicher, H. Z., P. A. Gabow, A. H. Moss, et al. 1981. Syndromes of toluene sniffing in adults. *Ann. Intern. Med.* 94:758–762.

27. Hodgson, M. J., A. E. Heyl, and D. H. VanThiel. 1989. Liver disease associated with exposure to 1,1,1-trichloroethane. *Arch. Intern. Med.* 149:1793–1798.

28. Hoet, P., M. L. Graf, M. Bourdi, et al. 1997. Epidemic of liver disease caused by hydrochlorofluorocarbons used as ozone-sparing substitutes of chlorofluorocarbons. *Lancet* 350:556–559.

29. Taher, S. M., R. J. Anderson, R. McCartney, et al. 1974. Renal tubular acidosis associated with toluene "sniffing." *N. Engl. J. Med.* 290:765–768.

30. Moss, A. H., P. A. Gabow, W. D. Kaehny, et al. 1980. Fanconi's syndrome and distal renal tubular acidosis after glue sniffing. *Ann. Intern. Med.* 92:69–70.

31. Will, A. M., and E. H. McLaren. 1981. Reversible renal damage due to glue sniffing. *BMJ* 283:525–526.

32. Taverner, D., D. J. Harrison, and G. M. Bell. 1988. Acute renal failure due to interstitial nephritis induced by "glue-sniffing" with subsequent recovery. *Scott. Med. J.* 33:246–247.

33. Gupta, R. K., J. van der Meulen, and K. V. Johny. 1991. Oliguric renal failure due to glue-sniffing. *Scand. J. Urol. Nephrol.* 25:247–250.

34. Nielsen, H. K., L. Krusell, J. Baelum, et al. 1985. Renal effects of acute exposure to toluene. A controlled clinical trial. *Acta Med. Scand.* 218:317–321.

35. Smith, M. T. 1996. Overview of benzene-induced aplastic anemia. *Eur. J. Haematol.* 60:107–110.

36. Powars, D. 1965. Aplastic anemia secondary to glue sniffing. *N. Engl. J. Med.* 273:700–702.

37. Travis, L. B., C. Y. Li, Z. N. Zhang, et al. 1994. Hematopoietic malignancies and related disorders among benzene exposed workers in China. *Leuk. Lymphoma* 14:91–102.

38. King, M. D. 1982. Neurologic sequelae of toluene abuse. *Hum. Toxicol.* 1:281–287.

39. Cairney, S., P. Maruff, C. Burns, and B. Currie. 2002. The neurobehavioral consequences of petrol (gasoline) sniffing. *Neurosci. Behavior Rev.* 26:81–89.

40. Burns, T. M., B. F. Shneker, and V. C. Juel. 2001. Gasoline sniffing multifocal neuropathy. *Pediatr. Neurol.* 25:419–421.

41. Cairney, S., P. Maruff, C. B. Burns, et al. 2004. Neurological and cognitive impairment associated with leaded gasoline encephalopathy. *Drug Alcohol Depend.* 73:183–188.

42. Knox, J. W., and J. R. Nelson. 1966. Permanent encephalopathy from toluene inhalation. *N. Engl. J. Med.* 275:1494–1496.

43. King, M. D., R. E. Day, J. S. Oliver, et al. 1981. Solvent encephalopathy. *BMJ* 283:663–665.

44. Filley, C. M., R. K. Heaton, and N. L. Rosenberg. 1990. White matter dementia in chronic toluene abuse. *Neurology* 40:532–534.

45. Winek, C. L., W. W. Wahba, and L. Rozin. 1995. Accidental death by nitrous oxide inhalation. *Forensic Sci. Int.* 73:139–141.

46. Suruda, A. J., and J. D. McGlothlin. 1990. Fatal abuse of nitrous oxide in the workplace. *J. Occup. Med.* 32:682–684.
47. Yamashita, M., A. Matsuki, and T. Oyama. 1984. Illicit use of modern volatile anesthetics. *Can. Anaesth. Soc. J.* 31:76–79.
48. Ngai, S. H. 1980. Effects of anesthetics on various organs. *N. Engl. J. Med.* 302:564–566.
49. Mayhew, J. 1983. Cardiovascular collapse associated with nitrous oxide administration. *Can. Anaesth. Soc. J.* 30:226.
50. Zainea, M., W. F. C. Duvernoy, A. Chauhan, et al. 1994. Acute myocardial infarction in angiographically normal coronary arteries following induction of general anesthesia. *Arch. Intern. Med.* 154:2495–2498.
51. Kaplan, H. G., J. Bakken, L. Quadracci, and W. Schubach. 1979. Hepatitis caused by halothane sniffing. *Ann. Intern. Med.* 90:797–798.
52. Weimann, J. 2003. Toxicity of nitrous oxide. *Best Pract. Res. Clin. Anaesthesiol.* 17:47–61.
53. Butzkueven, H., and J. O. King. 2000. Nitrous oxide myelopathy in an abuser of whipped bream bulbs. *J. Clin. Neurosci.* 7:73–75.
54. Miller, M. A., V. Maritnez, R. McCarthy, and M. M. Patel. 2004. Nitrous oxide "whippit" abuse presenting as clinical B12 deficiency and ataxia. *Am. J. Emerg. Med.* 22:124.
55. Jenkins, J., and A. C. Milne. 1984. Convulsive reaction following enflurane anesthesia. *Anaesthesia* 39:44–45.
56. Horne, M. K., M. R. Waterman, L. M. Simon, et al. 1979. Methemoglobinemia from sniffing butyl nitrite. *Ann. Intern. Med.* 91:417–418.
57. Bradberry, S. M., R. M. Whittington, D. A. Parry, and J. A. Vale. 1994. Fatal methemoglobinemia due to inhalation of isobutyl nitrite. *J. Toxicol. Clin. Toxicol.* 32:179–184.
58. Wright, R. O., W. J. Lewander, and A. D. Woolf. 1999. Methemoglobinemia: Etiology, pharmacology, and clinical management. *Ann. Emerg. Med.* 34:646–656.
59. Hoegl, L., E. Thoma-Greber, J. Poppinger, and M. Röcken. 1999. Butyl nitrite-induced acrocyanosis in an HIV-infected patient. *Arch. Dermatol.* 135:90–91.
60. Covalla, J. R., C. V. Strimlan, and J. G. Lech. 1981. Severe tracheobronchitis from inhalation of an isobutyl nitrite preparation. *Drug Intell. Clin. Pharm.* 15:51–52.
61. Chu, P. L., W. McFarland, S. Gibson, et al. 2003. Viagra use in a community-recruited sample of men who have sex with men, San Francisco. *J. Acquir. Immune Defic. Syndr.* 33:191–193.
62. Graves, T. D. 2003. Acute haemolytic anemia after inhalation of amyl nitrite. *J. R. Soc. Med.* 96:594–595.
63. Stalnikowicz, R., Y. Amitai, and Y. Bentur. 2004. Aphrodisiac drug-induced hemolysis. *J. Toxicol. Clin. Toxicol.* 42:313–316.
64. Ostrow, D. G., E. D. Beltran, J. G. Jospeph, et al. 1993. Recreational drug use and sexual behaviour in the Chicago MACS/CCS cohort of homosexually active men. *J. Subst. Abuse* 5:311–325.
65. Brennan, R. O., and D. T. Durack. 1981. Gay compromise syndrome. *Lancet* 318:1338–1339.

66. Dinwiddie, S. H., C. F. Zorumski, and E. H. Rubin. 1987. Psychiatric correlates of chronic solvent abuse. *J. Clin. Psychiatry* 48:334–337.

67. Skuse, D., and S. Burrell. 1982. A review of solvent abusers and their management by a child psychiatric out-patient service. *Human Toxicol.* 1:321–329.

68. Dinwiddie, S. H., T. Reich, and C. R. Cloninger. 1990. Solvent use and psychiatric comorbidity. *Br. J. Addict.* 85:1647–1656.

13

Anabolic Steroids and Athletes

BACKGROUND

Much recent media attention has focused on the use of anabolic steroids by professional athletes. This chapter focuses on anabolic steroids, but other performance-enhancing drugs that have been used by athletes will be discussed briefly at the end.

The anabolic or "muscle-building" effects of testosterone were first recognized in the 1930s. Initially, testosterone was used for its androgen (masculinizing) effects in the treatment of hypogonadism. Later uses included the treatment of anemia, burns, and malnutrition. However, as early as the 1940s, weightlifters started using testosterone for its anabolic (muscle-building) effects to enhance athletic performance. This was followed by the synthesis of new compounds related to testosterone that are longer-acting (testosterone enthanate and testosterone cypionate), are orally active (methyl-testosterone and stanozolol), are more potent (nandrolone), have less conversion to estrogen resulting in less gynecomastia (methandrostenolone), have fewer androgen effects (oxandrolone and oxymetholone), and are more difficult to detect by drug testing. Routes of use include injection, transdermal (as gels or creams), and oral. A list of commonly abused anabolic steroids can be found in Table 13.1. By the 1970s, the use of anabolic steroids had become so widespread among amateur athletes, including adolescents, that they were banned from Olympic competition in 1975 (1). The United States Drug Enforcement Agency classified them as scheduled drugs in 1991.

Anabolic steroids promote growth of skeletal muscle and increase lean body mass (2). They are anti-catabolic and can convert a negative nitrogen balance to a positive balance by improving utilization of dietary protein and increasing protein synthesis (3). Oxandrolone, an oral synthetic anabolic steroid, and testosterone are prescribed for involuntary weight loss and wasting related to HIV (4). In this setting, anabolic steroids are safe to prescribe, with low abuse potential (5).

When used by athletes, anabolic steroids are used in cycles of weeks or months. "Stacking" (use of more than one preparation) and "pyramiding" (dosages gradually increased and then tapered) are common patterns of administration. Dosages used are much greater than those administered for therapeutic purposes, and abusers often achieve circulating androgen levels up to 100 times higher than normal levels of an adult male (6). Some users fulfill DSM-IV criteria for psychoactive substance abuse and dependence (7).

EPIDEMIOLOGY

A household survey on drug abuse conducted in 1995 estimated that there were more than one million current or former users of anabolic steroids in the United States (8). More than 300,000 individuals had used within the previous year. The median age of first use was 18. During 2003, 1.8% of adults ages 19–28 reported using anabolic steroids at least once in their lifetime, 0.5% reported use within the past year, and 0.2% reported use within the previous month (9). In a study of high school football players, prevalence of anabolic steroid use was 6.3% (10). A 2003 study found that 2.5% of eighth graders, 3.0% of tenth graders, and 3.5% of twelfth graders reported using steroids at least once in their lifetimes (11).

Table 13.1.   Commonly abused anabolic steroids

Trade Name	Generic
Injectable	
Deca-Durabolin	Nandrolone decanoate
Delatestryl	Testosterone enanthate
Depo-testosterone	Testosterone cypionate
Durabolin	Nandrolone phenpropionate
Equipoise	Boldenone undecyclenate
Finajet	Trenbolone acetate
Oreton	Testosterone propionate
Parabolin	Trebolone
Primabolin depot	Methenolone enanthate
Oral	
Anadrol	Oxymetholone
Anavar	Oxandrolone
Dianabol	Methandrostenolone
Halotestin	Fluoxymestrone
Maxibolin	Ethylestrenol
Nilevar	Norethandrolone
Primobolan	Methenolone acetate
Proviron	Mesterolone
Teslac	Testolactone
Winstrol	Stanozolol
Transdermal	
Androderm	Testosterone
Androgel	Testosterone

DRUG EFFECTS

Acute Effects

Acute experimental administration of single doses of testosterone to eugonadal individuals produces no acute psychoactive effect (**12**). In this regard, testosterone is unlike all other drugs of abuse. How anabolic steroids produce dependence is not well understood (13).

Chronic Effects

Testosterone is mostly bound to plasma proteins and in this form is not biologically active. The metabolites of testosterone, such as dihydroxytestosterone, are responsible for changes in intracellular protein production and the anabolic effects. With continuous use of short-acting anabolic steroids or use of a long-acting ester, total body weight increases, partly because of salt and water retention and also because of a true increase in lean body mass. Many users also take diuretics to counter the fluid retention effects of anabolic steroids.

Most studies show that body weight increases by an average of 2–5 kilograms as a result of short-term (less than 12 weeks) use of anabolic steroids (14, 15). This increase in body weight is due to an increase in muscle mass, with increases proportional to amount of anabolic steroid used and the intensity of exercise training (16). Changes in muscle mass have been shown to result in increased strength (2, 17).

Many individuals who use anabolic steroids chronically feel an increased level of aggression. The mechanism by which anabolic steroids increase aggressiveness is unclear, with one study suggesting an association between aggressiveness and changes in free thyroxine (18).

Overdose

There are no reports of anabolic steroid overdose in the literature. "Steroid rage" with violence has been reported in individuals who have been using increasing amounts of anabolic steroids over several weeks.

Withdrawal

Despite claims of individuals developing dependence on anabolic steroids (6, 7), there is no classification "anabolic steroid dependence" in DSM-IV (19). Furthermore, there is no evidence of a typical withdrawal syndrome from anabolic steroids. Anecdotally, there are a variety of withdrawal symptoms linked to cessation of use of anabolic steroids. These symptoms include mood swings, fatigue, restlessness, drug craving, loss of appetite, insomnia, reduced sex drive, the desire to take more steroids, and depression (6).

DIAGNOSIS

Specific inquiry related to use of anabolic steroids should be pursued in athletes and bodybuilders. A survey of 80 weight lifters found that 56% had never revealed their use of anabolic steroids to a physician (20). Presence of androgen-induced side effects outlined below should also raise suspicion for the diagnosis of anabolic steroid abuse.

MEDICAL COMPLICATIONS

The most common and almost uniformly noted medical complications of anabolic steroid use are the direct result of excess exogenous androgens. In men, this causes the suppression of endogenous androgen production with resultant testicular atrophy, decreased sperm count, and infertility (21). Many users of anabolic steroids also inject human chorionic gonadotropin or use oral clomiphene to prevent testicular atrophy and maintain fertility. In women, excess androgen produces hoarse voice, amenorrhea or dysmenorrhea, hirsutism, and clitoral hypertrophy. Excess androgens also typically cause acne and alopecia. In adolescents, excess exogenous androgens cause premature fusion of epiphyses of long bones with stunting of growth.

Pulmonary Complications

There are no reported pulmonary complications of anabolic steroid use. Anabolic steroids do not increase aerobic capacity.

Cardiovascular Complications

The literature for cardiovascular complications of anabolic steroid use has been limited to case reports and small series. Complications reported include myocardial infarction (22–25), atrial fibrillation (26), and dilated cardiomyopathy (27). Episodes of sudden and premature death in elite weight lifters and bodybuilders have been attributed to anabolic steroids (28–30). However, these athletes commonly have evidence of left ventricular hypertrophy on echocardiography, even in the absence of anabolic steroid use (31, 32). Anabolic steroids potentially increase the risk of myocardial infarction as a result of lowering levels of HDL cholesterol (33–35).

Gastrointestinal Complications

Liver abnormalities are most commonly reported in association with the use of oral anabolic steroids, as these drugs require hepatic metabolism (36, 37). There are case reports of liver complications that include elevations in liver enzymes (37, 38), cholestasis (37), peliosis hepatitis (formation of blood-filled sacs in the liver) (39), and hepatic carcinoma (40). However, elevations in liver enzymes generally do not occur in users who do not use oral anabolic steroids (37, 41). Users of anabolic steroids with pre-existing liver disease (i.e., related to alcohol or hepatitis C) may be especially prone to developing liver complications (42).

Renal Complications

Renal complications related to anabolic steroid use appear to be rare. There are two reports of renal cell carcinoma in bodybuilders using anabolic steroids (43, 44).

Neuromuscular Complications

There are case reports of musculoskeletal injury attributed to the use of anabolic steroids, including bone fractures (45) and tendon injuries (46, 47). Additionally, rhabdomyolysis has been reported in a bodybuilder using anabolic steroids (48).

Psychiatric Complications

The most reported behavioral change caused by anabolic steroids is aggression, or "roid rage" (49, 50). These findings have been reported in women as well as men (51). However, increased aggression does not develop in all users (52). At baseline, individuals who become hypomanic and aggressive do not differ from those who do not become more aggressive (52). There are also case reports of depression (53) and suicide (54) attributed to anabolic steroid use. However, many users of anabolic steroids abuse other drugs including alcohol, cocaine, amphetamines, marijuana, and opiates (55).

TREATMENT

There are no reports in the literature related to drug treatment specific to anabolic steroid abuse. In a survey of 175 treatment centers, only 19% of those responding had ever treated a client using anabolic steroids and almost all of these individuals also abused other drugs (56). Patients should be clinically followed for the possible development of withdrawal symptoms such as fatigue, restlessness, or depression. Counseling needs to focus on addressing the reasons anabolic steroids were used (i.e., physical appearance and athletic performance). For individuals abusing other substances in addition to anabolic steroids, traditional psychosocial substance abuse treatment, including 12-step self-help groups, is warranted.

OTHER DRUGS

Most media attention on athletes has focused on anabolic steroids, but performance-enhancing drugs include many other drugs used not only to improve strength but also to improve endurance and accuracy. The World Anti-Doping Code is the international standard for establishing the evolving list of drugs banned in international sports competitions, including the Olympics (57). A summary of the code is found in Table 13.2. In addition to the drugs listed, beta-blockers are prohibited in some sports where accuracy is important, including archery, curling, gymnastics, shooting, and diving.

The list of drugs has evolved over the last few years as athletes have made further attempts to gain the additional slight advantage to go from an elite athlete to the best. In sports such as sprinting, where the difference between winning and losing may be one-hundredth of a second, athletes have been particularly prone to using performance-enhancing drugs. In the 1980s, many long-distance runners started using blood products and erythropoietin to improve endurance. As more drugs were added to the banned list, athletes

Table 13.2.   World Anti-Doping Code prohibited drug list

Anabolic androgenic steroids (including over-the-counter DHEA)

Erythropoietin

Growth hormone

Gonadotrophins

Corticotrophin

Beta-2 agonists (except if special permission to use by inhalation for asthma)

Antiestrogens (clomiphene, tamoxifen, raloxifene)

Diuretics

Blood products and blood substitutes

Drugs that enhance oxygen uptake (perfluorochemicals, efaproxiral)

Stimulants (amphetamines, modafinil, strychnine, ephedrine)

Narcotics (except codeine and hydrocodone)

Cannabinoids

Glucocorticoids (except topical)

Probenecid

turned to ways to evade getting caught. Antiestrogens, go-nadotrophins, and clomiphene were used by male athletes to avoid the gynecomastia and infertility problems associated with anabolic steroids. Diuretics and probenecid were used to rapidly clear drugs prior to testing. Nevertheless, many drugs, including growth factors, are still difficult to detect, and as long as some athletes are so driven to do whatever it takes to win, use of performance-enhancing drugs will continue.

REFERENCES

1. Bahrke, M. S., and C. E. Yesalis. 2004. Abuse of anabolic andro-genic steroids and related substances in sport and exercise. *Curr. Opin. Pharmacol.* 4:614–620.
2. Bhasin, S., T. W. Storer, N. Berman, et al. 1996. The effects of sup-raphysiologic doses of testosterone on muscle size and strength in normal men. *N. Engl. J. Med.* 335:1–7.
3. Sheffield-Moore, M. 2000. Androgens and the control of skeletal muscle protein synthesis. *Ann. Med.* 32:181–186.
4. Strawford, A., T. Barbieri, M. Van Loan, et al. 1999. Resistance exercise and supraphysiologic androgen therapy in eugonadal men with HIV-related weight loss: A randomized controlled trial. *JAMA* 281:1282–1290.
5. Gold, J., H. A. High, Y. Li, et al. 1996. Safety and efficacy of nan-drolone decanoate for treatment of wasting in patients with HIV infection. *AIDS* 10:745–752.
6. Brower, K. J., G. A. Eliopulous, F. C. Blow, et al. 1990. Evidence for physical and psychological dependence on anabolic andro-genic steroids in eight weight lifters. *Am. J. Psychiatry* 147:510 512.
7. Kashkin, K. B., and H. D. Kleber. 1989. Hooked on hormones: An anabolic steroid addiction hypothesis. *JAMA* 262:3166–3170.
8. Yesalis, C. E., N. J. Kennedy, A. N. Kopstein, and M. S. Bahrke. 1993. Anabolic-androgenic steroid use in the United States. *JAMA* 270:1217–1221.
9. National Institute on Drug Abuse and University of Michigan. 2004. *Monitoring the future National survey results on drug use, 1975–2003, Volume II: College students and adults ages 19–45.* Available at http://www.monitoringthefuture.org
10. Stilger, V. G., and C. E. Yesalis. 1999. Anabolic-androgenic steroid use among high school football players. *J. Commun. Health* 24:131–145.
11. National Institute on Drug Abuse and University of Michigan. 2003, December. *Monitoring the future—2003 data from in-school surveys of 8th, 10th and 12th grade students.*
12. Fingerhood, M. I., J. T. Sullivan, M. P. Testa, and D. R. Jasinski. 1997. Abuse liability of testosterone. *J. Psychopharmacol.* 11:65–69. *Ten males, with a history of opioid abuse but no his-tory of anabolic steroid abuse, received intramuscular testos-terone (50, 100, and 200 mg), morphine (10 mg), or placebo for five consecutive days. Testosterone, unlike morphine, produced no pharmacological effects that are associated with other drugs of abuse.*
13. Wood, R. I. 2004. Reinforcing aspects of androgens. *Physiol. Behav.* 83:279–289.

14. Hervey, G. R., I. Hutchinson, A. V. Knibbs, et al. 1976. "Anabolic" effects of methandienone in men undergoing athletic training. *Lancet* 308:699–702.

15. Hervey, G. R., A. V. Knibbs, L. Burkinshaw, et al. 1981. Effects of methandienone on the performance and body composition of men undergoing athletic training. *Clin. Sci.* 60:457–461.

16. Bhasin, S. 2000. The dose-dependent effects of testosterone on sexual function and on muscle mass and function. *Mayo Clin. Proc.* 75:S70–S75.

17. Giorgi, A., R. P. Weatherby, and P. W. Murphy. 1999. Muscular strength, body composition and health responses to the use of testosterone enanthate: A double blind study. *J. Sci. Med. Sport* 2:341–355.

18. Daly, R. C., T. P. Su, P. J. Schmidt, et al. 2003. Neuroendocrine and behavioral effects of high-dose anabolic steroid administration in male normal volunteers. *Psychoneuroendocrinology* 28:317–331.

19. American Psychiatric Association. 2000. *Diagnostic and statistical manual of mental disorders.* 4th ed. (DSM IV-TR). Washington, DC: American Psychiatric Association.

20. Pope, H. G., G. Kanayama, M. Ionescu-Pioggia, and J. I. Hudson. 2004. Anabolic steroid users' attitudes towards physicians. *Addiction* 99:1189–1194.

21. Torres-Calleja, J., M. Gonzalez-Unzaga, R. DeCelis-Carrillo, et al. 2001. Effect of androgenic anabolic steroids on sperm quality and serum hormone levels in adult male bodybuilders. *Life Sci.* 68:1769–1774.

22. Fisher, M., M. Appleby, D. Rittoo, and L. Cotter. 1996. Myocardial infarction with extensive intracoronary thrombus induced by anabolic steroids. *Br. J. Clin. Pract.* 50:180–181.

23. Sullivan, M. L., C. M. Martinez, P. Gennis, et al. 1998. The cardiac toxicity of anabolic steroids. Prog. Cardiovasc. Dis. 41:1–15.

24. Ferenchick, G. S., and S. Adelman. 1992. Myocardial infarction associated anabolic steroids use in a previously healthy 37-year-old weight lifter. *Am. Heart J.* 124:507–508.

25. Palatini, P., F. Giada, G. Garavelli, et al. 1996. Cardiovascular effects of anabolic steroids in weight-trained subjects. *J. Clin. Pharmacol.* 36:132–140.

26. Sullivan, M. L., C. M. Martinez, and E. J. Gallagher. 1999. Atrial fibrillation and anabolic steroids. *J. Emerg. Med.* 17:851–857.

27. Ferrera, P. C., D. L. Putnam, and V. P. Verdile. 1997. Anabolic steroid use as the possible precipitant of dilated cardiomyopathy. *Cardiology* 88:218–220.

28. Parssinen, M., U. Kujala, E. Vartiainen, et al. 2000. Increased premature mortality of competitive powerlifters suspected to have used anabolic agents. *Int. J. Sports Med.* 21:225–227.

29. Hausmann, R., S. Hammer, and P. Betz. 1998. Performance-enhancing drugs (doping agents) and sudden death: A case report and review of the literature. *Int. J. Legal Med.* 111:261–264.

30. Luke, J. L., A. Farb, R. Virmani, et al. 1990. Sudden cardiac death during exercise in a weight lifter using anabolic androgenic steroids: Pathological and toxicological findings. *J. Forensic Sci.* 35:1441–1447.

31. Wright, J. N., and D. Salem. 1995. Sudden cardiac death and the "athlete's heart." *Arch. Intern. Med.* 155:1473–1480.

32. Dickerman, R. D., F. Schaller, and W. J. McConathy. 1998. Left ventricular wall thickening does occur in elite power athletes with or without anabolic steroid use. *Cardiology* 90:145–148.

33. Urhausen, A., A. Torstein, and K. Wilfried. 2003. Reversibility of the effects on blood cells, lipids, liver function and hormones in former anabolic-androgenic steroid abusers. *J. Steroid Biochem. Molec. Biol.* 84:369–375. *This cohort study of 32 bodybuilders compared 17 current users of anabolic steroids with 15 former users (had not used anabolic steroids for at least 1 year). HDL levels were 43+11 mg/dl in ex-users and 17+11 mg/dl in current users, p < .0001. ALT and AST were 65+55 U/l and 38+27 U/l, respectively, in users and 24+10 U/l and 18+11 U/l, respectively, in ex-users, p < .0001.*

34. Glazer, G. 1991. Atherogenic effects of anabolic steroids on serum lipid levels. *Arch. Intern. Med.* 151:1925–1933.

35. Hartgens, F., G. Rietjens, H. A. Keizer, et al. 1984. Severe depression of high-density lipoprotein cholesterol levels in weight lifters and body builders by self-administered exogenous testosterone and anabolic-androgenic steroids. *Metabolism* 33:971–975.

36. Soe, K. L., M. Soe, and C. Gluud. 1992. Liver pathology associated with the use of anabolic-androgenic steroids. *Liver* 12:73–79.

37. Ishak, K. G., and H. J. Zimmerman. 1987. Hepatotoxic effects of the anabolic androgenic steroids. *Semin. Liver Dis.* 7:230–236.

38. Freed, D. L., A. J. Banks, D. Longson, et al. 1975. Anabolic steroids in athletics: Crossover double-blind trial on weightlifters. *BMJ* 2:471–473.

39. Cabasso, A. 1994. Peliosis hepatis in a young adult bodybuilder. *Med. Sci. Sports Exerc.* 26:2–4.

40. Kosaka, A., H. Takahashi, Y. Yajima, et al. 1996. Hepatocellular carcinoma associated with anabolic steroid therapy: Report of a case and review of the Japanese literature. *J. Gastroenterol.* 31:450–454.

41. Kuipers, H., J. A. G. Wijnen, F. Hartgens, et al. 1991. Influence of anabolic steroids on body composition, blood pressure, lipid profile and liver function in bodybuilders. *Int. J. Sports Med.* 12:413–418.

42. Wilson, J. D. 1988. Androgen abuse by athletes. *Endocr. Rev.* 9:181–199.

43. Bryden, A. A. G., P. J. N. Rothwell, and P. H. O'Reilly. 1995. Anabolic steroid abuse and renal cell carcinoma. *Lancet* 346:1306–1307.

44. Martorana, G., S. Concetti, F. Manferrari, et al. 1999. Anabolic steroid abuse and renal cell carcinoma. *Clin. Urol.* 162:2089.

45. Tannenbaum, S. D., and H. Rosler. 1989. Proximal humeral fracture in weight lifter using anabolic steroids. *Arch. Phys. Med. Rehabil.* 70:A89.

46. Laseter, J. T., and J. A. Russell. 1991. Anabolic steroid-induced tendon pathology: A review of the literature. *Med. Sci. Sports Exerc.* 23:1–3.

47. Liow, R., and S. Tavares. 1995. Bilateral rupture of the quadriceps tendon associated with anabolic steroids. *Br. J. Sports Med.* 29:77–79.

48. Bolgiano, E. B. 1994. Acute rhabdomyolysis due to body building exercise: Report of a case. *J. Sports Med. Phys. Fitness* 34:76–78.

49. Su, T. P., M. Pagliaro, P. J. Schmidt, et al. 1993. Neuropsychiatric effects of anabolic steroids in male normal volunteers. *JAMA* 269:2760–2764.

50. Thiblin, I., and T. Parlklo. 2002. Anabolic androgenic steroids and violence. *Acta Psychiatr. Scand. Suppl.* 412:125–128.

51. Gruber, A. J., and H. G. Pope. 2000. Psychiatric and medical effects of anabolic-androgenic steroid use in women. *Psychother. Psychosom.* 69:19–26.

52. Pope, H. G., E. M. Kouri, and J. I. Hudson. 2000. Effects of supraphysiologic doses of testosterone on mood and aggression in normal men: A randomized controlled trial. *Arch. Gen. Psychiatry* 57:133–140. *Fifty-six men were randomized to testosterone cypionate in doses up to 600 mg/week or placebo for 6 weeks, followed by 6 weeks of no treatment, followed by 6 weeks of crossover treatment. Among 50 subjects who completed the study, six became mildly hypomanic and two became markedly hypomanic, with minimal effects in the other 42. The 8 "responders" and 42 "nonresponders" did not differ on baseline demographic, psychological, or physiological measures.*

53. Pope, H. G., and D. L. Katz. 1994. Psychiatric and medical effects of anabolic-androgenic steroid use. A controlled study of 160 athletes. *Arch. Gen. Psych.* 51:375–382.

54. Thiblin, I., B. Runeson, and J. Rajs. 1999. Anabolic androgenic steroids and suicide. *Ann. Clin. Psychiatry* 11:223–231.

55. Fudala, P. J., R. M. Weinreb, J. S. Calarco, et al. 2003. An evaluation of anabolic-androgenic steroid users over a period of 1 year: Seven case studies. *Ann. Clin. Psychiatry* 15:121–130.

56. Clancy, G. P., and W. R. Yates. 1992. Anabolic steroid use among substance abusers in treatment. *J. Clin. Psychiatry* 53:97–100.

57. World Anti-Doping Agency. The World Anti-Doping Code—The 2005 Prohibited List. Available at http://www.wada-ama.org

14

Prescription Drug Abuse

BACKGROUND

Prescription drug abuse is a growing problem that includes the improper prescribing of medications and drug diversion. A related term "nonmedical use of a prescription drug" is defined as "using a psychotherapeutic drug, even once that was not prescribed for you or that you took only for the experience or feeling it caused." Over the past few years, the street value and prevalence of diverted prescription drugs have increased dramatically.

In rural communities that never had problems with illicit drugs, the use of diverted prescription drugs, especially long-acting oxycodone (OxyContin), is epidemic. An additional concern has been the explosion of overseas-based online pharmacies that will fill prescriptions for controlled substances without a prescription (1, 2). Of the prescription drug classes reported by the federal government, opioids are consistently the class with the greatest nonmedical use, with resultant abuse and dependence problems. How to deal with the increasing problem of prescription opioid abuse without interfering with legitimate use has no clear answer.

EPIDEMIOLOGY

Prescription and over-the-counter (OTC) drugs were the primary substances of abuse for 4% of the 1.9 million treatment admissions reported to the Treatment Episode Data Set (TEDS) in 2002 (3). Prescription drugs in TEDS are grouped as prescription narcotics (e.g., oxycodone), prescription stimulants (e.g., methylphenidate), tranquilizers (e.g., diazepam), and sedatives (e.g., chloral hydrate). OTC drugs include cough syrup (dextromethorphan), diphenhydramine (Benadryl), and decongestants (Sudafed). Of the more than 78,000 admissions for primary prescription or OTC drug abuse in 2002, 55% (43,100 admissions) were for prescription narcotics, 28% (22,000 admissions) for prescription stimulants, 10% (8200 admissions) for tranquilizers, 6% (4500 admissions) for sedatives, and less than 1% (600 admissions) for OTC medications. An additional 100,000 admissions listed prescription or OTC drugs as their secondary or tertiary substances of abuse. Females comprised a larger proportion of prescription and OTC drug admissions (46%) than for other substances (30%), with data for specific categories showing females comprising 47% for prescription narcotics, 44% for prescription stimulants, 50% for tranquilizers, 51% for sedatives, and 42% for OTC drugs.

Primary care providers are the main prescribers of controlled drugs. Despite concerns over unscrupulous doctors who write inappropriate prescriptions for controlled substances, only a small number of doctors registered with the DEA are ever targeted by a DEA investigation. In fiscal year 2001, there were 923,829 doctors registered by the DEA, of whom only 831 (0.09%) were investigated (4). These investigations resulted in actions against 0.08% of the registrants (739 doctors) and led to the arrest of only 92 doctors. However, there are likely providers not targeted by the DEA who knowingly or unknowingly put a large number of scheduled drugs on the illicit market.

ABUSED PRESCRIPTION DRUGS

The benzodiazepines and narcotics are the most commonly abused controlled drugs. Long-term use of these drugs is sometimes appropriate. However, regular use will result in physical dependence. Non-pharmacological modalities should always be used to increase the interval between doses, decrease the required dosage, and permit intermittent use of these drugs if possible.

Pain Relievers

In 2003, an estimated 31.2 million Americans over the age of 12 had ever used a pain reliever for a nonmedical use, up from 29.6 million in 2002. Specific pain relievers with statistically significant increases in lifetime use from 2002 to 2003 were hydrocodone (including Vicodin, Lortab, and Lorcet), from 17.6 million to 21.4 million; short-acting oxycodone (including Percocet, Percodan, or Tylox), from 9.7 million to 10.8 million; OxyContin, from 1.9 million to 2.8 million; methadone, from 0.9 million to 1.2 million; and tramadol (Ultram), from 52,000 to 186,000 (5). An estimated 11 million of the 13.7 million individuals who used oxycodone had never used heroin. Importantly, over the same time interval there was no change in heroin use. Among lifetime oxycodone-"only" users, 7.2% met criteria for current opiate dependence or abuse. Prescription opiate abuse has become much more common among patients presenting for methadone maintenance treatment, with one study reporting 83% of new admissions reporting prescription opiate abuse (6).

It should be noted that tramadol, an "opioid-like" drug, is not a scheduled drug, but there are reports of abuse and dependence, especially in individuals with a history of substance abuse (7). The rates of abuse are relatively low and did not change when the generic formulation of tramadol was marketed (8). In patients with a history of drug use and intolerance to nonsteroidal anti-inflammatory drugs, tramadol poses less risk than the controlled narcotics (9). Special mention should also be made of butorphanol, a schedule IV narcotic available for intranasal use. Butorphanol is most commonly prescribed for acute pain relief in patients unable to take oral medication, including patients with migraine headaches and associated nausea. When originally approved for use, intranasal butorphanol was not controlled, but reports of abuse and dependence caused it to become scheduled (10).

Available data reports that the rates of opioid abuse in chronic pain patients on long-term opioid therapy ranges from 3.2 to 18.9% (11). One study suggests that most patients without a history of substance abuse problems do not abuse opioids prescribed to them for relief of chronic pain (12). However, more controlled prospective studies are needed.

Several strategies have been developed by the pharmaceutical industry to reduce the abuse risk of opioid pain medications. One strategy is to control the rate and extent of delivery of the opioid medication into the bloodstream and/or central nervous system (CNS), as the rate of drug onset in the CNS influences abuse liability (i.e., transdermal delivery systems and controlled-release oral formulations). These systems typically provide a gradual onset and sustained delivery of medication. Drug formulations with gradual onset are generally associated with reduced abuse liability, when compared with rapid-onset or immediate-release formulations. The diversion or abuse of the fentanyl transdermal system is thought to be uncommon, but there have been case reports of abusers swallowing or chewing the patch (13) or extracting the fentanyl from the patch for intravenous use (14).

Sustained-release formulations do not necessarily ensure low abuse liability if users can circumvent the intended slow-release feature. Such tampering has been noted with sustained-release oxycodone (OxyContin), as by crushing or dissolving an OxyContin tablet the entire dose intended for slow release can be made immediately available and used as a bolus by intranasal or injection routes. Such formulations need to be redesigned so that they are not vulnerable to being altered to an immediate-release form. Additionally, mixing oral opiates with the opioid antagonist naloxone would deter abuse by injection (but not by other routes); this is done with a sublingual formulation of buprenorphine. If an opioid-dependent person then injected the product, naloxone would precipitate an aversive withdrawal reaction; however, if the medication were taken orally, a negligible amount of naloxone would be ingested.

Sedatives

The prescribing of all sedatives should be done with a plan that includes a clear therapeutic goal and an endpoint. Risk of abuse (even for the new non-benzodiazepine sleep medications zolpidem, eszopiclone, and zaleplon) is greatest in individuals with other substance abuse. Specific issues related to abuse liability of sedatives are discussed in Chapter 6.

Stimulants

In 2003, 20.8 million Americans aged 12 or older (8.8% of that population) had used prescription-type stimulants non-medically at least once in their lifetime (15). An estimated 378,000 persons in the United States met the diagnostic criteria for dependence on or abuse of stimulants in the past year. Lifetime use of methamphetamines was reported by 12.3 million (5.2% of the population), prescription diet pills (phentermine and sibutramine) by 8.7 million (3.6%), methylphenidate (Ritalin) by 4.2 million (1.8%), and dextroamphetamine (Dexedrine) by 2.6 million (1.1%). Abuse of these drugs is discussed in Chapter 9.

Other Prescription Drugs

Noncontrolled prescription drugs with reports of abuse include clonidine, muscle relaxants, tricyclic antidepressants, bupropion, tramadol (discussed earlier), and antiemetics.

Clonidine is mostly abused by individuals with opiate dependence; some abuse is for alleviating symptoms of opiate dependence (see Chapter 7), but much abuse occurs in individuals continuing to abuse opiates (16) and also in individuals receiving methadone maintenance (17). In some communities, a high level of clonidine abuse with frequent drug diversion has warranted the advice to health care providers not to use clonidine at all as an antihypertensive. Abuse has been reported with the clonidine patch as well, with case reports of hypotension from chewing and swallowing the patch (18).

Muscle relaxants are abused to take advantage of their common side effect of sedation, and there are reports of overdose from all them. All published case reports of muscle relaxant abuse are related to carisoprodol (discussed in Chapter 6), but the others (cyclobenzaprine [Flexeril], methocarbamol [Robaxin], and metaxalone [Skelaxin]) should generally be avoided in individuals with other substance abuse.

Antiemetics (promethazine and prochlorperazine) are abused by opiate-dependent individuals to counter the nausea and stomach-turning side effects of opiates and to potentiate the euphoric effects of opiates. When prescribing these drugs to individuals with a history of opiate dependence, the prescription should be written carefully (see below) with avoidance of refills.

Patients with addiction commonly have sleep problems and depression resulting in them receiving prescriptions for tricyclic antidepressants. Most reports of abuse and intoxication from these drugs have been related to amitriptyline (Elavil) (19). Patients on methadone maintenance have an especially high rate of amitriptyline abuse (20). Some patients even seek out the drug because of the brand name and the thought that the drug will make them "high," when in fact it makes them sedated.

There are also reports of abuse of the antidepressant bupropion, generally by the intranasal route (21), with one report of abuse complicated by a seizure (22). There has also been a report of intranasal abuse of the atypical antipsychotic quetiapine among prisoners in Los Angeles (23).

Over-the-Counter (OTC) Drugs

Most of the recent attention related to abuse of over-the-counter drugs has focused on the use of pseudoephedrine to manufacture methamphetamine. Many pharmacies have restricted sales of pseudoephedrine and taken bottles off open shelves. The most directly abused over-the-counter drugs are dextromethorphan-containing cough syrups and the antihistamines diphenhydramine (Benadryl) and dimenhydrinate (Dramamine). Case reports of dextromethorphan abuse have generally been in adolescents (24). Individuals after ingesting large amounts (8 ounces or more) of dextromethorphan-containing cough syrup may experience euphoria, disorientation, and hallucinations (25). Withdrawal symptoms develop in some individuals and consist of insomnia and dysphoria. Symptoms of overdose include altered mental status, ataxia, and nystagmus; deaths from overdose have been reported (26). Dimenhydrinate, therapeutically used for motion sickness, is composed of diphenhydramine plus the methylxanthine 8-chlorotheophylline in equimolar ratios. Dimenhydrinate can cause euphoria, visual and tactile hallucinations, and sedation (27, 28). The antimuscarinic properties of diphenhydramine become more prominent at high doses, and these properties, which cause hallucinations and euphoria, are likely responsible for the abuse potential (29).

MARKERS OF ABUSE

Health care providers must be vigilant to avoid being "duped" by acquiescing to demanding patients. Although no one behavior is grounds for denying patients a potentially therapeutic agent, providers should be vigilant and take note of these signs.

Table 14.1.   Generally inappropriate prescribing practices

Prescription of scheduled drugs from two or more practitioners simultaneously

Prescribing the same scheduled drug to several members of a family

Prescribing drugs of high abuse liability to someone with addiction without a clear plan

Prescribing multiple scheduled drugs for the same purpose

Prescribing scheduled drugs to friends or family members

Prescribing three or more scheduled drugs to a patient

Practitioners should be suspicious of patients who

1. have a history of substance abuse,
2. have a history of violent behavior,
3. insist on a controlled drug on the first visit,
4. have new problems related to work, school, or family and friends,
5. obtain prescriptions from multiple providers or switch providers frequently,
6. demand one specific medication (or refuse generic preparations) as the only one that will work,
7. run out of medication before the time that would be expected,
8. make flattering comments like "You are the only person who understands me,"
9. lose prescriptions or medications (patients rarely lose their blood pressure medication),
10. have slurred speech or unexplained cognitive impairment.

There are a number of other behaviors that are strong indicators of abuse, including forging or altering prescriptions, selling medication obtained by prescription, and overdosing on prescription medication. Patients who show these signs should not be prescribed controlled substances except for compelling indications and under strict supervision. Prescribing practices that may be illegal, dangerous, or inappropriate are listed in Table 14.1. Even though schedule III, IV, V, and VI drugs may be refilled five times within 6 months (schedule II drugs may not be refilled), giving refills for drugs in these classes should be carefully considered.

STRATEGIES TO AVOID PRESCRIPTION DRUG ABUSE

Some of the most difficult issues in primary care are related to prescribing medications for anxiety, pain, and sleep. These issues are even more complicated and anxiety-provoking (for the primary care provider) when they involve a patient with a history of addiction. In general, the following rules should be followed:

1. When treating anxiety, always try non-benzodiazepines first, and if benzodiazepines are prescribed, use them for a short, defined time period. If a patient requires chronic, regular use of a benzodiazepine, it would be best that this be done under the supervision of a mental health specialist.

2. Treat short-term severe acute pain with appropriate pain medicines, including opiates, but be clear about the expectations and have an endpoint. For patients in recovery, discuss the implications of giving an opiate. Some patients would rather tolerate the pain than run the risk of relapse.

3. When treating chronic pain, always combine modalities, including non-pharmacological (e.g., physical therapy, acupuncture, and exercise) and non-opiate medications, before adding opiates. If using opiates, focus on using long-acting medications to prevent emergence of symptoms and use a pain contract (see Figure 14.1). If you feel uncomfortable with your approach, consult a pain management specialist.

4. Do not prescribe benzodiazepines to treat insomnia in individuals with a history of addiction.

5. Although we all like to please our patients, do not be afraid to say no. Stick with your original plan: If you sense a patient is pressuring you to prescribe a medication that you would not prescribe otherwise, "turn the tables" and tell them that you feel pressured to do something you feel is not appropriate.

To avoid possible abuse, medications with abuse liability should be prescribed on a fixed schedule and, if possible, with a therapeutic

---

PAIN CONTRACT

1. I understand that the aim of pain management is to improve my quality of life and increase the amount of activity I can perform.

2. I understand that it is unlikely that all of my pain will be relieved.

3. I agree to pursue any/all non-medication therapies that may improve my pain.

4. I understand that narcotic pain medications used over long periods of time cause dependence and if stopped abruptly may result in withdrawal symptoms.

5. I agree to have only one provider prescribe all of my narcotic pain medications.

6. I agree to always take my pain medication as prescribed. Any changes in dose must be made by agreement with my provider.

7. I am responsible for my prescriptions lasting the appropriate amount of time. I understand I will not receive additional medication ahead of time.

_____

Patient Signature

_____

Provider Signature

Figure 14-1.   A sample pain contract.

endpoint. This strategy improves control of symptoms, minimizes the emergence of symptoms (rather than reacting to symptoms after they occur), and avoids patient focus on immediate relief. Medications should be prescribed for short periods during treatment of acute problems. Patients should be seen for reassessment at frequent intervals and telephone refills should be avoided. If possible, long-acting medications should be used rather than short-acting ones. When providers practice in a group setting, clear instructions for refills should be on patient charts and the practice should have strict rules that on-call physicians do not call in prescriptions for scheduled drugs, even though the DEA does allow schedule III, IV, and V drugs to be called in to pharmacies.

Because of the risk of theft of prescription blanks or the alteration of prescriptions, all prescription pads should be safeguarded. Regular prescriptions should be marked "not for scheduled drugs." Prescription blanks for scheduled drugs should be kept locked separately. Prescriptions should be written clearly, and the number of pills to be dispensed and the number of refills should be written out (not just a number). If no refills are intended, "No Refills" should be clearly written to avoid altering of a prescription to allow refills. Additionally, the dose may need to be written out as a word, as for example a "10" can easily be changed to a "40." All prescribing of scheduled drugs should be documented clearly in the chart.

REFERENCES

1. St George, B. N., J. R. Emmanuel, and K. L. Middleton. 2004. Overseas-based online pharmacies: A source of supply for illicit drug users? *Med. J. Austr.* 180:118–119.

2. Romero, C. E., J. D. Baron, A. P. Knox, et al. 2004. Barbiturate withdrawal following Internet purchase of Fioricet. *Arch. Neurol.* 61:1111–1112.

3. Substance Abuse and Mental Health Services Administration. Treatment Episode Data Set (TEDS). Available at http://www. drugabusestatistics.samhsa.gov.

4. Zacny, J., G. Bigelow, P. Compton, et al. 2003. College on Problems of Drug Dependence taskforce on prescription opioid non-medical use and abuse: Position statement. *Drug Alcohol Depend.* 69:215–232.

5. Substance Abuse and Mental Health Services Administration. 2004. Results from the 2003 National Survey on Drug Use and Health: National Findings (Office of Applied Studies, NSDUH Series H-25, DHHS Publication No. SMA 04-3964). Rockville, MD.

6. Brands, B., J. Blake, B. Sproule, et al. 2004. Prescription opioid abuse in patients presenting for methadone maintenance treatment. *Drug Alcohol Depend.* 73:199–207. *Retrospective review of 178 admissions (mean age 34.5, 65% male); 83% had been using prescription opioids. Four groups were identified: 24% had used prescription opioids only; 24% used prescription opioids initially and heroin later; 35% used heroin first and prescription opioids subsequently; and 17% had used heroin only. Those that used prescription opioids only or initially were more likely to have ongoing pain problems and to be involved in psychiatric treatment.*

7. Woody, G. E., E. C. Senay, A. Geller, et al. 2003. An independent assessment of MEDWatch reporting for abuse/dependence and withdrawal from Ultram (tramadol hydrochloride). *Drug Alcohol Depend.* 72:163–168.

8. Cicero, T. J., J. A. Inciardi, E. H. Adams, et al. 2005, May 12. Rates of abuse of tramadol remain unchanged with the introduction of new branded and generic products: Results of an abuse monitoring system, 1994–2004. *Pharmacoepidemiol. Drug Saf.* (E-pub. ahead of print).

9. Preston, K. L., D. R. Jasinski, and M. Testa. 1991. Abuse potential and pharmacological comparison of tramadol and morphine. *Drug Alcohol Depend.* 27:7–17.

10. Fisher, M. A., and S. Glass. 1997. Butorphanol (Stadol): A study in problems of current drug information and control. *Neurology* 48:1156–1160.

11. Fishbain, D. A., H. L. Rosomoff, and R. S. Rosomoff. 1992. Drug abuse, dependence, and addiction in chronic pain patients. *Clin. J. Pain* 8:77–85.

12. Portenoy, R. K., and K. M. Foley. 1986. Chronic use of opioid analgesics in non-malignant pain: Report of 38 cases. *Pain* 25:171–186.

13. Nevin, J. 2004. Drug update: Fentanyl patch abuse. *Emerg. Med. Serv.* 33:24–25.

14. Tharp, A. M., R. E. Winecker, and D. C. Winston. 2004. Fatal intravenous fentanyl abuse: Four cases involving extraction of fentanyl from transdermal patches. *Am. J. Forensic Med. Pathol.* 25:178–181.

15. Substance Abuse and Mental Health Services Administration. The NSDUH Report: Stimulant Use 2003. Available at http://www.oas.samhsa.gov

16. Dennison, S. J. 2001. Clonidine abuse among opiate addicts. *Psychiatr. Q.* 72:191–195.

17. Beuger, M., A. Tommasello, R. Schwartz, and M. Clinton. 1998. Clonidine use and abuse among methadone program applicants and patients. *J. Subst. Abuse Treat.* 15:589–593.

18. Rapko, D. A., and D. A. Rastegar. 2003. Intentional clonidine patch ingestion by 3 adults in a detoxification unit. *Arch. Intern. Med.* 163:367–368.

19. Prahlow, J. A., and J. E. Landrum. 2005. Amitriptyline abuse and misuse. *Am. J. Forensic Med. Pathol.* 26:86–88.

20. Cohen, M. J., R. Hanbury, and B. Stimmel. 1978. Abuse of amitriptyline. *JAMA* 240:1372–1373. *Survey of 346 persons in a methadone maintenance program; 86 (25%) admitted taking amitriptyline for the purpose of achieving euphoria and 34% had a positive urine screen for amitriptyline at least once during a 5-month interval.*

21. Khurshid, K. A., and D. H. Decker. 2004. Bupropion insufflation in a teenager. *J. Child Adolesc. Psychopharm.* 14:157–158.

22. Welsh, C. J., and S. Doyon. 2002. Seizure induced by insufflation of bupropion. *N. Engl. J. Med.* 347:951.

23. Pierre, J. H., I. Shnayder, D. A. Wirshing, and W. C. Wirshing. 2004. Intranasal quetiapine abuse. *Am. J. Psychiatr.* 161:1718.

24. Murray, S., and T. Brewerton. 1993. Abuse of over-the-counter dextromethorphan by teenagers. *South. Med. J.* 86:1151–1153.

25. Wolfe, T. R., and E. M. Caravati. 1995. Massive dextromethorphan ingestion and abuse. *Am. J. Emerg. Med.* 13:174–176.

26. Rammer, L., P. Holmgren, and H. Sandler. 1988. Fatal intoxication by dextromethorphan: A report on two cases. *Forensic Sci. Int.* 37:233–236.

27. Malcolm, R., and W. C. Miller. 1972. Dimenhydrinate (Dramamine) abuse: Hallucinogenic experiences with a proprietary antihistamine. *Am. J. Psychiatr.* 128:1012–1013.

28. Halpert, A. G., M. C. Olmstead, and R. J. Beninger. 2002. Mechanisms and abuse liability of the anti-histamine dimenhydrinate. *Neurosci. Biobehav. Rev.* 26:61–67.

29. Dilsaver, S. C. 1988. Antimuscarinic agents as substances of abuse: A review. *J. Clin. Psychopharmacol.* 8:14–22.

15

Medical Care for the Addicted Patient

BACKGROUND

Addiction is a chronic illness that is associated with a long list of medical conditions and complications that health care providers must deal with. Moreover, there are special challenges in providing this care to this population. In this section, we will discuss some of these issues. We will begin with the medical complications of injection drug use; complications associated with particular substances are addressed in the individual chapters on those substances. We will then discuss some issues that arise in caring for individuals on methadone maintenance and treating pain in opioid addicts. Finally, we will address some of the challenges that can arise from dealing with "difficult" patients and suggest strategies for dealing with them.

MEDICAL COMPLICATIONS OF INJECTION DRUG USE

Many of the medical complications that addicts acquire are due to the use of needles to administer the drug. According to the *2003 National Survey on Drug Use and Health* (NSDUH), an estimated 3.7 million Americans have used (at some time in their lives) a needle to inject a drug that was not prescribed (1.5% of those aged 12 and older) (1). Injection drug use is risky; in a cohort of injection drug users in Scotland followed from 1980 to 2001, the average annual mortality was 2.3%. Overdose was the primary cause of death early on and was overtaken by the complications of HIV infection in the late 1980s; mortality from HIV declined after 1996 and hepatitis C subsequently became a significant cause of mortality (2).

Infectious Complications

The most serious dangers to the health of injection drug users are infectious complications, particularly those associated with sharing needles. Hepatitis B, hepatitis C, and human immunodeficiency virus (HIV) infection are spread among addicts through this route. Other infectious complications will be covered in the subsequent organ system-based sections.

Hepatitis B

Epidemiological studies indicate that injection drug users are at high risk for acquiring hepatitis B (HBV); in one study of users in Baltimore, 80% were HBV seropositive, and this was associated with needle-sharing and duration of use but not with high-risk sexual behavior (3). Most who acquire hepatitis B have a clinical illness with nausea, vomiting, and jaundice that resolves within a few weeks. In contrast to hepatitis C, only a minority develop persistent infection and remain infectious to others; in one case series, this occurred in about 2% of addicts with acute hepatitis B (4). Detection of hepatitis B surface antigen (HBsAg) generally identifies the chronically infected, but one study found evidence of occult hepatitis B infection in almost half of a cohort of hepatitis C-infected injection drug users; the clinical significance of this finding has not been established (5).

Needle exchange programs appear to reduce the risk of hepatitis B transmission (6). All addicts who are not hepatitis B–infected or immune (i.e., do not have positive hepatitis B surface antigen or surface antibody) should be offered hepatitis B vaccine.

Hepatitis C

Hepatitis C virus (HCV) infection is very common among injection drug users. In one study of subjects in a detoxification program, 71% of the heroin users had HCV antibodies (7). Another study of injection drug users in San Francisco found that 95% were anti-HCV positive (8). Non-injection drug users are at substantially lower risk of hepatitis C (about 5% in one cohort) (9), but they still have a higher prevalence than the 2% seen in the general U.S. population (10); HCV can be found in nasal secretions, so sharing of implements for snorting is a potential route of transmission (11).

Acute hepatitis C is usually asymptomatic, but some do develop an acute self-limited illness with jaundice; this is actually a good prognostic sign, since those with symptomatic acute hepatitis C are more likely to clear the virus (12). Overall, about 85% become chronically infected; those who do clear the virus spontaneously can be reinfected but are at lower risk than others (13). Carriers of HCV are generally asymptomatic but may develop complications such as essential mixed cryoglobulinemia, which can lead to systemic vasculitis, peripheral neuropathy, and glomerulonephritis (14). Over the long term, chronic HCV infection can lead to cirrhosis and hepatocellular carcinoma. In one cohort of 1667 anti-HCV-positive injection drug users who had used for a median of 13.7 years at entry and were followed for a median of 8.8 years, the rate of end-stage liver disease was 3 per 1000 person-years; while 9% of the deaths in this cohort were due to liver disease, 40% were due to complications of HIV, 19% due to overdose, and 12% due to bacterial infections (15).

The current standard treatment for HCV is pegylated interferon with ribavirin; in clinical trials, sustained response rates are approximately 50% with genotype 1 and 75% with other genotypes (2, 3, and 4) (16). Most drug users have genotype 1. For those who are coinfected with HIV, the prognosis is worse and the response rates are lower. Many practitioners are reluctant to treat addicts who have HCV; however, at least in one recent study, their rates of sustained response were as good as matched non-drug-using controls (17). However, those who do have a sustained response are still at risk for reacquiring the infection if they share needles again.

For those who develop liver failure from HCV, liver transplantation is the only treatment option. While almost all programs consider active drug use a contraindication for transplantation, many also exclude those on methadone maintenance treatment (18). However, one study of 36 liver transplant recipients on methadone maintenance treatment (followed for an average of 4 years) reported outcomes comparable to the national average; all of these subjects were drug and alcohol free for at least 6 months prior to transplantation (19).

The risk of transmission of HCV may be reduced by cleaning syringes and needles with bleach (20). Needle exchange programs may also help reduce the risk of HCV transmission (6).

HIV Infection

In the United States, injection drug use has been an important route of transmission of HIV infection. Of the 385,000 Americans known to be living with AIDS in 2002, 122,000 (32%) were injection drug users; furthermore, many of those who acquire HIV through heterosexual exposure do so from contact with injection drug users (21). The prevalence of HIV infection among injection drug users has been found to be as high as 20% in one study (22). On the other hand, while the number of new AIDS diagnoses has been fairly stable from 2000 to 2003, those associated with injection drug use appear to be gradually declining (23).

The acquisition of HIV infection is usually followed by a mild to severe flu-like illness that has been called the "acute retroviral syndrome." The most common signs and symptoms of primary HIV infection are fever, malaise, myalgia, pharyngitis, and rash. The syndrome is nonspecific and cannot be differentiated from other acute viral illnesses on the basis of signs or symptoms alone (24). Patients commonly do not seek medical attention, and even when they do, primary HIV infection is often not recognized. HIV antibody is negative during this phase of the illness, but acute infection can be diagnosed by measurement of HIV p24 antigen or mRNA level ("viral load").

The acute phase of HIV infection is followed by a prolonged asymptomatic phase that generally lasts several years. During this phase, there is a gradual decline in immunity and infected persons are at higher risk for community-acquired pneumonia and tuberculosis but not for the opportunistic infections that are seen only in immunocompromised hosts. The final phase of this illness, the acquired immunodeficiency syndrome (AIDS), is when the immune system is so impaired that the host is at risk for opportunistic infections; this stage is generally defined as a CD4 count below 200 or the presence of an opportunistic infection (for example, *Pneumocystis* pneumonia). Injection drug users do not appear to be at any higher risk for progression to AIDS (25), but they are at high risk for other infections, particularly pneumonia and endocarditis (26).

The introduction of potent three-drug combinations of antiretroviral medications in 1996 ("highly active antiretroviral therapy," or HAART) has dramatically improved survival and quality of life for those who have access to these medications (27). While those who acquired the infection through injection drug use do benefit from treatment (28), there are indications that they may not benefit as much as others do. Some have observed that success rates with HAART (as defined by complete suppression of HIV) are poorer with injection drug users than with other patients (29); this is probably due to poorer adherence with these unforgiving regimens.

Needle exchange programs may help to reduce the risk of HIV transmission (30), and some have advocated that physicians write prescriptions for needles and syringes for addicts who would not otherwise have access to them. Patients on methadone maintenance appear to be at lower risk for acquiring the infection than drug users who are not in treatment (31).

Syphilis and Other STDs

Although injection drug use does not directly cause sexually transmitted diseases (STDs), these infections are a concern among this population because of an association between injection drug use and risky behaviors, such as having multiple partners, commercial sex work, or exchanging sex for drugs or money. This appears to be particularly a concern for those who use the stimulants cocaine and methamphetamine (32). A number of studies indicate that injection drug users are at increased risk for syphilis (33), particularly those who trade sex for money or drugs (34). Injection drug use also appears to be associated with an increased risk of other STDs, such as gonorrhea (35) and chlamydia (36). It is probably prudent to routinely test injection drug users for these STDs (i.e., serum RPR/VDRL and urine, endocervical, or endourethral specimen for gonorrhea and chlamydia); at the very minimum, these individuals should be questioned about their sexual practices and those who engage in high-risk sexual behavior tested (and counseled).

Cutaneous Complications

Injection drug users are at high risk for developing skin and soft tissue infections. In one community-based study of injection drug users in San Francisco, 32% reported having an abscess or cellulitis; many of them had treated themselves by lancing the abscess or taking antibiotics they had purchased on the street. In this study, subcutaneous or intramuscular injection ("skin-popping") and less experience with use were associated with these infections (37). In a case-control study of injection drug users, development of an abscess that required drainage was associated with skin-popping and use of speedballs (heroin and cocaine mixture); cleaning the skin with alcohol appeared to have a protective effect (38). Many injection drug users treat themselves with antibiotics they purchase on the street. As a result, they are at increased risk of carrying—and being infected with—antibiotic-resistant organisms (39). For those who have recurrent soft tissue infections, intranasal mupirocin may help eradicate carriage of staph aureus and prevent further infections, though this has not been demonstrated in a clinical trial (40).

While the treatment of cellulitis and abscesses is relatively straightforward, injection drug users are also at risk for necrotizing soft tissue infections that require much more aggressive surgical management and may be difficult to recognize on clinical exam. A study of patients treated at San Francisco General Hospital over 5 years reported that among 3560 injection drug users who underwent incision and drainage of an abscess, 30 (0.8%) of these were found to have necrotizing soft tissue infections and required wide debridement or amputation—20% of them died (41).

Injection drug users are also at risk for developing chronic wounds in the upper or lower extremities. Treatment requires cessation of the drug use and (often prolonged) wound care; skin grafting may be helpful in some cases.

Neuromuscular Complications

Botulism

Although botulism is generally a food-borne illness, the organism can also be introduced through subcutaneous injection and has been seen in injection drug users (42). The organism, *C. botulinum,* produces an endotoxin that blocks transmission at the neuromuscular junction, leading to descending paralysis and even death. Treatment is generally supportive; botulinum anti-toxin may be beneficial.

Tetanus

Tetanus is caused by a toxin-producing anaerobic bacteria, *Clostridium tetani,* that can result in localized or generalized muscles spasms. The spores of this organism are present in soil and can enter the body through cutaneous wounds. One of the first (if not *the* first) descriptions of intravenous drug use in the medical literature was an 1876 report of a woman who developed tetanus as a result (43). While tetanus is quite rare in the United States (about 40 cases/year), injection drug users have been noted to be at risk and accounted for 15% of the cases (44). Tetanus can be prevented by immunization; the disease is generally seen in those who have not been adequately vaccinated.

Pulmonary Complications

Injection drug users who inject talc-containing crushed tablets are at risk for pulmonary granulomatosis, which may lead to pulmonary hypertension (45) and chronic obstructive lung disease (46). This complication has been generally (but not exclusively) associated with intravenous methylphenidate (Ritalin) use.

Injection heroin users have been noted to sometimes develop non-cardiogenic pulmonary edema, generally in the setting of overdose. In one series, of 1278 heroin overdoses treated at one hospital, 27 (2.1%) developed pulmonary edema as a complication and nine required mechanical ventilation; most recovered within 24 hours (47). In addition, users who inject into their neck are at risk for pneumothorax (48).

Cardiovascular Complications

Endocarditis

Endocarditis is one of the most serious complications of injection drug use. In one prospective study of 2529 injection drug users, the incidence of endocarditis was 7 cases/1000 person-years and was higher among those with HIV infection, a history of previous endocarditis, and women (49). Cocaine use in particular also appears to increase the risk of this complication (50). Endocarditis is a concern when evaluating an injection drug user with an acute febrile illness. Unfortunately, clinical history, examination, and routine laboratory tests are not reliable for ruling out this potentially lethal complication, and we must rely on blood cultures (51, 52). *Staph aureus* is by far the most common organism (about 70% of cases) followed by streptococci (8%) (53). The tricuspid valve is infected in about 50% of these cases, followed by the aortic valve (25%) and mitral valve (20%). Endocarditis may be complicated by septic emboli to the lungs (in right-sided infections) or to the brain, extremities, kidneys, or viscera (in left-sided cases). Persons with endocarditis may also develop osteomyelitis or septic arthritis, and the pain from these complications may be the presenting symptom of this illness (54). The risk of mortality is increased with large vegetations (>2.0

cm) (55), aortic valve involvement (56), and severe immunosup-pression due to HIV infection (i.e., CD4 count <200) (57).

The standard treatment for endocarditis is 2–6 weeks of in-travenous antibiotics, the type of antibiotic and duration de-pending on the organism, location, and presence of other complications. Oral antibiotics may be an option in some right-sided cases if intravenous treatment is not feasible (58). Surgery is generally indicated for severe valvular insufficiency, persist-ent systemic embolization, or persistent sepsis from a ring or myocardial abscess. In one series of surgical treatment for 80 in-jection drug users with endocarditis, 30-day surgical mortality was 7.5% and 5-year survival was 70% (59).

Simple measures, such as cleaning the skin, may reduce the risk of endocarditis in injection drug users (60). Of course, the most effective prevention measure is effective addiction treat-ment.

Myocarditis

Injection drug users also appear to be at risk for myocarditis, which can lead to cardiomyopathy and even sudden death (61).

Vascular Complications

Injection drug users are also at risk for endovascular compli-cations in locations other than the cardiac valves. These include venous thrombosis (62), septic thrombophlebitis, or infected pseudoaneurysms (63). Injection drug users may also develop ar-terial thrombosis and upper-extremity ischemia from inadver-tent injection into an artery (64, 65).

Renal Complications

In the 1970s and 1980s, an association was observed between injection heroin use and nephrotic syndrome (so-called heroin nephropathy), sometimes leading to end stage renal disease. These patients were generally African-American men and patho-logic evaluation revealed sclerosing glomerulonephritis (66). The etiology of this condition has never been clearly established and may well have been due to an adulterant mixed with the heroin; it appears that the problem has declined since then (67), but it may still account for some new cases of end-stage renal disease (68). Hepatitis C may also be responsible for some of the renal disease seen in injection drug users (69).

Addicts who inject into their subcutaneous tissues, generally when veins are no longer accessible (so-called skin-poppers), can develop chronic skin infections or wounds that may lead to amyloidosis and renal failure (70). In addition, addicts who overdose may develop renal failure due to rhabdomyolysis and myoglobinuria (71).

MEDICAL CARE OF PATIENTS ON METHADONE

Methadone maintenance has become a common treatment modality for opioid dependence; there are approximately 150,000 Americans receiving methadone from almost 700 treat-ment programs (72). Some individuals remain on this treatment for years and even decades. In this section, we will try to address a number of special issues that arise in caring for individuals on methadone maintenance. These include long-term medical complications, drug interactions, pain management, and treatment of hospitalized patients on methadone.

Medical Complications

Patients on stable doses of methadone maintenance generally develop a tolerance to the side effects, particularly sedation and respiratory depression. Opioids are associated with relatively few long-term sequelae. However, there are a number of medical complications that are particularly problematic for patients who are on long-term methadone maintenance; these include constipation, hypogonadism, prolonged QT interval, and cognitive impairment. Constipation is briefly discussed in the chapter on opioids.

Experimental and clinical studies have shown that opioids can produce hypogonadotropic hypogonadism; they appear to do this via suppression of gonadotropin-releasing hormone (GnRH) (73). This results in low testosterone levels, impotence, and osteoporosis in men and amenorrhea or irregular menstrual cycles and infertility in women. This effect appears to be dose-dependent (74) and is especially common among individuals receiving intrathecal opioids for pain management (75).

A number of studies have reported that the synthetic opioids methadone and levacetylmethadol (LAAM) are associated with a dose-dependent prolongation of the QT interval (76). This has been linked with reports of syncope and arrhythmia (specifically, torsades de pointes) in some patients (77, 78). In one series of 17 patients on methadone who developed torsades de pointes, the mean dose was 397 mg/day (range 65–1000 mg) and only three had structural heart disease (79). The use of cocaine may trigger this arrhythmia in some individuals on methadone (80). There is also evidence that protease inhibitors, used for the treatment of HIV infection, may also prolong the QT interval, and there are case reports of torsades de pointes associated with their use; some were also on methadone, suggesting that the risk may be increased by the concurrent use of the two agents (**81**).

Another possible complication of methadone maintenance is cognitive impairment. A study of subjects on methadone maintenance (mean dose of 67 mg) found significantly impaired performance on cognitive tests when compared with healthy, non-drug-abusing controls; psychomotor slowing appeared to be the most prominent impairment (82). A follow-up study comparing these with abstinent drug abusers found that their performance fell in between the non-drug abusers and those on methadone, suggesting that the observed impairments on methadone are not entirely due to prior drug use (83). On the other hand, a study of simulated driving performance of individuals on methadone, levomethadyl acetate (LAAM), and buprenorphine maintenance found no impairment when compared with non-drug-using controls; however, the methadone doses in this study were relatively modest (mean 48 mg) (84). Of note, a recent study of opioid addicts who were given buprenorphine found minimal (if any) cognitive effects (85), but more research needs to be done on its effects in comparison with methadone.

Drug Interactions

Practitioners who care for patients on methadone maintenance must be aware of possible drug interactions. The most obvious of these is the use of other opioids or opioid antagonists. Table 15.1 lists some other drugs that may affect the serum levels or drug effects of methadone. Methadone is metabolized by the cytochrome P450 system; the isoenzymes CYP3A4, CYP2C8, and CYP2D6 appear the most important in this process (86). However, there is a great deal of genetic variation in the p450 activity that leads to variations in drug effects and the impact of drug-drug interactions (87). Nevertheless, inhibitors of these enzymes may increase methadone levels, and inducers of these enzymes will tend to lower levels. Levomethadyl acetate (LAAM), which is also used for opioid maintenance treatment, is likewise metabolized by the p450 system (88), so these interactions should be taken into consideration for individuals on this treatment as well. In many

Table 15.1.   Drugs that may interact with methadone

Drugs That May *Increase* Methadone Effects/Levels

Antibiotics
 Ciprofloxacin (Cipro)
 Macrolide antibiotics— erythromycin, clarithromycin (Biaxin), azithromycin (Zithromax), etc.

Antifungal Agents
 Azoles—fluconazole (Diflucan), itraconazole (Sporanox), ketoconazole (Nizoral), etc.

Antidepressants
 Fluvoxamine (Luvox)
 Paroxetine (Paxil)
 Sertraline (Zoloft)

Others
 Cimetidine (Tagamet)

Drugs That May *Decrease* Methadone Effects/Levels

Antibiotics
 Rifampin (Rifadin, Rimactane)
 Rifapentine (Priftin)

Antiretroviral Agents
 Efavirenz (Sustiva)
 Fosamprenavir (Lexiva)
 Nevirapine (Viramune)
 Nelfinavir (Viracept)
 Ritonavir (Norvir, Kaletra)

Table 15.1. *Continued*

Drugs That May *Decrease* Methadone Effects/Levels

Antiepileptic Agents

Carbamazepine (Carbatrol, Tegretol)

Fosphenytoin (Cerebyx)

Phenytoin (Dilantin, Phenytek)

Phenobarbital

Opioid Antagonists

Buprenorphine (Buprenex, Subutex, Suboxone)

Pentazocine (Talwin)

Naloxone (Narcan)

Naltrexone (Revia)

Nalmefene (Revex)

Other Agents

Ammonium Chloride

Metyrapone

Risperidone (Risperdal)

Note: Brand names are in parentheses. Many of these interactions are not clinically significant; see text for more details.

cases, these interactions produce only modest changes and are not clinically significant. However, in other cases, individuals may experience withdrawal symptoms or toxicity and dose modification may be necessary.

These drug interactions are particularly important for HIV-infected opioid addicts on methadone who require antiretroviral treatment; the non-nucleoside reverse transcriptase inhibitors (NNRTIs) efavirenz (**89**) and nevirapine (**90**) lower methadone levels and frequently precipitate withdrawal symptoms. Furthermore, a number of protease inhibitors appear to reduce serum methadone levels, including ritonavir, nelfinavir, and amprenavir (and its prodrug, fosamprenavir) (91), but this does not appear to be as clinically significant. The antimicrobial rifampin, which is frequently used for treatment of tuberculosis, also appears to lower methadone levels and has been reported to precipitate withdrawal symptoms (**92**); however, a related agent, rifabutin, does not seem to have this effect (93). In addition, a number of antiepileptic drugs (phenytoin [94], phenobarbital [95], and carbamazepine [96]) reduce methadone levels and have been reported to cause withdrawal symptoms. Fosphenytoin, which is a prodrug of phenytoin, probably has a similar effect. Finally, the antipsychotic risperidone has been reported to have caused withdrawal in two individuals on methadone maintenance (97).

On the other hand, a number of drugs may increase methadone levels by inhibiting its metabolism. This effect, which is generally mild and of limited clinical significance, has been noted with

SSRI antidepressants sertraline (**98**) and paroxetine (99) but appears to be most significant with fluvoxamine (100). In contrast, another SSRI, fluoxetine, does not appear to have any effect on methadone levels (101). The azole antifungal agents (ketoconazole, fluconazole, itraconazole, voriconazole) are cytochrome p450 inhibitors (102) and may increase methadone levels; however, we were unable to find any reports that indicate that this effect is clinically significant and, in our own clinical practice, we have not observed any opioid toxicity among patients on methadone who required antifungal treatment. The macrolide antibiotics (especially erythromycin) are also P450 inhibitors and may increase methadone levels, but again we have not been able to find any reports on the clinical significance of this interaction for patients on methadone and have not observed any ill effects with the use of clarithromycin or azithromycin in this population. Finally, the antibiotic ciprofloxacin has been reported (in one case) to have led to clinically significant opioid toxicity in an individual on chronic methadone (103).

While there is no medication that is absolutely contraindicated for an individual on methadone (except the opioid antagonists naltrexone, nalmefene, or naloxone outside of the setting of overdose), practitioners should remain vigilant for possible interactions and coordinate care with the patient's methadone program when there is a potential for interaction. Measuring trough serum methadone levels may be helpful to determine whether a dose adjustment is needed, especially when a patient reports continued withdrawal symptoms despite a dose increase. However, methadone levels do not always correlate with its therapeutic effect; while one study found no correlation between trough levels of methadone (or its metabolite) and withdrawal symptoms or illicit heroin use (104), another study suggested that a level of 100 ng/ml is generally adequate (105).

A number of other medications do not interact directly with methadone metabolism but should be avoided in patients on methadone maintenance. First and foremost among these are the benzodiazepines, which enhance the effects (and toxicity) of methadone and are frequently abused by individuals on methadone maintenance (**106**). Some individuals may have an anxiety disorder or some other condition that requires chronic benzodiazepine use, but it is probably best that this be done only under the close supervision of a mental health professional. Clonidine is also abused by individuals on methadone and should be avoided, even for those who have hypertension. The antiemetics promethazine (Phenergan) and prochlorperazine (Compazine) also potentiate the sedative effects of methadone and should also be avoided.

Pain Management

The approach to the treatment of pain in patients on methadone maintenance is generally the same as with other patients, with a few caveats. In general, practitioners should avoid prescribing opioids, particularly for patients with chronic pain, since there is a substantial risk of abuse or diversion. Chronic severe pain is a common problem among clients on methadone programs, and many of them take prescribed opioids in addition to their methadone (107). There is some evidence that use of chronic opioids may induce hyperalgesia and relative pain intolerance (108). In general, it is best to focus on non-pharmacological treatments and non-opioid analgesics for treatment of chronic pain. If these are not effective, an increase in methadone dosage may help, particularly if the program allows them to split their dose (i.e., divide it into two or three doses). Many programs are willing to work with primary care practitioners to help their clients and will allow take-home dosages if the client has been compliant with the treatment program.

Caring for Hospitalized Patients on Methadone Maintenance

A number of issues arise in the management of patients on methadone who are hospitalized or require surgery. In general, patients on methadone who require surgery or hospitalization should be continued on their regular dose after this has been confirmed by their program. They can be given supplemental opioid analgesics, if necessary; however, their methadone dose should not be altered without coordinating changes with their treatment program. Patients on methadone have high tolerance to opioids and generally require higher-than-usual doses at more frequent intervals. Buprenorphine and pentazocine should be avoided in patients on methadone because they may precipitate withdrawal syndrome due to their antagonistic effects.

If the patient is unable to take oral medications, methadone can be given parenterally; two-thirds of the regular daily dose can be given intramuscularly in two divided doses (109). For example, someone on 100 mg per day of methadone could be given 30 mg intramuscularly twice daily instead.

TREATING PAIN IN THE OPIOID ADDICT

Treating pain in opioid addicts is a difficult task for even the most experienced health care providers. On one hand, it is wrong to make someone needlessly suffer because of his or her addiction. On the other hand, health care providers should be conscious of the fact that opioid addicts may be abusing or diverting the medication they are given and that the nature of addiction is such that addicts will often go to great lengths to obtain these drugs. Health care providers should resist the temptation to *punish* addicts for their addiction by denying them adequate palliative treatment. It is important to remember that withholding opioid analgesics from an opioid addict will not cure them of their addiction and that needlessly giving them opioids will not make their addiction worse.

In general, we believe that the best policy is to "trust but verify"; in other words, give the patient the benefit of the doubt and do your best to treat their pain, but be vigilant for signs of abuse and willing to act when a patient shows these signs. As with other patients, depending on the nature of the problem, it may be appropriate to begin treatment with opioids, or to start with other agents and then move on to opioids if they are not effective. In the inpatient setting, the dosage can be titrated quickly and the patient's response assessed. However, in the ambulatory setting, assessment of response is more difficult and the risk of diversion much higher. When prescribing opioids to someone with active opioid addiction or to someone who is in recovery, it is important to be honest and up front about your concerns and to understand the patient's expectations and be clear about your expectations at the beginning of treatment. A "pain contract" may be a useful tool to document this discussion (see Figure 14.1). It is probably prudent to give limited amounts of medication for shorter periods of time and assess these patients more frequently. As with other patients, providers should be on the lookout for signs of prescription drug abuse; this is discussed further in the chapter on this topic (Chapter 14).

For active opioid addicts with acute pain (an acute fracture, for example), intravenous administration of an opioid such as morphine would be appropriate. Patient-controlled analgesia (PCA) is often very effective. Given their high tolerance to opioids, addicts may require higher doses of medication than others do and will be less susceptible to the side effects. If the pain is expected to last more than a few days, it would be appropriate to begin a long-acting opioid. In general, we find that it is best to minimize the use of "as-needed medication" and to rely more on long-acting medication or standing doses of medications to provide better symptom control and avoid a focus on immediate relief. The patient should always be included in the decision-making process and be informed of any changes in advance.

Buprenorphine is generally not a good choice for treatment of acute pain, but it may be utilized in some situations where detoxification is a concurrent goal—for example, an opioid addict with an abscess or cellulitis who wishes to be detoxified. An intramuscular dose of 0.3 mg of buprenorphine, or a 4 mg sublingual dose, is roughly equivalent to 10 mg of morphine. In cases where the patient is experiencing severe pain or where detoxification is not a goal (for example, an addict on methadone maintenance), buprenorphine would not be the treatment of choice.

Treating opioid addicts who have chronic pain is a more difficult task. One strategy is to enroll them in a methadone maintenance program so that they can receive opioids in a controlled and supervised manner. Methadone is generally not effective for 24 hours as an analgesic, so this may need to be supplemented by other medications. Addicts who earn take-home dosages for good behavior can split their dose to get more even analgesic effect. Buprenorphine also has analgesic effect, but current guidelines recommend against its use for treatment of chronic pain. In our experience, it can provide some relief to individuals who have mild to moderate pain (osteoarthritis of the knees, for example), but it would probably not be effective for individuals who require high doses of opioids for pain relief.

DEALING WITH DIFFICULT PATIENTS

Ideally patients and care providers are allied in a mutually agreed-upon quest for common goals. However, there are times (not infrequently) when this does not occur; in some of these cases, the patient may evoke feelings of frustration and even anger among care providers. These individuals are often called "difficult" (or "problem") patients and frequently consume a great deal of health care providers' time and energy ("the thick chart syndrome"). There are a number of conditions that are associated with being a "difficult patient," including somatoform disorder, anxiety or panic disorder, dysthymia or depression, and alcohol abuse or dependence (110). Unrecognized personality disorders appear to be quite common among these patients (111). Substance abuse is a fairly common problem among these difficult patients, at least partly because of the association between substance use and personality disorders.

There is little empirical data on how best to manage difficult patients, but there are some commonsense strategies that we feel are helpful. First, it is important to establish rapport and win the trust of the patient. This means listening and showing empathy for the patient's problems no matter how trivial they may seem; trying to downplay or dismiss their complaints is a setup for an adversarial relationship. It is also important to understand the patient's goals and expectations; this does not mean that you have to acquiesce to all their demands, but you cannot come up with a mutually acceptable plan of action unless you address their concerns.

Managing Manipulative Behavior

All patients should be treated with honesty and respect. It is natural for patients to bring certain expectations and desires to their interactions with health care professionals, and there is nothing wrong with them pursuing these goals, especially when this is done through open and honest dialogue. In general, "manipulative behavior" is when patients use "inappropriate" tactics to achieve their goals, such as lying, deception, threats (or flattery), and so on. Generally this occurs when patients feel that their goals and agenda are at odds with their health care providers'. Most health care providers are trained to work with patients and do what is best for them, but many are ill prepared to deal with situations where the patient appears to be working at odds with these goals.

Manipulative behavior is probably more common among addicts, but these individuals should not be stereotyped in this fashion. Manipulative behavior is a characteristic of individuals with personality disorder (particularly borderline, narcissistic, and antisocial personality disorders) (112) and, as noted above, substance abuse is also associated with this disorder. There are probably a number of other reasons why addicts may resort to manipulative behavior. Addiction is a powerful force and the compulsion to continue this leads addicts to behave in ways they would probably not otherwise. As a result, addicts may employ lying and deception in their interactions with others, either to obtain their substance of choice or to hide their addiction. Furthermore, there is often a mistrust of health care professionals among addicts, and they may feel that they can get the care they need only through manipulative behaviors. It is important to remember that manipulative behavior may be "appropriate" and normal for persons who are dealing with a hostile system.

As with any problem, prevention is the best strategy. We feel that a number of measures can help prevent this kind of behavior. The first preventive measure is to address their addiction and its complications in a nonjudgmental and compassionate manner; this will help patients to be honest and forthright about their addiction and should help lower barriers for them to seek help for their addiction when they need it. The second preventive measure is to be honest and up front with the patient; this will help to foster trust. This may seem overly obvious and many health care practitioners would argue that they are always honest, but we have observed many situations where this has not been the case. When dealing with addicts who appear to be making unreasonable demands, some practitioners find it easier to avoid these patients and make decisions without speaking to them; we have even seen situations where patients have been deceived about the medications they are receiving. We believe that this approach just increases mistrust and encourages further manipulative behavior. As noted earlier, "manipulation" is a natural and normal response to a hostile and authoritarian system, so creating that sort of environment will only foster manipulative behavior.

However, even when treated with respect and honesty, some patients may still choose to use manipulative behavior to get what they want. This sort of behavior often creates feelings of anger among care providers. It is important to always keep focused on the best interests of the patient, even when you are upset or frustrated with them, and to resist the temptation to punish them. The first step in dealing with a manipulative or demanding patient is to step back and consider whether the patient may have legitimate unmet needs; this does not condone manipulative behavior, but these needs should be addressed. For example, a patient who demands more pain medication and is labeled as "drug-seeking" may, in fact, be undertreated. When dealing with patients who are being manipulative, it is best to directly address this behavior with them; identify the specific problem behavior and tell them why you find it unacceptable, and then try to develop a mutually acceptable plan for their subsequent treatment and how their problems will be dealt with in the future. It may be helpful to write down your agreement with the patient to document this discussion and reinforce its importance with him or her. It is also important that members of the health care team be in agreement with one another about the treatment plan and that one person be responsible for important decisions (to avoid "splitting").

At times, the level of behavior may be such that it would be appropriate to terminate your relationship with the patient (for example, personal threats), but it is important that this be done only when there is no other option and not just to get rid of a difficult patient. In these situations, it is essential that the patient be given assistance to find another source of care and be provided continued care until that transfer can occur.

Refusal of Care

Sometimes the disagreement between health care providers and patients can lead to situations where the patient refuses to comply with the recommended treatment. A number of studies indicate that patients with substance abuse problems are less likely to comply with recommended treatment (113). Furthermore, alcohol- and drug-related problems are associated with leaving hospitals against medical advice (114, 115). This is of particular concern during situations where the patient has an acute life-threatening illness and refuses to comply with a potentially lifesaving treatment. One example is the injection drug user hospitalized for endocarditis who wishes to leave the hospital and refuses to complete a course of intravenous antibiotics. The first step should be to try to understand why the patient wishes to leave and to see if (reasonable) accommodations can be made so that the patient can complete his or her treatment. Very often, refusal of care occurs during time of conflict or disagreement between patient and care providers, and the temptation to simply rid oneself of a problem patient must be resisted. In addition, it is important to assess whether the patient is competent to make this decision and able to understand the risks and options. If so, the patient should be informed of the risks he or she is taking and this discussion carefully documented. If the patient still insists on leaving, the patient should not be abandoned; alternative treatment should be offered (for example, oral antibiotics) and the patient given the option to return for further treatment.

Assessment of a patient's competence or decision-making capacity is always difficult; there is not a clear line that separates "competence" from "incompetence" or, for that matter, "treatment" from "nontreatment." Moreover, there are issues particular to addicts that further complicate these decisions. The first problem is acute intoxication or delirium; this is particularly an issue for alcoholics. In these situations, it may be best to hold the patient until the acute phase has cleared, especially if the patient has an acute medical problem. The second problem is the limited ability of someone who has an addiction to make rational and appropriate choices, even when he or she is not intoxicated or delirious. Some have argued that addicts who wish to leave against medical advice when under treatment for a life-threatening illness are, almost by definition, incompetent, since their addiction prevents them from making rational choices (116). On the other hand, we all make choices that may seem "irrational" to others or may be motivated by forces beyond our control. For example, we generally respect the wishes of those who refuse blood transfusion on religious grounds, even though this may not seem "rational" to us. Nonetheless, involuntary commitment may be an option if it is felt that the patient is at great risk and is not competent to make decisions regarding his or her care, or it may be used when an individual is a potential hazard to others, such as a person with tuberculosis who does not comply with treatment. However, this should always be the last resort and must be balanced with consideration for patient autonomy.

REFERENCES

1. Substance Abuse and Mental Health Services Administration. 2004. Results from the 2003 National Survey on Drug Use and

Health: National Findings (Office of Applied Studies, NSDUH Series H-25, DHHS Publication No. SMA 04-3964). Rockville, MD.

2. Copeland, L., J. Budd, J. R. Robertson, and R. A. Elton. 2004. Changing patterns in causes of death in a cohort of injecting drug users, 1980-2001. *Arch. Intern. Med.* 164:1214–1220.

3. Levine, O. S., D. Vlahov, J. Koehler, et al. 1995. Seroepidemiology of hepatitis B virus in a population of injection drug users. Association with drug injection patterns. *Am. J. Epidemiol.* 142:331–341.

4. Gjeruldsen, S. R., B. Myrang, and S. Opjordsmoen. 2003. A 25-year follow-up study of drug addicts hospitalised for acute hepatitis: Present and past morbidity. *Eur. Addict. Res.* 9:80–86.

5. Torbenson, M., R. Kannangai, J. Astemborski, et al. 2004. High prevalence of occult hepatitis B in Baltimore injection drug users. *Hepatology* 39:51–57.

6. Hagan, H., D. C. DesJarlais, S. R. Friedman, et al. 1995. Reduced risk of hepatitis B and hepatitis C among injection drug users in the Tacoma Syringe exchange program. *Am. J. Pub. Health* 85:1531–1537.

7. Fingerhood, M. I., D. R. Jasinski, and J. T. Sullivan. 1993. Prevalence of hepatitis C in a chemically dependent population. *Arch. Intern. Med.* 153:2025–2030.

8. Lorvick, J., A. H. Kral, K. Seal, et al. 2001. Prevalence and duration of hepatitis C among injection drug users in San Francisco, Calif. *Am. J. Pub. Health* 91:46–47.

9. Koblin, B. A., S. H. Factor, Y. Wu, and D. Vlahov. 2003. Hepatitis C virus infection among noninjecting drug users in New York City. *J. Med. Virol.* 70:387–390.

10. Alter, M. J., D. Kruszon-Moran, O. V. Nainan, et al. 1999. The prevalence of hepatitis C virus infection in the United States, 1988 through 1994. *N. Engl. J. Med.* 341:556–562.

11. McMahon, J. M., M. Simm, D. Milano, and M. Clatts. 2004. Detection of hepatitis C virus in the nasal secretions of an intranasal drug-user. *Ann. Clin. Microbiol. Antimicrob.* 3:6

12. Gerlach, J. T., H. M. Diepolder, R. Zachoval, et al. 2003. Acute hepatitis C: High rate of both spontaneous clearance and treatment-induced viral clearance. *Gastroenterology* 125:80–88.

13. Mehta, S. H., A. Cox, D. R. Hoover, et al. 2002. Protection against persistence of hepatitis C. *Lancet* 359:1478–1483.

14. Gumber, S. C., and S. Chopra. 1995. Hepatitis C: A multifaceted disease. Review of extrahepatic manifestations. *Ann. Intern. Med.* 123:615–620.

15. Thomas, D. L., J. Astemborski, R. M. Rai, et al. 2000. The natural history of hepatitis C: Host, viral, and environmental factors. *JAMA* 284:450–456.

16. Fried, M. W., M. L. Shiffman, K. R. Reddy, et al. 2002. Peginterferon alpha-2a plus ribavarin for chronic hepatitis c virus infection. *N. Engl. J. Med.* 347:975–982.

17. Van Thiel, D. H., A. Anantharaju, and S. Creech. 2003. Response to treatment of hepatitis C in individuals with a recent history of intravenous drug abuse. *Am. J. Gastroenterol.* 98:2281–2288.

18. Koch, M., and P. Banys. 2001. Liver transplantation and opioid dependence. *JAMA* 285:1056–1058.

19. Liu, L. U., T. D. Schiano, N. Lau, et al. 2003. Survival and risk of recidivism in methadone-dependent patients undergoing liver transplantation. *Am. J. Transplant.* 3:1273–1277.

20. Kapadia, F., D. Vlahov, D. C. DesJarlais, et al. 2002. Does bleach disinfection of syringes protect against hepatitis C infection among young adult injection drug users? *Epidemiology* 13:738–741.

21. Centers for Disease Control and Prevention. 2002. *HIV/AIDS Surveillance Report* 14:1–20.

22. Garfein, R. S., D. Vlahov, N. Galai, et al. 1996. Viral infections in short-term injection drug users: The prevalence of the hepatitis C, hepatitis B, human immunodeficiency, and human T-lymphotrophic viruses. *Am. J. Pub. Health* 86:655–661.

23. Centers for Disease Control and Prevention. 2004. Diagnoses of HIV/AIDS—32 states 2000–2003. *MMWR* 53:1106–1110.

24. Daar, E. S., S. Little, J. Pitt, et al. 2001. Diagnosis of primary HIV-1 infection. *Ann. Intern. Med.* 135:25–29.

25. Chaisson, R. E., J. C. Kerully, and R. D. Moore. 1995. Race, sex, drug use, and the risk of progression of human immunodeficiency virus disease. *N. Engl. J. Med.* 333:751–756.

26. Selwyn, P. A., P. Alcabes, D. Hartel, et al. 1992. Clinical manifestations and predictors of disease progression in drug users with human immunodeficiency virus infection. *N. Engl. J. Med.* 327:1697–1709.

27. Detels, R., A. Muñoz, G. McFarlane, et al. 1998. Effectiveness of potent antiretroviral therapy on time to AIDS and death in men with known HIV infection duration. *JAMA* 280:1497–1503.

28. Whitman, S., J. Murphy, M. Cohen, and R. Sherer. 2000. Marked declines in human immunodeficiency virus-related mortality in Chicago in women, African Americans, Hispanics, young adults, and injection drug users, from 1995 through 1997. *Arch. Intern. Med.* 160:365–369.

29. Lucas, G. M., R. E. Chiasson, and R. D. Moore. 1998. Highly active antiretroviral therapy in a large urban clinic: Risk factors for virologic failure and adverse drug reactions. *Ann. Intern. Med.* 131:81–87.

30. Heimer, R., E. H. Kaplan, K. Khoshnood, et al. 1995. Needle exchange decreases the prevalence of HIV-1 proviral DNA in returned syringes in New Haven, Connecticut. *Am. J. Med.* 98:596–598.

31. Novick, D. M., H. Joseph, T. S. Croxson, et al. 1990. Absence of antibody to human immunodeficiency virus in long-term, socially rehabilitated methadone maintenance patients. *Arch. Intern. Med.* 150:97–99.

32. Hudgins, R., J. McCusker, and A. Stoddard. 1995. Cocaine use and risky injection and sexual behaviors. *Drug Alcohol Depend.* 37:7–14.

33. Gourevitch, M. N., D. Hartel, E. E. Schoenbaum, et al. 1996. A prospective study of syphilis and HIV infection among injection drug users receiving methadone in the Bronx, NY. *Am. J. Pub. Health* 86:1112–1115.

34. López-Zetina, J., W. Ford, M. Weber, et al. 2000. Predictors of syphilis seroreactivity and prevalence of HIV among street recruited injection drug users in Los Angeles County, 1994–6. *Sex. Transm. Inf.* 76:462–469.

35. Upchurch, D. M., W. E. Brady, C. A. Reichart, E. W. Hook III. 1990. Behavioral contributions to acquisition of gonorrhea in pa-

tients attending an inner city sexually transmitted disease clinic. *J. Infect. Dis.* 161:938–941.

36. Latka, M., J. Ahern, R. S. Garfein, et al. 2001. Prevalence, incidence, and correlates of chlamydia and gonorrhea among young adult injection drug users. *J. Subst. Abuse* 13:73–88.

37. Binswanger, I. A., A. H. Kral, R. N. Blumenthal, et al. 2000. High prevalence of abscesses and cellulitis among community-recruited injection drug users in San Francisco. *Clin. Infect. Dis.* 30:579–581.

38. Murphy, E. L., D. DeVita, H. Liu, et al. 2001. Risk factors for skin and soft-tissue abscesses among injection drug users: A case control study. *Clin. Infect. Dis.* 33:35–40.

39. Charlebois, E. D., D. R. Bangsberg, N. J. Moss, et al. 2002. Population-based community prevalence of methicillin-resistant Staphylococcus aureus in the urban poor of San Francisco. *Clin. Infect. Dis.* 34:425–433.

40. Kluytmans, J. A., and H. F. Wertheim. 2005. Nasal carriage of Staphylococcus aureus and prevention of nosocomial infections. *Infection* 33:3–8.

41. Callahan, T. E., W. P. Schecter, and J. K. Horn. 1998. Necrotizing soft tissue infection masquerading as cutaneous abscess following illicit drug injection. *Arch. Surg.* 133:812–819.

42. Merrison, A. F., K. E. Chidley, J. Dunnett, and K. A. Sieradzan. 2002. Wound botulism associated with subcutaneous drug use. *BMJ* 325:1020–1021.

43. Anonymous. 1876. Tetanus after hypodermic injection of morphia. *Lancet* 108:873.

44. Pascual, F. B., E. L. McGinley, L. R. Zanardi, et al. 2003. Tetanus surveillance—United States 1998–2000. *MMWR* 52(SS08):1–8.

45. Arnett, E. N., W. E. Battle, J. V. Russo, and W. C. Roberts. 1976. Intravenous injection of talc-containing drugs intended for oral use. A cause of pulmonary granulomatosis and pulmonary hypertension. *Am. J. Med.* 60:711–718.

46. Sherman, C. B., I. D. Hudson, and D. J. Pierson. 1987. Severe precocious emphysema in intravenous methylphenidate (Ritalin) abusers. *Chest* 92:1085–1087.

47. Sporer, K. A., and E. Dorn. 2001. Heroin-related noncardiogenic pulmonary edema: A case series. *Chest* 120:1628–1632.

48. Lewis, J. W., N. Groux, J. P. Elliot, et al. 1980. Complications of attempted central venous injections performed by drug abusers. *Chest* 78:613–617.

49. Wilson, L. E., D. L. Thomas, J. Astemborski, et al. 2002. Prospective study of infective endocarditis among injection drug users. *J. Infect. Dis.* 185:1761–1766.

50. Chambers, H. F., D. L. Morris, M. G. Täuber, and G. Modin. 1987. Cocaine use and the risk for endocarditis in intravenous drug users. *Ann. Intern. Med.* 106:833–836.

51. Marantz, P. R., M. Linzer, C. L. Feiner, et al. 1987. Inability to predict diagnosis in febrile drug abusers. *Ann. Intern. Med.* 106:823–828.

52. Samet, J. H., A. Shevitz, J. Fowle, and D. E. Singer. 1990. Hospitalization decision in febrile intravenous drug users. *Am. J. Med.* 89:53–57.

53. Moreillon, P., and Y. Que. 2004. Infective endocarditis. *Lancet* 363:139–149.

54. Sapico, F. L., J. A. Liquete, and R. J. Sarma. 1996. Bone and joint infections in patients with infective endocarditis: Review of a 4-year experience. *Clin. Infect. Dis.* 22:783–787.

55. Hecht, S. R., and M. Berger. 1992. Right-sided endocarditis in intravenous drug users: Prognostic features in 102 episodes. *Ann. Intern. Med.* 117:560–566.

56. Matthew, J., T. Addai, A. Anand, et al. 1995. Clinical features, site of involvement, bacteriologic findings, and outcome of infective endocarditis in intravenous drug users. *Arch. Intern. Med.* 155:1641–1648.

57. Ribera, E., J. Miró, E. Cortés, et al. 1998. Influence of human immunodeficiency virus 1 infection and degree of immunosuppression in the clinical characteristics and outcome of infective endocarditis in intravenous drug users. *Arch. Intern. Med.* 158:2043–2050.

58. Heldman, A. W., T. V. Hartert, S. C. Ray, et al. 1996. Oral antibiotic treatment of right-sided staphylococcal endocarditis in injection drug users: Prospective randomized comparison with parenteral therapy. *Am. J. Med.* 101:68–76.

59. Mathew, J., G. Abreo, K. Namburi, et al. 1995. Results of surgical treatment for infective endocarditis in intravenous drug users. *Chest* 106:73–77.

60. Vlahov, D., M. Sullivan, J. Astemborski, and K. E. Nelson. 1992. Bacterial infections and skin cleaning prior injections among intravenous drug users. *Pub. Health Rep.* 107:595–598.

61. Turnicky, R. P., J. Goodin, J. E. Smialek, et al. 1992. Incidental myocarditis with intravenous drug use: The pathology, immunopathology, and potential implications for human immunodeficiency virus-associated myocarditis. *Hum. Pathol.* 23:138–143.

62. Lisse, J. R., C. P. Davis, and M. E. Thurmond-Anderle. 1989. Upper extremity deep venous thrombosis: Increased prevalence due to cocaine abuse. *Am. J. Med.* 87:457–458.

63. Johnson, J. E., C. E. Lucas, A. M. Ledgerwood, and L. A. Jacobs. 1984. Infected pseudoaneurysm. A complication of drug addiction. *Arch. Surg.* 119:1097–1098.

64. Charney, M. A., and P. J. Stern. 1991. Digital ischemia in clandestine intravenous drug users. *J. Hand Surg.* [Am] 16:308–310.

65. Silverman, S. H., and W. W. Turner. 1991. Intraarterial drug abuse: New treatment options. *J. Vasc. Surg.* 14:111–116.

66. Cunningham, E. E., J. R. Brentjens, M. A. Zielezny, et al. 1980. Heroin nephropathy. A clinicopathologic and epidemiologic study. *Am. J. Med.* 68:47–53.

67. Friedman, E. A., and T. K. Tao. 1995. Disappearance of uremia due to heroin-associated nephropathy. *Am. J. Kidney Dis.* 25:689–693.

68. Perneger, T. V., M. J. Klag, and P. K. Whelton. 2001. Recreational drug use: A neglected risk factor for end-stage renal disease. *Am. K. Kid. Dis.* 38:49–56.

69. do Sameiro Faria, M., S. Sampaio, V. Faria, and E. Carvalho. 2003. Nephropathy associated with heroin abuse in Caucasian patients. *Nephrol. Dial. Transplant.* 18:2308–2313.

70. Neugarten, J., G. R. Gallo, J. Buxbaum, et al. 1986. Amyloidosis in subcutaneous heroin abusers ("skin poppers" amyloidosis). *Am. J. Med.* 81:635–640.

71. Rice, E. K., N. M. Isbel, G. J. Becker, et al. 2000. Heroin overdose and myoglobinuric acute renal failure. *J. Clin. Nephrol.* 54:449–454.

72. Substance Abuse and Mental Health Services Administration. 2004. Alcohol and Drug Services Study (ADSS). The National Treatment System: Outpatient Methadone Facilities. Office of Applied Studies. Rockville, MD.

73. Abs, R., J. Verhelst, J. Maeyaert, et al. 2000. Endocrine consequences of long-term intrathecal administration of opioids. *J. Clin. Endocrin. Metabol.* 85:2215–2222.

74. Mendelson, J. H., J. E. Mendelson, and V. D. Patch. 1975. Plasma testosterone levels in heroin addiction and during methadone maintenance. *J. Pharmacol. Exp. Ther.* 192:211–217.

75. Finch, P. M., L. J. Roberts, L. Price, et al. 2000. Hypogonadism in patients treated with intrathecal morphine. *Clin. J. Pain* 16:251–254.

76. Martell, B. A., J. H. Arnsten, B. Ray, and M. N. Gourevitch. 2003. The impact of methadone on cardiac conduction in opiate users. *Ann. Intern. Med.* 139:154–155.

77. Krantz, M. J., I. B. Kutinsky, A. D. Robertson, and P. S. Mehler. 2003. Dose-related effects of methadone on QT prolongation in a series of patients with torsades de pointes. *Pharmacotherapy* 23:802–805.

78. Gil, M., M. Sal, I. Anguera, et al. 2003. QT prolongation and torsades de pointes in patients infected with human immunodeficiency virus and treated with methadone. *Am. J. Card.* 92:995–997.

79. Krantz, M. J., L. Lewkowiez, H. Hays, et al. 2002. Torsades de pointes associated with very-high-dose methadone. *Ann. Intern. Med.* 137:501–504

80. Krantz, M. J., S. B. Rowan, and P. S. Mehler. 2005. Cocaine-related torsade de pointes in a methadone maintenance patient. *J. Addict. Dis.* 24:53–60.

81. Anson, B. D., J. G. R. Weaver, M. J. Ackerman, et al. 2005. Blockade of HERG channels by HIV protease inhibitors. *Lancet* 365:682–686. *Lopinavir, ritonavir, nelfinavir, and saquinavir were found to cause dose-dependent blockade of HERG channels, which can lead to QT prolongation.*

82. Mintzer, M. Z., and M. L. Stitzer. 2002. Cognitive impairment in methadone maintenance patients. *Drug Alcohol Depend.* 67:41–51.

83. Mintzer, M. Z., M. L. Copersino, and M. L. Stitzer. 2005. Opioid abuse and cognitive performance. *Drug Alcohol Depend.* 78:225–230.

84. Lenné, M. G., P. Dietze, G. R. Rumbold, et al. 2003. The effects of the opioid pharmacotherapies methadone, LAAM and buprenorphine, alone and in combination with alcohol, on simulated driving. *Drug Alcohol Depend.* 72:271–278.

85. Mintzer, M. Z., C. J. Correia, and E. C. Strain. 2004. A dose-effect study of repeated administration of buprenorphine/naloxone on performance in opioid-dependent volunteers. *Drug Alcohol Depend.* 74:205–209.

86. Wang, J. S., and C. L. DeVane. 2003. Involvement of CYP3A4, CYP2C8 and CYP2D6 in the metabolism of (R)- and (S)-methadone in vitro. *Drug Metab. Dispos.* 31:742–747.

87. Rogers, J. F., A. N. Nafziger, and J. S. Bertino. 2002. Pharmacogenetics affects dosing, efficacy, and toxicity of cytochrome p450-metabolized drugs. *Am. J. Med.* 113:746–750.

88. Moody, D. E., S. L. Walsh, D. E. Rollins, et al. 2004. Ketoconazole, a cytochrome p450 3A4 inhibitor, markedly increases concentrations of levo-acetyl-alpha-methadol in opioid naïve individuals. *Clin. Pharmacol. Ther.* 76:154–166.

89. Clarke, S. M., F. M. Mulcahy, J. Tija, et al. 2001. Pharmacokinetics of methadone in HIV-positive patients receiving the non-nucleoside reverse transcriptase inhibitor efavirenz. *Br. J. Clin. Pharmacol.* 51:213–217. *In 11 patients, the mean methadone area under the curve (AUC) was reduced by over 50% after starting efavirenz. Nine reported withdrawal symptoms; the mean methadone dose increase required was 22% (15–30 mg/day).*

90. Clarke, S. M., F. M. Mulcahy, J. Tija, et al. 2001. Pharmacokinetic interactions of nevirapine and methadone and guidelines for use of nevirapine to treat injection drug users. *Clin. Infect. Dis.* 33:1595–1597. *In eight subjects, the mean methadone area under the curve (AUC) was reduced by over 50% after starting nevirapine; six reported withdrawal symptoms. The mean methadone dose increase required was 16%.*

91. Hendrix, C. W., J. Wakeford, M. B. Wire, et al. 2004. Pharmacokinetics and pharmacodynamics of methadone enantiomers after coadministration with amprenavir in opioid-dependent subjects. *Pharmacotherapy* 24:1110–1121.

92. Kreek, M. J., J. W. Garfield, C. L. Gutjahr, and L. M. Giusti. 1976. Rifampin-induced methadone withdrawal. *N. Engl. J. Med.* 294:1104–1106. *Among 86 patients with tuberculosis on methadone maintenance, 30 received rifampin and 21 (70%) developed withdrawal symptoms; none of the 56 who received regimens that did not include rifampin developed withdrawal symptoms.*

93. Brown, L. S., R. C. Sawyer, R. Li, et al. 1996. Lack of pharmacologic interaction between rifabutin and methadone in HIV-infected former injecting drug users. *Drug Alcohol Depend.* 43:71–77.

94. Tong, T. G., S. M. Pond, M. J. Kreek, et al. 1981. Phenytoin-induced methadone withdrawal. *Ann. Intern. Med.* 94:349–351.

95. Liu, S. J., and R. I. Wang. 1984. Case report of barbiturate-induced enhancement of methadone metabolism and withdrawal syndrome. *Am. J. Psychiatry* 141:1287–1288.

96. Kuhn, K. L., J. A. Halikas, and K. D. Kemp. 1989. Carbamazepine treatment of cocaine dependence in methadone maintenance patients with dual opiate-cocaine addiction. *NIDA Res. Monogr.* 95:316–317.

97. Wines, J. D., Jr., and R. D. Weiss. 1999. Opioid withdrawal during risperidone treatment. *J. Clin. Psychopharmacol.* 19:265–267.

98. Hamilton, S. P., E. V. Nunes, M. Janal, and L. Weber. 2000. The effect of sertraline on methadone plasma levels in methadone-maintenance patients. *Am. J. Addict.* 9:63–69. *Thirty-one depressed patients on methadone were randomly assigned to sertraline or placebo and followed for 12 weeks. Those on sertraline had an increase in serum methadone levels during the first 6 weeks; this declined toward baseline during the second 6 weeks. None had any signs or symptoms of toxicity.*

99. Begre, S., U. von Bardeleben, D. Ladewig, et al. 2002. Paroxetine increases steady-state concentrations of (R)-methadone in CYP2D6 extensive but not poor metabolizers. *J. Clin. Psychopharmacol.* 22:211–215.

100. Alderman, C. P., and P. A. Frith. 1999. Fluvoxamine-methadone interaction. *Aust. N.Z. J. Psychiatry* 33:99–101.

101. Batki, S. L., L. B. Manfredi, P. Jacob III, and R. T. Jones. 1994. Fluoxetine for cocaine dependence in methadone maintenance: Quantitative plasma and urine cocaine/benzoylecgonine concentrations. *J. Clin. Psychopharmacol.* 13:243–250.

102. Venkatakrishnan, K., L. L. von Moltke, and D. J. Greenblatt. 2000. Effects of the antifungal agents on oxidative drug metabolism: Clinical relevance. *Clin. Pharmacokinet.* 38:111–180.

103. Herrlin, K., M. Segerdahl, L. L. Gustafsson, and E. Kalso. 2000. Methadone, ciprofloxacin, and adverse drug reactions. *Lancet* 356:2069–2070.

104. Torrens, M., C. Castillo, L. San, et al. 1998. Plasma methadone concentrations as an indicator of opioid withdrawal symptoms and heroin use in a methadone maintenance program. *Drug Alcohol Depend.* 52:193–200.

105. Bell, J., V. Seres, P. Bowron, et al. 1988. The use of serum methadone levels in patients receiving methadone maintenance. *Clin. Pharmacol. Ther.* 43:623–629.

106. Iguchi, M. Y., L. Handelsman, W. K. Bickel, and R. R. Griffiths. 1993. Benzodiazepine and sedative use/abuse by methadone maintenance clients. *Drug Alcohol Depend.* 32:257–266. *Five hundred forty-seven clients in methadone programs in Baltimore, Philadelphia, and NYC were asked about sedative use; overall, 84% reported using these agents at one time and 50% reported using in the last 6 months. Among the benzodiazepines, diazepam, lorazepam, and alprazolam were frequently used to get a "high" or sold for money.*

107. Rosenblum, A., H. Joseph, C. Fong, et al. 2003. Prevalence and characteristics of chronic pain among chemically dependent patients in methadone maintenance and residential treatment facilities. *JAMA* 289:2370–2378.

108. Compton, P., V. C. Charuvastra, and W. Ling. 2001. Pain intolerance in opioid-maintained former opiate addicts. Effect of long-acting maintenance agent. *Drug Alcohol Depend.* 63:139–146.

109. Fultz, J. M., and E. C. Senay. 1975. Guidelines for the management of hospitalized narcotic addicts. *Ann. Intern. Med.* 82:815–818.

110. Hahn, S. R., K. Kroenke, R. L. Spitzer, et al. 1996. The difficult patient: Prevalence, psychopathology, and functional impairment. *J. Gen. Intern. Med.* 11:1–8.

111. Schafer, S., and D. P. Nowlis. 1998. Personality disorders among difficult patients. *Arch. Fam. Med.* 7:126–129.

112. Bowers, L. 2003. Manipulation: Searching for an understanding. *J. Psychiatric Ment. Health Nurs.* 10:329–334.

113. Gebo, K. A., J. Keruly, and R. D. Moore. 2003. Association of social stress, illicit drug use, and health beliefs with nonadherence to antiretroviral therapy. *J. Gen. Intern. Med.* 18:104–111.

114. Saitz, R., W. A. Ghali, and M. A. Moskowitz. 1999. Characteristics of patients with pneumonia who are discharged from hospitals against medical advice. *Am. J. Med.* 107:507–509.
115. Anis, A., H. Sun, D. P. Guh, et al. 2002. Leaving hospital against medical advice among HIV-positive patients. *CMAJ* 167:633–637.
116. Treisman, G. J., A. F. Angelino, and H. E. Hutton. 2001. Psychiatric issues in the management of patients with HIV infection. *JAMA* 286:2857–2864.

16

Psychiatric Illness and Addiction

BACKGROUND

Psychiatric illness and addiction are common problems and are often found concurrently in persons who are seeking care. Moreover, having one disorder increases the risk for—and complicates the treatment of—the other disorder. Those with co-occurring psychiatric and substance use disorders—the so-called "dual-diagnosed" patient—offer unique challenges for practitioners. These patients tend to be overrepresented among the homeless and incarcerated; they are also at high risk for human immunodeficiency virus (HIV) infection and other serious medical illnesses.

In this chapter, we will briefly review the association between psychiatric illness and the abuse of different substances. We will also try to address the ways in which each affects the treatment strategies and outcomes of the other. Unfortunately, there is little high-quality evidence to guide practitioners in the treatment of these persons, since most studies of addiction treatment and psychiatric illnesses exclude those with co-occurring disorders. It is beyond the scope of this book to review the diagnosis and management of psychiatric illnesses, and we will focus our discussion on the ways in which they intersect with addiction and addiction treatment. The Substance Abuse and Mental Health Services Administration (SAMHSA) has issued treatment guidelines for individuals with co-occurring substance use and mental disorders (1); this is a useful resource for those who want more information and guidance on this complicated topic and can be obtained free of charge through their Web site (www.samhsa.gov).

EPIDEMIOLOGY

A number of studies have shown that individuals with psychiatric illness have higher rates of substance abuse and those who abuse substances are at increased risk of psychiatric illness. Most of this data comes from studies of persons who are seeking care for psychiatric illness or addiction, and for this reason, it may overestimate the actual prevalence of co-occurring disorders and their association. Nonetheless, epidemiological data indicates that persons with drug or alcohol dependence are at increased risk for psychiatric disorders, and vice versa. In the Epidemiologic Catchment Area (ECA) study, conducted in the United States between 1980 and 1984, among those with a psychiatric disorder, the odds ratio (OR) of a substance use disorder was 2.7, and among those with a substance use disorder, the odds of a psychiatric disorder was 3.0 (2). This association was found for all major substances and psychiatric diagnoses; Table 16.1 provides data from this study on the lifetime prevalence rates of mental disorders and odds of substance abuse and dependence associated with each. Similarly, the 2003 National Survey of Drug Use and Health (NSDUH) reported that 21.3% of adults with a serious mental illness were also dependent on or abused alcohol or illicit drugs, compared to 7.9% of those without (3). Studies from other countries have also found an association between substance use disorders and mental disorders (4).

The aforementioned studies did not include nicotine addiction (i.e., smoking) in their analyses. Nonetheless, nicotine addiction also appears to be associated with mental illness; in one study, among those with nicotine dependence, the 12-month prevalence of mood disorder was 21% (OR: 3.3), anxiety disorder 22% (OR: 2.7), and personality disorder 32% (OR: 3.3) (5).

There are a number of possible reasons for the association between mental illness and addiction. The first explanation is that mental illness and addiction have common risk factors and etiologies; these may be genetic or environmental. The second is that addiction may lead to mental illness; it is clear that the use of a variety of substances, particularly when habitual, leads to changes in the brain that may persist even after use of the substance had

Table 16.1. Lifetime prevalence of alcohol or illicit drug abuse or dependence among persons with mental disorders

Mental Disorder	Overall Lifetime Prevalence of Disorder	Lifetime Prevalence of Substance Abuse or Dependence	Odds Ratio*
Schizophrenia	1.5%	47.0%	4.6
Antisocial personality disorder	2.6%	83.6%	29.6
Anxiety disorders	14.6%	23.7%	1.7
Obsessive-compulsive disorder	2.5%	32.8%	2.5
Affective disorders	8.3%	32.0%	2.6
Any mental disorder	16.2%	28.9%	2.7

* Odds of substance abuse or dependence among those with the mental disorder (compared with those without the disorder).

Source: Regier, D. A., et al. 1990. *JAMA* 264:2511–2518.

ceased. However, a recent systematic review of studies of the association between illicit drug use and psychosocial harm did not find that the evidence supported a causal relationship (6). The third possible reason is that psychiatric illness leads to addiction and that these individuals may be "self-treating" their illness with these substances. Finally, the self-limited acute effects of a substance (or withdrawal from it) may be mistaken for a long-standing psychiatric illness (7). These hypotheses are not mutually exclusive, and it is possible that some or all of these processes contribute to the observed association.

In the following sections we will review the relationship between specific psychiatric conditions and substance use disorders.

AFFECTIVE DISORDERS

The affective disorders, including major depression and bipolar disorder, are associated with substance use disorders. In a study of individuals presenting for outpatient treatment of major depression, 27.3% were nicotine dependent, 6.1% abused or were dependent on alcohol, and 4.6% abused or were dependent on other drugs; overall, 33% had a current substance use disorder and 60% had one at some point during their lifetime (8). In a study of individuals seeking care for illicit drug or alcohol dependence, 29% had depression (9). In an epidemiological study (the ECA study—discussed earlier) (2), affective disorders were found to be associated with increased lifetime risk of abuse of alcohol (OR: 1.9), cocaine (OR: 5.9), opiates (OR: 5.0), amphetamines (OR: 5.7), barbiturates (OR: 6.6), and hallucinogens (OR: 5.9). The risk of substance use disorders was particularly high for those with bipolar disorder, with an odds ratio of 6.6, compared to 1.9 for unipolar depression.

Depression

The features of depression include low mood, decreased energy, feelings of low self-worth or guilt, and changes in appetite, weight, or sleep. Depression has been found to be associated with poorer drug treatment outcomes in a variety of settings (10). On the other hand, drug treatment alone is often associated with improvements in depressive symptoms (11, 12). A number of studies have addressed the treatment of patients with co-occurring depression and substance use disorders. A small study of depressed alcoholics reported that cognitive-behavioral therapy was effective for treatment of depressive symptoms and reducing alcohol use (13). A recent study of desipramine for depressed cocaine addicts reported that it was effective for depression but did not have any effect on cocaine use (14). This is consistent with the findings of a recent meta-analysis of studies of pharmacological treatment of depression in patients with drug or alcohol dependence. This study concluded that antidepressant medication is effective for treatment of depression in this situation but has a limited effect on substance abuse outcomes, suggesting that these individuals still need targeted addiction treatment (15). This analysis also found high rates of improvement of depression in the placebo arms, suggesting that many will improve without antidepressant treatment. Moreover, the antidepressant treatment effect seemed to be greatest when it was targeted to individuals who were still depressed after at least a week of abstinence. For treatment-seeking addicts who are depressed, this finding supports the practice of initially treating the addiction and then addressing depression if symptoms persist once abstinence (or maintenance) is achieved. It also reinforces the importance of screening depressed individuals for addiction and addressing this problem directly.

Bipolar Disorder

The bipolar disorders are characterized by alternating periods of depression and mania (bipolar I) or hypomania (bipolar II). As noted earlier, bipolar disorder has a strong association with addiction; in the ECA study, those with bipolar disorder had an increased lifetime risk of alcohol abuse or dependence (43.6%; OR: 5.1), as well as illicit drug abuse or dependence (33.6%; OR: 8.3) (2). In a study of 288 outpatients with bipolar disorder, 4% had a current substance use disorder and 42% had a lifetime history; the lifetime prevalence was highest for alcohol (33%) followed by marijuana (16%), non-cocaine stimulants (9%), cocaine (9%), opiates (7%), and hallucinogens (6%) (16). It is possible that some of the association is due to misdiagnosis of individuals who are experiencing the effects of the drugs they are using; for example, stimulant users may exhibit signs such as mood swings, irritability, and insomnia that may be mistakenly attributed to bipolar disorder rather than drug use (17).

A number of studies indicate that persons with bipolar disorder and a concurrent drug or alcohol problem often have more severe presentation of mania (18) and slower remission (19). Bipolar patients with concurrent substance abuse seem to have a more severe disease course and are more likely to be hospitalized for their psychiatric illness (20); furthermore, psychiatric treatment has been found to be less effective (21), probably at least partly due to poorer compliance with medications (22). Bipolar patients with concurrent substance abuse disorders are also at higher risk for suicide attempts (23).

The optimal treatment approach for substance-abusing bipolar patients has yet to be established (24), but there is some evidence supporting an integrated approach that addresses both problems simultaneously, though most of this is from observational studies (25). One small controlled study of integrated group therapy for patients with bipolar disorder and substance dependence reported that this treatment approach was associated with significantly improved addiction outcomes (**26**).

A number of pharmacological agents may be beneficial for bipolar patients with substance dependence. A randomized controlled trial of valproate for bipolar patients with alcoholism reported improved drinking measures over 24 weeks; however, there was no significant benefit in terms of psychiatric outcomes (**27**). A small study of bipolar adolescents with a substance dependence reported that lithium significantly reduced drug use over a 6-week period (**28**). The atypical antipsychotic quetiapine may help bipolar patients reduce their cocaine (**29**) and alcohol

(30) use, but this has yet to be tested in a controlled clinical trial. Likewise, observational data suggests that lamotrigine may be beneficial for cocaine-dependent bipolar patients (**31**).

ANXIETY DISORDERS

The anxiety disorders are characterized by persistent and excessive anxiety and worry; they include simple phobias as well as panic, generalized anxiety, and post-traumatic stress disorder (covered in following section). As with other mental disorders, anxiety disorders are associated with substance abuse and dependence. In the ECA study, the lifetime prevalence of anxiety disorders was 14.6%, and almost one-fourth of them (23.7%) had a substance use disorder at some point in their lives (OR: 1.7). Among the anxiety disorders, substance abuse or dependence appears to be more strongly associated with panic disorder (OR: 2.9) than with simple phobias (OR: 1.6) (2). Other studies have found associations between anxiety disorders and smoking (32), alcoholism (33), and marijuana use (34). Furthermore, in a study of patients with severe affective disorders (major depression or bipolar disorder), the presence of a coexisting anxiety disorder was associated with abuse of a number of substances, including opioids, sedatives, cocaine, and other stimulants (35).

There is little data on the optimal treatment of individuals with concurrent anxiety and substance use disorders. In general, benzodiazepines are to be avoided because of their abuse potential; a number of non-habit-forming medications have been studied. A pilot study of subjects with co-occurring social anxiety and alcohol use disorder reported that paroxetine was effective for treatment of social anxiety but did not reduce alcohol use (36). A study of buspirone for anxious alcoholics reported some benefits in terms of anxiety and alcohol use (**37**). On the other hand, a study of buspirone for anxiety among opioid addicts on methadone failed to show any benefit in terms of anxiety or substance abuse (**38**).

POST-TRAUMATIC STRESS DISORDER (PTSD)

Post-traumatic stress disorder (PTSD) is an anxiety disorder that follows a traumatic event and is characterized by persistent intrusive thoughts, avoidance of stimuli related to the trauma, and symptoms of increased arousal. A number of studies have found an association between PTSD and substance use disorders. For example, in one study of cocaine-dependent outpatients participating in a treatment study, 30% of the women and 15% of the men met diagnostic criteria for PTSD (39). In another study of adolescents in residential substance abuse treatment programs, 12% of the males and 40% of the females were judged to have PTSD (40). Longitudinal data suggests that exposure to traumatic events alone does not increase the risk of subsequent substance use disorders but that the minority of trauma survivors who develop PTSD are at increased risk, particularly for prescription psychoactive drug abuse or dependence (41).

A number of treatment approaches may be effective at preventing the development of PTSD and helping those with PTSD and substance use disorders. A study of trauma survivors who were randomly assigned to usual care versus a "stepped collaborative care" (which included case management, as well as psychological and psychiatric care, if needed) reported that the intervention significantly reduced the risk of PTSD and of alcohol dependence or abuse over 12 months (42).

Cognitive-behavioral therapy may be effective for persons with PTSD and substance use disorders. One study of 18 incarcerated women with PTSD and substance abuse reported improvement in PTSD symptoms and substance abuse after 12 weeks of twice-weekly cognitive-behavioral therapy sessions (43). Another study comparing two different cognitive-behavioral approaches with usual care reported that both treatments were associated with significant improvements in PTSD symptoms and substance abuse; however, the approach designed specifically for individuals with substance abuse and PTSD ("seeking safety") was not shown to be more effective than standard relapse prevention (44).

There is little data on pharmacological treatment of co-occurring PTSD and substance use disorders. In one randomized controlled trial, the antidepressant sertraline was not found to be effective (**45**).

SCHIZOPHRENIA

Schizophrenia is a severe, incapacitating mental illness characterized by distorted thoughts, perceptions, beliefs, and sensations; features include delusions, hallucinations, agitation, or catatonia. Like other mental illnesses, schizophrenia is associated with substance use disorders. Nicotine dependence appears to be particularly prevalent among schizophrenics (46). In fact, this has led some to postulate that smoking may have beneficial effects for those with schizophrenia or that smoking may be a risk factor for the development of schizophrenia. One study of Israeli military recruits found that those who smoked at age 18 were more likely to subsequently be hospitalized with a diagnosis of schizophrenia (relative risk: 1.94) (47). In contrast, a study of Swedish military conscripts, which was able to take other risk factors into account, found no such association and reported a *lower* risk of schizophrenia associated with smoking (48).

There are similar concerns regarding an association between marijuana use and schizophrenia. A cohort study of Swedish conscripts found an association between self-reported marijuana use and subsequent risk of inpatient admission for schizophrenia (adjusted odds ratio: 1.5), though only 20% of those who developed schizophrenia had ever used marijuana (49).

A study of 83 hospitalized psychotic patients (most were schizophrenic) found that about half met criteria for substance abuse or dependence. The substance-abusing patients were not significantly different in any demographic factors but were more likely to report a family history of substance abuse. Symptom measures on admission were not significantly different, but the substance-abusing patients had less severe psychopathology at the time of discharge, despite a lack of difference in length of stay or amounts of neuroleptic medications they received (50). This suggests that substance-abusing schizophrenic patients do as well as (if not better than) other patients with standard inpatient treatment.

In terms of outpatient management, an integrated treatment program that included motivational interviewing, cognitive-behavioral therapy, and family therapy was found to be superior to standard care for patients with schizophrenia and substance use disorders in one study (**51**). There is little other data on optimal treatment strategies for patients with coexisting schizophrenia and substance use disorders.

PERSONALITY DISORDERS

Personality disorders are persistent, inflexible, and maladaptive behavior patterns that cause significant impairment or distress. The personality disorders are divided into three clusters. Cluster A includes "odd or eccentric" personality disorders (paranoid, schizoid, schizotypal). Cluster B includes borderline, antisocial, histrionic, and narcissistic personality disorders. Cluster C includes dependent, avoidant, and obsessive-compulsive personality disorders.

Personality disorders appear to have a strong association with illicit drug and alcohol abuse and dependence (2). Nicotine dependence has also been found to be associated with personality disorders (5). Furthermore, among those with an Axis I psychiatric disorder (mood, psychotic, or anxiety disorders), the presence of a coexisting personality disorder (particularly borderline personality disorder) is associated with an increased risk for substance use disorders (52). Substance use disorders are most strongly associated with the cluster B borderline and antisocial personality disorders. Borderline personality disorder is characterized by unstable mood and self-image, as well as volatile interpersonal relationships. Antisocial personality disorders are characterized by chronic irresponsible and antisocial behavior (illegal activities, recklessness, aggression, poor academic and job performance); these individuals often feel victimized and have limited capacity for intimacy. Some of the association between these disorders and substance abuse may be artifactual, since the impulsive behaviors and illicit activity associated with drug abuse contribute to the diagnostic criteria for these disorders (53).

Substance abuse seems to have a detrimental effect on the disease course and treatment of personality disorders. In a study of 290 patients with borderline personality disorder who were followed for 6 years, 62% had a substance use disorder at baseline and this factor was associated with a significant delay in time to remission (54). Moreover, substance abusers with personality disorders are at increased risk for other complications. For example, in a study of 615 heroin users, personality disorders (borderline and antisocial) were associated with overdose, attempted suicide, and needle sharing (55). As would be expected, injection drug users with personality disorders are at increased risk for acquiring HIV infection (56).

Personality disorders also appear to have a deleterious effect on addiction treatment outcomes. In one study of 266 alcoholics, antisocial personality disorder was associated with poorer treatment outcomes at 1 year (57). Similarly, in a prospective cohort study of 2616 patients with substance use disorders, personality disorder was associated with deterioration after 1 year, more so than any other psychiatric disorder (58). On the other hand, a study of therapeutic community treatment outcomes reported that those with antisocial personality disorder did as well as those without (59).

There is little data on the optimal treatment of substance abusers with personality disorders. It has been postulated that those with antisocial personality disorders respond best to highly structured treatment with rewards for desirable behavior (i.e., contingency management). In a study of 120 opioid- and cocaine-dependent persons on methadone maintenance comparing contingency management and cognitive-behavioral therapy, those with antisocial personality disorder seemed to respond best to contingency management (**60**). However, a preliminary study of 40 opioid addicts with antisocial personality disorder, who were enrolled in methadone maintenance, failed to demonstrate better outcomes with a contingency management approach (**61**).

There is little data on treatment of patients with borderline personality and substance use disorders. A cognitive-behavioral approach called *dialectical behavior therapy* has been investigated in two small studies (total of 50 subjects). This treatment approach attempts to combine directive, problem-oriented, and supportive techniques, balancing acceptance with change. Unfortunately, these studies failed to demonstrate that this approach is significantly better than standard addiction treatment or simple supportive therapy (62, 63).

ATTENTION DEFICIT HYPERACTIVITY DISORDER

Attention deficit hyperactivity disorder (ADHD) is characterized by inattention, hyperactivity, and impulsivity. A few studies have reported high rates of ADHD among substance abusers. For example, in one study of 298 treatment-seeking cocaine abusers, 35% met criteria for this disorder (64). Those with ADHD do appear to be at increased risk for substance use disorders, but this may be limited to those with coexisting conduct disorder or bipolar disorder (65).

One concern that has been raised is whether the use of stimulants for treatment of ADHD increases the risk for subsequent substance use disorders, especially stimulant abuse. However, a 16-year follow-up study of a randomized controlled trial of stimulants for children with learning disabilities found that those who received methylphenidate did not have an increased risk of subsequent substance use disorders (66). An observational study of hyperactive children and adolescents who were followed for 13 years found that those who were treated with stimulants did have an increased risk of ever using cocaine (but not other substances); this association was no longer significant when they controlled for severity of illness and the presence of conduct disorder (67). A meta-analysis of this question concluded that stimulant therapy is actually associated with a reduced risk of subsequent substance use disorders (68).

The presence of ADHD may have some impact on addiction treatment outcomes. A study of cocaine abusers admitted to a therapeutic community reported that those with ADHD were more likely to drop out of the program (69). On the other hand, a study of opioid addicts entering methadone maintenance found that those with ADHD were no different in terms of treatment retention or illicit drug use (70).

A number of studies have investigated the use of a variety of pharmacological agents for treatment of substance abusers with ADHD; in general, these studies show beneficial effects on ADHD, but most fail to demonstrate significant improvements in substance use disorders. A few preliminary studies suggest that methylphenidate improves ADHD symptoms and may reduce drug use when given to cocaine addicts with ADHD (71, **72**, 73). A trial of another stimulant, pemoline, for substance-abusing adolescents with ADHD and conduct disorder reported an improvement in ADHD symptoms, but not in substance use (74). Diversion of prescription stimulants by patients with ADHD is a concern; in one study of adolescents in a residential addiction treatment program, 31% had a current ADHD diagnosis and 20% of them reported illicit diversion of medication (75). Some experts recommend that pharmacotherapy for individuals with ADHD and substance use disorders begin with medications with low likelihood of abuse or diversion, such as antidepressants or atomoxetine (76).

A number of other medications may be beneficial. The antidepressant bupropion was reported to be effective (for ADHD) in an uncontrolled trial of 13 adolescents with substance use disorders and ADHD (77). A study of 11 adults with cocaine dependence and ADHD reported reductions in cocaine use after 12 weeks of treatment with bupropion (78). Another antidepressant, venlafaxine, appeared to be beneficial in a 12-week trial of treatment of 10 alcohol- or cocaine-abusing patients with ADHD (79). These small studies offer some promising leads, but more research needs to be done before any specific treatment can be recommended for individuals with these co-occurring disorders.

EATING DISORDERS

The eating disorders, anorexia and bulimia, share a preoccupation with being overweight. Anorexics often severely restrict their caloric intake or exercise excessively, are underweight, and display physical signs of malnutrition. Bulimics often alternate eating with starvation or purging and are usually of normal weight. Both groups may abuse appetite suppressants, diuretics, and laxatives to achieve their goals. A number of studies report high rates of substance use disorders among individuals with eating disorders. Those with coexisting personality disorder (cluster B) and eating disorder appear to be at highest risk for substance abuse or dependence (80). The association between eating and substance use disorders appears to be primarily among those with a bulimic (as opposed to anorexic) pattern (81). In fact, in one study of adolescents with eating disorders, those with a restrictive (anorexic) pattern had lower rates of substance use disorders than their (non-eating-disordered) peers (82).

In addition, high rates of eating disorders have been reported among individuals seeking care for substance use disorders. One study of women in residential treatment reported that 14% had a concurrent eating disorder and that the rates were highest among cocaine addicts and lowest among opioid addicts (83). Another study of women in alcohol treatment reported that 26% had a "probable eating disorder" (84). On the other hand, a study of over 4000 alcoholic men and women found that the women had lifetime rates of 1.4% and 6.2% for anorexia and bulimia, respectively, and 1.4% of the men had bulimia (85). This study concluded that bulimia does occur at a higher-than-expected rate among alcoholics, but it is not common and other concurrent psychiatric disorders may account for this association.

There is some evidence that education may help prevent substance abuse and disordered eating. A 2002 Cochrane review concluded that there was not sufficient evidence for the effectiveness of any intervention in preventing eating disorders (86). However, a recent study of a peer-led educational intervention for adolescent female athletes reported that those who received the intervention were more likely to engage in healthy eating behaviors and had fewer new users of diet pills and other "body-shaping substances" (amphetamines, anabolic steroids, and muscle-building supplements) (87). We were unable to find any studies on the treatment of persons with coexisting eating and substance use disorders.

REFERENCES

1. Center for Substance Abuse Treatment. 2005. Substance Abuse Treatment for Persons with Co-Occurring Disorders. Treatment Improvement Protocol (TIP) Series 42. DHHS Publication no. (SMA) 05-3992. Rockville, MD: Substance Abuse and Mental Health Services Administration.
2. Regier, D. A., M. E. Farmer, D. S. Rae, et al. 1990. Comorbidity of mental disorders with alcohol and other drug abuse. Results from the Epidemiologic Catchment Area study. JAMA 264:2511–2518.
3. Substance Abuse and Mental Health Services Administration. 2004. Results from the 2003 National Survey on Drug Use and Health: National Findings (Office of Applied Studies, NSDUH Series H-25, DHHS Publication No. SMA 04-3964). Rockville, MD.
4. Merikangas, K. R., R. L. Mehta, B. E. Molnar, et al. 1998. Comorbidity of substance use disorders with mood and anxiety disorders: Results of the international consortium in psychiatric epidemiology. Addict. Behav. 23:893–907.
5. Grant, B. F., D. S. Hasin, P. Chou, et al. 2004. Nicotine dependence and psychiatric disorders in the United States. Results from the National Epidemiologic Survey on Alcohol and Related Conditions. Arch. Gen. Psychiatry. 61:1107–1115.
6. Macleod, J., R. Oakes, A. Copello, et al. 2004. Psychological and social sequelae of cannabis and other illicit drug use by young people: A systematic review of longitudinal, general population studies. Lancet 363:1579–1588.

7. Cohen, S. I. 1995. Overdiagnosis of schizophrenia: Role of alcohol and drug misuse. *Lancet* 346:1541–1542.

8. Zimmerman, M., I. Chelminski, and W. McDermut. 2002. Major depressive disorder and axis I comorbidity. *J. Clin. Psychiatry* 63:187–193.

9. Mertens, J. R., Y. W. Lu, S. Parthasarathy, et al. 2003. Medical and psychiatric conditions of alcohol and drug treatment patients in an HMO. *Arch. Intern. Med.* 163:2511–2517.

10. Rousnaville, B. J., T. R. Kosten, M. M. Weissman, and H. D. Kosten. 1986. Prognostic significance of psychopathology in treated opiate addicts. A 2.5-year follow-up study. *Arch. Gen. Psychiatry* 43:739–745.

11. Kosten, T. R., C. Morgan, and T. A. Kosten. 1990. Depressive symptoms during buprenorphine treatment of opioid abusers. *J. Subst. Abuse Treat.* 7:51–54.

12. Strain, E. C., M. L. Stitzer, and G. E. Bigelow. 1991. Early treatment time course of depressive symptoms in opiate addicts. *J. Nerv. Ment. Dis.* 179:215–221.

13. Brown, R. A., D. M. Evans, I. W. Miller, et al. 1997. Cognitive-behavioral treatment for depression in alcoholism. *J. Consult. Clin. Psychol.* 65:715–726.

14. McDowell, D., E. V. Nunes, A. M. Seracini, et al. 2005. Desipramine treatment of cocaine-dependent patients with depression: A placebo-controlled trial. *Drug Alcohol Depend.* [Epub ahead of print]. *One hundred eleven cocaine addicts with depression were randomized to desipramine (up to 300 mg/day) or placebo; after 12 weeks, those on desipramine had a higher rate of depression response (51% vs. 32%), but cocaine response was not significantly better (45% vs. 38%).*

15. Nunes, E. V., and F. R. Levin. 2004. Treatment of depression in patients with alcohol or other drug dependence. A meta-analysis. *JAMA* 291:1887–1896.

16. McElroy, S. L., L. L. Altshuler, T. Suppes, et al. 2001. Axis I psychiatric comorbidity and its relationship to historical illness variables in 288 patients with bipolar disorder. *Am. J. Psychiatry* 158:420–426.

17. Levin, F. R., and G. Hennessy. 2004. Bipolar disorder and substance abuse. *Biol. Psychiatry* 56:738–748.

18. Salloum, I. M., J. R. Cornelius, J. E. Mezzich, and L. Kirisci. 2002. Impact of concurrent alcohol misuse on symptom presentation of acute mania at initial presentation. *Bipolar Disord.* 4:418–421.

19. Goldberg, J. F., J. L. Garno, A. C. Leon, et al. 1999. A history of substance abuse complicates remission from acute mania in bipolar disorder. *J. Clin. Psychiatry* 60:733–740.

20. Cassidy, F., E. P. Ahearn, and B. J. Carroll. 2001. Substance abuse and bipolar disorder. *Bipolar Disord.* 3:181–188.

21. O'Connell, R. A., J. A. Mayo, L. Flatow, et al. 1991. Outcome of bipolar disorder on long-term treatment with lithium. *Br. J. Psychiatry* 159:123–129.

22. Keck, P. E., Jr., S. L. McElroy, S. M. Strakowski, et al. 1998. 12-month outcome of patients with bipolar disorder following hospitalization for a manic or mixed episode. *Am. J. Psychiatry* 155:646–652.

23. Dalton, E. J., T. D. Cate-Carter, E. Mundo, et al. 2003. Suicide risk in bipolar patients: The role of co-morbid substance use disorders. *Bipolar Disord.* 5:58–61.

24. O'Brien, C. P., D. S. Charney, L. Lewis, et al. 2004. Priority actions to improve the care of persons with co-occurring substance abuse and other mental disorders: A call to action. *Biol. Psychiatry* 56:703–713.

25. Levin, F. R., and G. Hennessy. 2004. Bipolar disorder and substance abuse. *Biol. Psychiatry* 56:738–748.

26. Weiss, R. D., M. L. Griffin, S. F. Greenfield, et al. 2000. Group therapy for patients with bipolar disorder and substance dependence: Results of a pilot study. *J. Clin. Psychiatry* 61:361–367. *Forty-five bipolar substance-abusing patients admitted to a psychiatric hospital were assigned in sequential blocks to "integrated group therapy" (IGT) or regular care; the IGT participants were significantly older. ASI score in both groups improved; those in IGT were more likely to have >3 consecutive months of abstinence (62% vs. 21%).*

27. Salloum, I. M., J. R. Cornelius, D. C. Daley, et al. 2005. Efficacy of valproate maintenance in patients with bipolar disorder and alcoholism. *Arch. Gen. Psychiatry* 62:37–45. *Fifty-two bipolar alcoholics were randomized to valproate or placebo after detox. All received lithium and weekly individual counseling; 20 completed the trial. After 24 weeks, those on valproate had lower proportion of heavy drinking days (0.09 vs. 0.19) and delay in time to relapse to sustained heavy drinking (93 vs. 62 days). Psychiatric measures improved in both groups equally.*

28. Geller, B., T. B. Cooper, K. Sun, et al. 1998. Double-blind and placebo-controlled study of lithium for adolescent bipolar disorders with secondary substance dependency. *J. Am. Acad. Child Adolesc. Psychiatry* 37:171–178. *Twenty-five adolescent bipolar addicts were randomized to lithium or placebo; over 6 weeks, those on lithium had fewer positive urine drug screens (~10% vs. 40%).*

29. Brown, E. S., V. A. Nejtek, D. C. Perantie, and L. Bobadilla. 2002. Quetiapine in bipolar disorder and cocaine dependence. *Bipolar Disord.* 4:406–411. *Quetiapine was added to the treatment regimen of 17 cocaine-dependent bipolar outpatients. After 12 weeks, there was improvement in psychiatric measures and cocaine craving, but not cocaine use.*

30. Longoria, J., E. S. Brown, D. C. Perantie, et al. 2004. Quetiapine for alcohol and craving in bipolar disorder. *J. Clin. Psychopharmacol.* 24:101–102.

31. Brown, E. S., V. A. Nejtek, D. C. Perantie, et al. 2003. Lamotrigine in patients with bipolar disorder and cocaine dependence. *J. Clin. Psychiatry* 64:197–201. *Lamotrigine was added to the treatment regimen of 33 cocaine-dependent bipolar outpatients for 12 weeks. The 30 who completed had improvement in psychiatric measures and cocaine craving; cocaine use also declined, but not significantly so.*

32. Isensee, B., H. U. Wittchen, M. B. Stein, et al. 2003. Smoking increases the risk of panic: Findings from a prospective community study. *Arch. Gen. Psychiatry* 60:692–700.

33. Cheng, A. T. A., S. F. Gau, T. H. H. Chen, et al. 2004. A 4-year longitudinal study on risk factors for alcoholism. *Arch. Gen. Psychiatry* 61:184–191.

34. Patton, G. C., C. Coffey, J. B. Carlin, et al. 2002. Cannabis use and mental health in young people: Cohort study. *BMJ* 325:1195–1198.

35. Goodwin, R. D., D. A. Stayner, M. J. Chinman, et al. 2002. The relationship between anxiety and substance abuse among individuals with severe affective disorders. *Comp. Psychiatry* 43:245–252.

36. Randall, C. L., M. R. Johnson, A. K. Thevos, et al. 2001. Paroxetine for social anxiety and alcohol use in dual-diagnosed patients. *Depression Anxiety* 14:255–262.

37. Kranzler, H. R., J. A. Burleson, F. K. Del Boca, et al. 1994. Buspirone treatment of anxious alcoholics; a placebo-controlled trial. *Arch. Gen. Psychiatry* 51:720–731. *Sixty-one alcoholics with anxiety (after ≥ 7 days of abstinence) randomly received buspirone or placebo for 12 weeks; all received cognitive-behavioral therapy as well. Those assigned to buspirone were more likely to complete treatment (84% vs. 53%) and they tended to have lower anxiety scores; at 6-month follow-up they had fewer drinking days and a trend toward fewer drinks per day. The treatment appeared to be most beneficial for those with higher baseline anxiety scores.*

38. McRae, A. L., S. C. Sonne, K. T. Brady, et al. 2004. A randomized, placebo-controlled trial of buspirone for the treatment of anxiety in opioid-dependent individuals. *Am. J. Addict.* 13:53–63. *Thirty-six opioid addicts on methadone with anxiety were randomized to buspirone or placebo. After 12 weeks, there was no difference in anxiety or depression symptoms—or in measures of illicit drug use.*

39. Najavits, L. M., D. R. Gastfriend, J. P. Barber, et al. 1998. Cocaine dependence with and without PTSD among subjects in the National Institute on Drug Abuse Collaborative Cocaine Treatment Study. *Am. J. Psychiatry* 155:214–219.

40. Deykin, E. Y., and S. L. Buka. 1997. Prevalence and risk factors for posttraumatic stress disorder among chemically dependent adolescents. *Am. J. Psychiatry* 154:752–757.

41. Chilcoat, H. D., and N. Breslau. 1998. Posttraumatic stress disorder and drug disorders: Testing causal pathways. *Arch. Gen. Psychiatry* 55:913–917.

42. Zatzick, D., P. Roy-Byrne, F. Rivara, et al. 2004. A randomized effectiveness trial of stepped collaborative care for acutely injured trauma survivors. *Arch. Gen. Psychiatry* 61:498–506.

43. Zlotnick, C., L. M. Najavits, D. J. Rohsenow, and D. M. Johnson. 2003. A cognitive-behavioral treatment for incarcerated women with substance abuse disorder and posttraumatic stress disorder: Findings from a pilot study. *J. Subst. Abuse Treat.* 25:99–105.

44. Hien, D. A., L. R. Cohen, G. M. Miele, et al. 2004. Promising treatments for women with comorbid PTSD and substance use disorders. *Am. J. Psychiatry* 161:1426–1432.

45. Brady, K. T., S. Sonne, R. F. Anton, et al. 2005. Sertraline in the treatment of co-occurring alcohol dependence and posttraumatic

stress disorder. *Alcohol Clin. Exp. Res.* 29:395–401. *Ninety-four alcoholics with PTSD were randomized to 150 mg/day of sertraline or placebo. After 12 weeks, there was no difference in alcohol consumption or PTSD symptoms.*

46. Hughes, J. R., D. K. Hatsukami, J. E. Mitchell, and L. A. Dahlgren. 1986. Prevalence of smoking among psychiatric outpatients. *Am. J. Psychiatry* 143:993–997.

47. Weiser, M., A. Reichenberg, I. Grotto, et al. 2004. Higher rates of cigarette smoking in male adolescents before the onset of schizophrenia: A historical-prospective cohort study. *Am. J. Psychiatry* 161:1219–1223.

48. Zammit, S., P. Allebeck, C. Dalman, et al. 2003. Investigating the association between cigarette smoking and schizophrenia in a cohort study. *Am. J. Psychiatry* 160:2216–2221.

49. Zammit, S., P. Allebeck, S. Andreasson, et al. 2002. Self-reported cannabis use as a risk factor for schizophrenia in Swedish conscripts of 1969: Historical cohort study. *BMJ* 325:1199–1203.

50. Dixon, L., G. Haas, P. J. Weiden, et al. 1991. Drug abuse in schizophrenic patients: Clinical correlates and reasons for use. *Am. J. Psychiatry* 148:224–230.

51. Barrowclough, C., G. Haddock, N. Tarrier, et al. 2001. Randomized controlled trial of motivational interviewing, cognitive behavior therapy, and family intervention for patients with comorbid schizophrenia and substance use disorders. *Am. J. Psychiatry* 158:1706–1713. *Thirty-six patient-caregiver pairs were randomized to standard care or a 9-month intervention that included the elements in the title. After 12 months of treatment, those in the intervention arm had better Global Assessment of Functioning (GAF) scores (60 vs. 46) and were less likely to have a relapse (33% vs 67%). The integrated care group had greater improvement in abstinence rates, but these were not statistically significant.*

52. Grilo, C. M., S. Martino, M. L. Walker, et al. 1997. Controlled study of psychiatric comorbidity in psychiatrically hospitalized young adults with substance use disorders. *Am. J. Psychiatry* 154:1305–1307.

53. Dulit, R. A., M. R. Fyer, G. L. Haas, et al. 1990. Substance use in borderline personality disorder. *Am. J. Psychiatry* 147:1002–1007.

54. Zanarini, M. C., F. R. Frankenburg, J. Hennen, et al. 2004. Axis I comorbidity in patients with borderline personality disorder: 6-year follow-up and prediction of time to remission. *Am. J. Psychiatry* 161:2108–2114.

55. Darke, S., A. Williamson, J. Ross, et al. 2004. Borderline personality disorder, antisocial personality disorder and risk-taking among heroin users: Findings from the Australian Treatment Outcomes Study (ATOS). *Drug Alcohol Depend.* 74:77–83.

56. Brooner, R. K., L. Greenfield, C. W. Schmidt, and G. E. Bigelow. 1993. Antisocial personality disorder and HIV infection among intravenous drug abusers. *Am. J. Psychiatry* 150:53–58.

57. Rounsaville, B. J., Z. S. Dolinsky, T. F. Babor, and R. E. Meyer. 1987. Psychopathology as a predictor of treatment outcome in alcoholics. *Arch. Gen. Psychiatry* 44:505–513.

58. Moos, R. H., B. S. Moos, and J. W. Finney. 2001. Predictors of deterioration among patients with substance-use disorders. *J. Clin. Psychol.* 57:1403–1419.

59. Messina, N. P., E. D. Wish, J. A. Hoffman, and S. Nemes. 2002. Antisocial personality disorder and TC treatment outcomes. *Am. J. Drug Alcohol Abuse* 28:197–212.

60. Messina, N., D. Frarabee, and R. Rawson. 2003. Treatment responsivity of cocaine-dependent patients with antisocial personality disorder to cognitive-behavioral and contingency management interventions. *J. Consult. Clin. Psychol.* 71:320–329. *One hundred twenty opioid/cocaine addicts on methadone were randomized to (1) cognitive-behavioral therapy (CBT), (2) contingency management (CM), (3) both (CBT+CM), or (4) methadone alone (MM). The main outcome was cocaine-free urine, and the analysis was divided between those with and without antisocial personality disorder (ASPD). After 16 weeks of treatment, those without ASPD did best in the CM arms, but this effect was lost at 52-week follow-up. Those with ASPD did better initially with CM only; after 52 weeks, all three active treatments were about the same (but better than MM).*

61. Brooner, R. K., M. Kidorf, V. L. King, and K. Stoller. 1998. Preliminary evidence of good treatment response in antisocial drug abusers. *Drug Alcohol Depend.* 49:249–260. *Forty opioid addicts with antisocial personality disorder on methadone maintenance were randomized to contingency management (CM) or standard methadone treatment (MM); 10% on MM and 30% on CM failed to complete 3 months of treatment. Both groups improved over time, but those in the CM arm did not do significantly better.*

62. Linehan, M. M., H. Schmidt, L. A. Dimeff, et al. 1999. Dialectical behavior therapy for patients with borderline personality disorder and drug dependence. *Am. J. Addict.* 8:279–292.

63. Linehan, M. M., L. A. Dimeff, S. K. Reynolds, et al. 2002. Dialectical behavior therapy versus comprehensive validation therapy plus 12-step for the treatment of opioid dependent women meeting criteria for borderline personality disorder. *Drug Alcohol Depend.* 67:13–26.

64. Carroll, K. M., and B. J. Rounsaville. 1993. History and significance of childhood attention deficit disorder in treatment-seeking cocaine abusers. *Compr. Psychiatry* 34:75–82.

65. Biederman, J., T. Wilens, E. Mick, et al. 1997. Is ADHD a risk factor for psychoactive substance use disorders? Findings from a four-year prospective follow-up study. *J. Am. Acad. Child Adolesc. Psychiatry* 36:21–29.

66. Mannuzza, S., R. G. Klein, and J. L. Moulton. 2003. Does stimulant treatment place children at risk for adult substance abuse? A controlled, prospective follow-up study. *J. Child Adolesc. Psychopharmacol.* 13:273–282.

67. Barkley, R. A., M. Fischer, L. Smallish, and K. Fletcher. 2003. Does the treatment of attention-deficit/hyperactivity disorder contribute to drug use/abuse? A 13-year prospective study. *Pediatrics* 111:97–109.

68. Wilens, T. E., S. V. Faraone, J. Biederman, and S. Gunawardene. 2003. Does stimulant therapy of attention-deficit/hyperactivity

disorder beget later substance abuse? A meta-analytic review of the literature. *Pediatrics* 111:179–185.

69. Levin, F. R., S. M. Evans, S. K. Vosburg, et al. 2004. Impact of attention-deficit hyperactivity disorder and other psychopathology on treatment retention among cocaine abusers in a therapeutic community. *Addict. Behav.* 29:1875–1882.

70. King, V. L., R. K. Brooner, M. S. Kidorf, et al. 1999. Attention deficit hyperactivity disorder and treatment outcome in opioid abusers entering treatment. *J. Nerv. Ment. Dis.* 187:487–495.

71. Levin, F. R., S. M. Evans, D. M. McDowell, and H. D. Kleber. 1998. Methylphenidate treatment for cocaine abusers with adult attention-deficit/hyperactivity disorder: A pilot study. *J. Clin. Psychiatry* 59:300–305.

72. Schubiner, H., K. K. Saules, C. L. Arfken, et al. 2002. Double-blind placebo-controlled trial of methylphenidate in the treatment of adult ADHD patients with comorbid cocaine dependence. *Exp. Clin. Psychopharmacol.* 10:286–294. *Forty-eight cocaine-dependent adults with ADHD were randomized to methylphenidate (MTP) or placebo. After 12 weeks, those on MTP had better ADHD symptom relief, but no decline in cocaine craving or use.*

73. Somoza, E. C., T. M. Winhusen, T. P. Bridge, et al. 2004. An open-label pilot study of methylphenidate in the treatment of cocaine dependent patients with adult attention deficit/hyperactivity disorder. *J. Addict. Dis.* 23:77–92.

74. Riggs, P. D., S. K. Hall, S. K. Mikulich-Gilbertson, et al. 2004. A randomized controlled trial of pemoline for attention-deficit/hyperactivity disorder in substance-abusing adolescents. *J. Am. Acad. Child Adolesc. Psychiatry* 43:420–429.

75. Gordon, S. M., F. Tulak, and J. Troncale. 2004. Prevalence and characteristics of adolescents patients with co-occurring ADHD and substance dependence. *J. Addict. Dis.* 23:31–40.

76. Wilens, T. E. 2004. Impact of ADHD and its treatment on substance abuse in adults. *J. Clin. Psychiatry* 65(Suppl. 3):38–45.

77. Riggs, P. D., S. L. Leon, S. K. Mikulich, and L. C. Pottle. 1998. An open trial of bupropion for ADHD in adolescents with substance use disorders and conduct disorder. *J. Am. Acad. Child Adolesc. Psychiatry* 37:1271–1278.

78. Levin, F. R., S. M. Evans, D. M. McDowell, et al. 2002. Bupropion treatment for cocaine abuse and adult attention-deficit/hyperactivity disorder. *J. Addict. Dis.* 21:1–16.

79. Upadhyaya, H. P., K. T. Brady, G. Sethuraman, et al. 2001. Venlafaxine treatment of patients with comorbid alcohol/cocaine abuse and attention-deficit/hyperactivity disorder: A pilot study. *J. Clin. Psychopharmacol.* 21:116–117.

80. Grilo, C. M., D. F. Becker, K. N. Levy, et al. 1995. Eating disorders with and without substance use disorders: A comparative study of inpatients. *Compr. Psychiatry* 36:312–317.

81. Braun, D. L., S. R. Sunday, and K. A. Halmi. 1994. Psychiatric comorbidity in patients with eating disorders. *Psychol. Med.* 24:859–867.

82. Stock, S. L., E. Goldberg, S. Corbett, and D. K. Katzman. 2002. Substance use in female adolescents with eating disorders. *J. Adolesc. Health* 31:176–182.

83. Walfish, S., D. E. Stenmark, D. Sarco, et al. 1992. Incidence of bulimia in substance-misusing women in residential treatment. *Int. J. Addict.* 27:425–433.

84. Peveler, R., and C. Fairburn. 1990. Eating disorders in women who abuse alcohol. *Br. J. Addict.* 85:1633–1638.

85. Schuckit, M. A., J. E. Tipp, R. M. Anthenelli, et al. 1996. Anorexia nervosa and bulimia nervosa in alcohol-dependent men and women and their relatives. *Am. J. Psychiatry* 153:74–82.

86. Pratt, B. M., and S. R. Woolfenden. 2002. Interventions for preventing eating disorders in children and adolescents. *The Cochrane Database of Systematic Reviews.* Issue 2. Art. No.: CD002891.

87. Elliot, D. L., L. Goldberg, E. L. Moe, et al. 2004. Preventing substance use and disordered eating. Initial outcomes of the ATHENA program. *Arch. Pediatr. Adolesc. Med.* 158:1043–1049.

17

Special Populations

*with codependence are similar to those for treating an individual
with addiction—gaining acceptance of the diagnosis of codependence, motivating the patient to get help, and referring to Al-Anon
or Nar-Anon.*
Annotated References   *286*

ADOLESCENTS

For many individuals with substance use disorders, their problems begin during adolescence (1). Furthermore, adolescent substance abuse itself is a serious public health problem. Adolescents tend to not perceive harm from drug use and often lack insight into the problems that result from use. A 2001 survey showed that 56% of U.S. adolescents perceived no potential harm from having five or more drinks at one time (2). Public health risk results from these adolescents then going out and driving. Adolescents are often perceived as rebellious, distrusting authority figures and "testing the waters." Factors often associated with adolescent substance abuse are listed in Table 17.1. In caring for adolescents, medical providers must sensitively develop rapport and trust, in order to effectively screen, diagnose, and treat substance use disorders.

Epidemiology

According to the *2003 National Survey on Drug Use and Health*, 11.2% of 12- to 17-year-olds reported current use of illicit drugs (3). Approximately 30.5% of youths reported using an illicit drug at least once during their lifetime and 21.8% reported using an illicit drug within the past year. Overall, marijuana was the most used drug; 40.2% of high school students reported having used marijuana in their lifetime and 7.9% reported current marijuana use. Adolescents' use of heroin was low, with most use by non-injection routes—smoking or sniffing. The results for individual drugs are shown in Table 17.2. For overall reporting of illicit drug use, prevalence of use increased with age. Compared to previous years, the use of most drugs by adolescents was similar or less, with the exception of an increase in the use of MDMA (Ecstasy) (4).

Table 17.1.   Factors associated with adolescent substance abuse

Parent with substance abuse

Mood disorder

Learning disorder/poor school performance

Low self-esteem

Early sexual activity

Dysfunctional family/parenting

Drug/alcohol-using peers

Easy availability of drugs/alcohol in community

Table 17.2. Percent of 12- to 17-year-olds reporting drug use, 2003

Drug	Lifetime	Past Year	Past Month
Any Illicit Drug	30.5%	21.8%	11.2%
Marijuana/hashish	19.6	15.0	7.9
Inhalants	10.7	4.5	1.3
Hallucinogens	5.0	3.1	1.0
Cocaine	2.6	1.8	0.6
Methamphetamine	1.3	0.7	0.3
Ecstasy	2.4	1.3	0.4
LSD	1.6	0.6	0.2
PCP	0.8	0.4	0.1
Heroin	0.3	0.1	0.1
Prescription drug (nonmedical use)	13.4	9.2	4.0

Source: Substance Abuse and Mental Health Services Administration. *Results from the 2003 National Survey on Drug Use and Health: National Findings* (Office of Applied Studies, NSDUH Series H-25, DHHS Publication No. SMA 04 3964) Rockville, MD.

An estimated 718,000 (8.6%) youth aged 12 or 13 used inhalants in their lifetime (5). Of these, 35% also used another illicit drug. Inhalant use was the most common form of drug abuse for this age group. From this report, initiating inhalant use prior to the age of 13 was associated with increased risk of involvement in violence, criminal activity, developing dependence on another drug, and dropping out from school.

A survey of U.S. college students found that the lifetime prevalence of nonmedical prescription opioid use was 12%, past-year prevalence was 7%, and past-month prevalence was 3% (6). Residents of off-campus housing and fraternities or sororities were almost two times more likely than students living in same-sex residence halls to use prescription opioids non-medically. A similar study of high school seniors found that the rates of illicit use of Vicodin and OxyContin in the past year were 9.6% and 4.0%, respectively (7).

Screening and Diagnosis

The American Medical Association's *Guidelines for Adolescent Preventive Services* (GAPS) recommends yearly tobacco, alcohol, and drug screening for all adolescent patients (8). The American Academy of Pediatrics Committee on Substance Abuse recommends that all pediatricians "be able to evaluate the nature and extent of tobacco, alcohol, and other drug use among their patients . . . offer appropriate counseling about the risks of substance abuse and make an assessment as to whether additional counseling and referral may be needed." (9). However, only 45%

of pediatricians routinely ask their adolescent patients about alcohol or other drug use (10).

The medical interview of adolescents related to substance abuse should be done in private, without the presence of parents. Tools for assessing substance abuse in adolescents are limited, as it is often difficult to distinguish limited experimentation from problem use. The alcohol screening tools (CAGE, AUDIT, and MAST) used in adults are described in Chapter 5, and the TWEAK, developed for screening pregnant women for alcohol use, is discussed later in this chapter. Studies vary as to the effectiveness of these screening tools in adolescents, and they are specifically validated for alcohol. The CRAFFT test (Figure 17.1) is a reliable, easy-to-administer screening tool for substance abuse (not just alcohol) in adolescents (11–13). The CRAFFT can enable providers to identify adolescents with problem use that would not have otherwise been identified (14).

The diagnosis of substance abuse disorders in adolescents is generally the same as in adults. Obviously, for adolescents, any use of alcohol may be judged problematic, since alcohol use by adolescents is illegal. Unlike adults whose drug use may impact job performance, adolescent use may impact school performance. For adolescents, experimental use of drugs that changes into social use may in some instances result in an adverse consequence that motivates abstinence without the need for treatment. Most adolescent drug use fits into the DSM-IV diagnosis of abuse, with dependence much less common. It is very unusual for an adolescent to develop alcohol dependence such that abstinence results in significant alcohol withdrawal (15). Signs and symptoms related to substance abuse in adolescents may include weight loss, sleep disorder, memory/focusing problems, hoarse voice, unexplained injuries, nasal erythema (from sniffing), teary red eyes (from inhalants), and needle marks.

C—Have you ever ridden in a CAR driven by someone (including yourself) who was "high" or had been using alcohol or drugs?

R—Do you ever use alcohol or drugs to RELAX, feel better about yourself, or fit in?

A—Do you ever use alcohol/drugs while you are by yourself, ALONE?

F—Do your family or FRIENDS ever tell you that you should cut down on your drinking or drug use?

F—Do you ever FORGET things you did while using alcohol or drugs?

T—Have you gotten into TROUBLE while you were using alcohol or drugs?

* Two or more "yes" answers suggests a significant problem.

Figure 17.1.   The CRAFFT questions: A brief screening test for adolescent substance abuse.*

Effects of Substance Abuse

The common complications of substance abuse in adolescents are poor school performance, poor peer relations, family problems, and involvement with the juvenile justice system. According to the Federal Bureau of Investigation's report "Crime in the United States," there were 137,658 juveniles (under the age of 18) arrested by state and local law enforcement agencies for drug abuse violations during 2003, representing 11.7% of the drug arrests in which the offender's age was reported (16). In a 2002 report, 59.7% of male juvenile detainees and 45.9% of female juvenile detainees tested positive for drug use (17). Binge drinking among adolescents is associated with road accidents, homicides, and violence and increases the risk of contracting a sexually transmitted disease as well as becoming pregnant (18). Binge drinking commonly results in blackouts and amnesia for events. Deaths from binge drinking occur in adolescents who drink large amounts of high-proof alcohol quickly, resulting in respiratory depression.

In 2002, 97,029 adolescents in the United States sought emergency department treatment related to drug use, with marijuana mentioned 18,845 times, cocaine 9497 times, methamphetamine 1230 times, and heroin 813 times (19). Psychiatric illness, including behavioral disorders, learning disabilities, depression, and anxiety, generally precede the onset of substance abuse disorders (20–22). Suicide, a leading cause of mortality in adolescents, has been shown in several studies to be more common in adolescents with substance abuse than in nonusers (23, 24). Most medical complications of substance abuse seen in adults are less common in adolescents. For example, liver abnormalities related to alcohol are rarely seen in adolescents (25). Medical complications of specific drugs of abuse are discussed elsewhere in this book.

Treatment

Most adolescents do not require acute treatment of drug withdrawal. Treatment after cessation of use generally consists of supportive care. Treatment should start with office-based motivational interviewing as outlined in Chapter 3. There is little data on the effectiveness of brief intervention for adolescents, although it seems plausible that it could work for some adolescents (26). There is insufficient data to evaluate the effectiveness of self-help groups for the treatment of substance abuse in adolescents. Currently, most adolescents identified with substance abuse problems are referred for treatment and part of the treatment consists of group therapy that follows much of the philosophy of Alcoholics Anonymous and Narcotics Anonymous.

Adolescents' right to consent to treatment for substance abuse varies by state, and the age at which consent is allowed also varies (27). During 2002, there were 159,397 admissions to treatment facilities in the United States involving individuals ages 17 and younger. In 2002, approximately 68.7% of all admissions to treatment reported first use of drugs at age 18 or younger. Among the individuals ages 15 and younger admitted to treatment during 2002, 55.4% were being treated for primary abuse of marijuana. Most treatments for adolescent substance abuse disorders have been limited to psychosocial intervention, often involving individual and family therapy. Relapse rates are high, with one study of 157 adolescents (who completed inpatient treatment followed by outpatient treatment) showing a relapse rate of 79% at 12 months (28). Some studies report reduction in drug use rather than abstinence as the outcome measure (29). It is unclear how to interpret this as an outcome and how useful this measure is clinically.

For adolescents with legal problems, drug treatment often involves a juvenile drug court (30). The juvenile drug court is a recently introduced program model developed in response to a need to intervene more effectively in the substance abuse–delinquency cycle. Reports of positive experiences with adult drug courts helped trigger interest in adapting the drug court model for juveniles. Currently, little is known about the impact of juvenile drug courts.

There are few studies of pharmacotherapy in the treatment of addiction in adolescents. None of the medications used for alcohol use disorders in adults (disulfiram, acamprosate, and naltrexone) have been validated for treatment in adolescents. There is no recent data regarding maintenance therapy for the treatment of opiate dependence in adolescents. A 1979 study of heroin-dependent adolescents showed methadone maintenance to be more effective than other drug-free modalities (31). However, currently most methadone maintenance treatment programs exclude adolescents. There are no reports on the use of buprenorphine in adolescents.

PRISONERS

Drug users frequently commit crimes to obtain money for the drugs they use or are arrested in the midst of buying or selling illicit drugs. Drug laws in many states impose lengthy mandatory sentences on those who are arrested related to crack cocaine possession. Individuals with alcoholism are often arrested for vagrancy and disorderly conduct. Historically, many government officials have felt the way to deal with the drug problem is to criminalize all aspects of addiction. In contrast, more recently, many states have turned to mandatory court-ordered drug treatment as a better option. Nevertheless, a large proportion of individuals incarcerated in the United States are there because of a drug-related offense. In the federal prison system, 53.8% of inmates were incarcerated for drug-related offenses (32). Many of these individuals suffer from the medical complications outlined in Chapter 15.

Studies of newly incarcerated individuals show high rates of recent drug use at the time of incarceration. The 2003 Arrestee Drug Abuse Monitoring program reported that among male arrestees 73.9 % tested positive for illicit drugs or alcohol, with 30.1% for cocaine, 44.1% for marijuana, 4.7% for methamphetamine, and 5.8% for opiates (33). Statistics for female arrestees were similar, as 73.6% tested positive for illicit drugs or alcohol, with 35.3% for cocaine, 31.6% for marijuana, 8.8% for methamphetamine, and 6.6% for opiates.

The majority of inmates at the time of incarceration perceive a need for drug treatment, especially those who abuse opiates and cocaine (34). Despite the obvious need for prison-based drug treatment, surveys have found availability severely limited (35). According to Department of Justice statistics, less than 15% of inmates receive drug treatment while in prison (36), with only 40% of all correctional facilities nationwide (federal, state, and local) providing any type of treatment (37). Inmates dependent on opiates are forced to undergo withdrawal without medications, and those who had been receiving methadone maintenance cannot continue treatment while incarcerated at most facilities. Clearly, the prison system must do more to provide drug treatment to inmates and facilitate ongoing treatment at release in order to prevent the revolving door of incarceration that many inmates with addiction experience.

OLDER ADULTS

The full extent of substance abuse disorders in older adults is unknown. Most substance abuse problems in the elderly are related to alcohol. However, 25% of community-dwelling older adults use prescribed medications for insomnia, chronic pain, anxiety, and mood disorders (38). There are few studies on the use of illicit drugs by older adults.

Alcohol

Women drink less than men at all ages, and in population studies, the percentage of men and women who drink drops at age 60 (39–41). In a multicity study, prevalence of alcohol abuse in older adults ranged from 1.5% to 3.7% (42). In a study of 2105 residents of San Diego County over the age of 65, heavy drinking as defined by 12 or more cans of beer per week or 8 or more glasses of wine per week was present in 8.2% of residents ages 65–75 and 6.4% of residents over 75 (43). It is possible that this is due to a cohort effect; however, another study showed a decline in drinking of 2.7% per year by cross-sectional and longitudinal analyses, suggesting a true age-related decline rather than a cohort effect (44). Another study of drinking habits among 3448 persons over the age of 65 found that 16% of male drinkers consumed more than two drinks per day and 15% of women drinkers consumed more than one drink per day (45).

Alcoholism has been found in 21% of elderly medical inpatients and 14% of elderly patients being seen in an emergency room (46, 47). The prevalence of an alcohol disorder among elderly hospitalized individuals ranges from 8% to 23% (39, 48, 49). In a National Hospital Discharge Survey, an alcohol-related diagnosis was more common in individuals over the age of 65 than in those ages 25–44 (50).

In older adults, the diagnosis of alcoholism may be more difficult, as they are less likely to experience job loss or legal problems and more likely to be unemployed and isolated. A change in functional status related to drinking may help define a problem related to alcohol use. Self-report of alcohol use in the elderly may be unreliable, with recall amounts less than diary-recorded amounts (51).

The performance of the CAGE in elderly populations has been assessed in several studies. In a study of 323 general medical outpatients over the age of 60, a CAGE score ≥ 1 had a sensitivity of 86% and a specificity of 78% (52). Another study of 154 medical outpatients over the age of 64 found that a CAGE score ≥ 1 had a sensitivity and specificity of 88% (53). A study of 103 frail homebound elderly found that the CAGE had a sensitivity of 60% and a specificity of 100% (54). The CAGE may not effectively discriminate elderly patients currently drinking from those with a history of a drinking problem. Further questioning should distinguish current pattern of use from past use. The CAGE may also perform poorly in detecting elderly binge drinkers (55).

To aid further in the diagnosis of alcoholism in the elderly, a geriatric version of the MAST has been developed (Figure 17.2) (56). Greater than five "yes" answers indicates an alcohol problem with a sensitivity of 91–93% and a specificity of 65–84% when using DSM criteria as the gold standard (57, 58).

Elderly individuals with alcoholism tend to fall into two groups: "early-onset" and "late-onset"; two-thirds fall into the early-onset group (59–62). Those in the early-onset group have had ongoing alcoholism but have often avoided some of the usual morbidities. The late-onset individual may have had a recent stressful life event: loss of spouse, retirement, or a new impairment in activities of daily life. There are no significant differences in age, marital status, employment, or education between individuals in the early- and late-onset alcoholism groups (61, 62). Women represent a greater proportion of the late-onset group than of the early-onset group, but this may be related to the overall higher life expectancy of females (60). The early-onset group is more likely to drink to intoxication; more likely to have been in alcohol treatment in the past; more likely to have legal, financial, or job problems; and less likely to have social support (60, 61). The late-onset group is more likely to enter treatment as a result of a crisis, have symptoms of depression or loneliness, and be in denial.

In older adults, alcohol tends to cause dysphoria, rather than euphoria. Tolerance may decrease with aging due to changes in absorption and change in distribution of alcohol in the body (63, 64). Age-related decrease in gastric alcohol dehydrogenase increases the amount of alcohol that enters the bloodstream (65). This effect may be increased by the use of H2 blockers and proton pump inhibitors commonly prescribed in the elderly. There is no evidence that liver metabolism of alcohol is significantly changed with aging (66).

The complications of alcohol use in the elderly are mostly the same as those discussed in Chapter 5. However, because the elderly are more likely to be taking prescribed medications, there is increased risk of interactions between alcohol and these medications. There are additional aspects of medical complications specific to older adults that deserve mention. Alcohol-related liver disease as defined by fatty liver on liver biopsy is present in 90–100% of elderly individuals with alcoholism (67). The probability of cirrhosis increases with the duration of drinking. In the

	Yes	No
1. After drinking, have you ever noticed an increase in your heart rate or beating in your chest?	___	___
2. When talking with others, do you ever underestimate how much you actually drink?	___	___
3. Does alcohol make you sleepy so that you often fall asleep in your chair?	___	___
4. After a few drinks, have you sometimes not eaten or been able to skip a meal because you didn't feel hungry?	___	___
5. Does having a few drinks help decrease your shakiness or tremors?	___	
6. Does alcohol sometimes make it hard for you to remember parts of the day or night?	___	___
7. Do you have rules for yourself that you won't drink before a certain time of the day?	___	___
8. Have you lost interest in hobbies or activities you used to enjoy?	___	___
9. When you wake up in the morning, do you ever have trouble remembering part of the night before?	___	___
10. Does having a drink help you sleep?	___	___
11. Do you hide your alcohol bottles from family members?	___	___
12. After a social gathering, have you ever felt embarrassed because you drank too much?	___	___
13. Have you ever been concerned that drinking might be harmful to your health?	___	___
14. Do you like to end an evening with a nightcap?	___	___
15. Did you find your drinking increased after someone close to you died?	___	___
16. In general, would you prefer to have a few drinks at home rather than go out to social events?	___	
17. Are you drinking more now than in the past?	___	___
18. Do you usually take a drink to relax or calm your nerves?	___	___
19. Do you drink to take your mind off your problems?	___	___
20. Have you ever increased your drinking after experiencing a loss in your life?	___	___
21. Do you sometimes drive when you have had too much to drink?	___	___
22. Has a doctor or nurse ever said they were worried or concerned about your drinking?	___	___
23. Have you ever made rules to manage your drinking?	___	___
24. When you feel lonely, does having a drink help?	___	___

Scoring: 5 or more "yes" responses indicative of alcohol problem.

Figure 17.2. Michigan Alcoholism Screening Test—Geriatric Version (MAST-G) by the Regents of the University of Michigan, 1991. Source: Blow, F. C., K. J. Brower, J. E. Schulenberg, et al. 1992. The Michigan Alcoholism Screening Test—Geriatric version (MAST-G): A new elderly specific screening instrument. *Alcoholism: Clin. Exp. Res.* **16:372.**

first year after diagnosis of cirrhosis, the mortality rate is 50% in individuals over age 60, compared to 7% in those under age 60 (68). The prevalence of alcohol-related liver disease tends to increase with age, and 25% of cases are in individuals over the age of 60 (68). Psychiatric complications of alcoholism in the elderly are similar to those seen in younger individuals. However, suicide has been identified as a particularly significant complication of alcoholism in the elderly (69).

In the elderly, the onset of withdrawal may not occur until several days after cessation. Confusion rather than tremor is often the predominant clinical sign, and the severity and duration of withdrawal tend to increase with age (70). Delirium tremens should be part of the differential in any confused elderly patient, and the diagnosis may depend on interviewing family members.

Elderly alcoholics without a history of severe withdrawal and without comorbid medical conditions can be managed with supportive care at home. The elderly alcoholic with a history of severe withdrawal is best monitored in the inpatient setting. Additionally, the elderly are at increased risk of adverse effects from the pharmacological treatment of withdrawal, warranting close monitoring. Benzodiazepines, prescribed for treatment of withdrawal, may cause gait disturbance, cognitive impairment, and incontinence.

Only 15% of alcoholics over the age of 60 are receiving adequate treatment (71). Few treatment studies have included older patients. Evidence suggests that alcohol treatment outcome success is optimized when older patients receive age-specific treatment (72–74). Treatment plans for elderly alcoholics should focus on overcoming isolation and on establishing social supports (75).

Senior center involvement is often a way for the elderly alcoholic to find new interests, socialize, and spend time. Treatment outcomes in elderly alcoholics are comparable to those found in younger alcoholics (72), with individuals with late-onset alcoholism having a greater likelihood of maintaining abstinence (76). The pharmacological agents available for use in the treatment of alcoholism (disulfiram, acamprosate, and naltrexone) have not been studied adequately in the elderly. Drug interactions and comorbid medical conditions often limit the use of disulfiram in the elderly.

Illicit Drug Abuse

There are few studies examining the prevalence of illicit drug abuse in the elderly. Older adults are less likely to hustle and survive on the street in order to obtain illicit drugs. It is felt that most elderly heroin abusers were younger addicts that have survived. Less than 1% of individuals on methadone maintenance are over the age of 60 (77). It is unclear if this is related to treatment bias, as elderly heroin addicts are less likely to be arrested or prosecuted for crimes that force them into treatment. Additionally, the need for treatment may diminish, as in some individuals addiction wanes with age.

Sedatives

Depression in the elderly often presents with features of anxiety and may be inappropriately treated with sedatives rather than an antidepressant (78). Studies have shown that benzodi-azepine use increases with age and the elderly tend to be on higher doses (79). Use is greater among elderly women compared with elderly men (80). Morbidity related to benzodiazepine use in older adults is discussed in Chapter 6.

Prescription Opioids

The elderly frequently suffer from chronic pain related to de-generative disorders, including arthritis. Non-pharmacological measures often fail, and the use of nonsteroidal anti-inflamma-tory drugs may be contraindicated by other medical disorders. In most circumstances, opiates can be safely prescribed for chronic pain with good pain relief and improvement in functional status. Most patients are prescribed a stable dose of opiate for pain relief without the need for dose escalation related to tolerance. Adverse consequences most often occur when a drug is used for the wrong purpose, excessive dosages are used, or mental illness is present.

Treatment

Detoxification of elderly individuals from prescribed sedatives and opiate drugs follows the same principles as those used for younger individuals. Inpatient treatment is generally reserved for individuals with high potential for morbidity with withdrawal, lack of social support, major medical illness, or failure at attempted out-patient tapering or detoxification. The long-term treatment of eld-erly who have misused or abused prescription drugs should be individualized. An elderly person who has abused prescription nar-cotics is unlikely to benefit from attendance at an NA meeting dominated by young people who have abused heroin. Group ther-apy specific for the elderly should be sought. Primary care provider involvement is essential, both for counseling and for coordination of a treatment plan. Non-pharmacological treatment of chronic pain or insomnia plays an essential role in long-term success.

HEALTH PROFESSIONALS

The prevalence among health professionals of alcoholism is sim-ilar to that for the general population (81). Among physicians, use of illicit drugs is far less common than among the general popula tion (82). However, physician self-prescribing and self-medication with controlled substances occurs and must be viewed as problem-atic. Nurses have access to parenteral narcotics intended for pa-tients. In a survey of 5426 physicians, emergency medicine physicians used more illicit drugs, anesthesiologists used more opi-ates, and psychiatrists used more benzodiazepines, while pediatri-cians and surgeons had overall low rates of self-reported drug use (83). Other studies have also examined the problematic use of opi-ates by anesthesiologists, often by diversion in the hospital (84, 85).

Despite an overall low prevalence of addiction, many health care providers lose their ability to work because of chemical de-pendence and many more practice despite being impaired. Professional organizations have implemented programs to address impairment in the health professions. Intervention with appro-priate treatment as soon as an addiction problem is recognized is imperative. In caring for a health professional with addiction, the interviewing approach outlined in Chapter 3 should be utilized. It is especially important to show concern and address the often dominant issues of shame and low self-esteem.

The manifestations of impairment from substance abuse among health professionals are the same as those seen in other individuals. When one is concerned about impairment in a colleague, it is advisable to contact one or more close associates of that colleague to confirm the impairment. When caring for physicians with substance abuse, the treating physician should openly discuss the issue of "physician-patients" writing prescriptions for themselves—both in terms of abuse and attempts at self-medicating symptoms.

Persuasion of an impaired professional to accept the existence of a problem and agree to rehabilitation can be attempted by a concerned colleague. Such efforts are often initially met with anger and denial. Most physicians participating in state monitoring programs are not self-referred (86), and in fact, physicians in treatment have had a problem for a mean of 6 years prior to entering treatment (87). The involvement of a state's physician or nurse rehabilitation committee is generally required. A directory of these programs is available through the Web site www.fsphp.org. State boards will directly confront the impaired health provider using a formal intervention. The goal of this process is to provide help, usually mandating intensive inpatient treatment, with the requirement to complete treatment in order to maintain a professional license. There are few clinical trials on the optimal type or length of addiction treatment for health professionals. One study of 120 Oklahoma physicians found that 3 to 4 months of residential treatment was superior to 4 to 6 weeks of treatment (88). However, the more effective lengthy inpatient treatment is unlikely to be an option in most circumstances. After rehabilitation, individuals may seek self-help group meetings specifically aimed at professionals; they are available in most communities. In survey studies, health professionals' acceptance of self-help groups tends to be high (88, 89), and indeed one of the founders of AA was a physician.

As in other individuals, relapse to drug use is not uncommon in health care professionals. Use of opiates with coexisting psychiatric illness and a family history of substance abuse are identified risk factors for relapse in health care professionals (91). Overall success rates for physicians are quite high (92–94), with one study of 100 physicians in Georgia showing 77 abstinent at 5 years (95). This is probably due to the tremendous consequences associated with continued use (i.e., loss of livelihood) and the intensive treatment that health care professionals have access to (unlike most other addicts).

WOMEN

According to the *2003 National Survey of Drug Use and Health,* 54.1 million women (41.9% of all women) over the age of 12 reported using an illicit drug ever in their lives, 12.4% reported use in the past year, and 6.5% reported use in the past month (3). For past-year use, 8.2% had used marijuana, 1.6% cocaine, 1.2% hallucinogens, and 0.1% heroin. Arrestee records for 2003 show that 18.3% of those arrested in the United States for drug abuse–related crimes were women (33). For 2002, there were 553,874 emergency room visits related to drug use in women, the greatest number related to alcohol, followed by cocaine (96). In 2001, there were 7439 women in the United States reported with drug-induced deaths (97). In 2002, 565,354 women were admitted to drug treatment facilities in the United States, representing 30.1% of admissions (98). Sedatives were the only drug category for which more women than men were admitted into treatment.

In 2003, 43.2% of females (compared to 57.3% of males) aged 12 or older in the United States were current drinkers (3). Among females aged 18 or older, 46.0% reported current alcohol use. Women tend to drink more subtly and covertly. In part, this is related to society's considering drinking in public, especially in a tavern or bar, less acceptable in women than in men. Women most often drink at home, and women who are unmarried, divorced, or unemployed drink more (99). Alcoholic women are also more likely to have alcoholic spouses (100). The CAGE questionnaire (see Chapter 5), although originally validated on a group of men, has been validated for women (101, 102). An additional tool similar to the CAGE, the TWEAK (see Figure 17.3), was developed

---

Prior to administering TWEAK, drinkers are identified by a positive response to the question "Do you or have you ever consumed beer, wine, wine coolers, or drinks containing liquor (i.e., whiskey, rum, or vodka)?"

Points

(1–2) **Tolerance**—How many drinks can you hold? *OR* How many drinks do you need to feel high?

(1–2) **Worried**—Have close friends or relatives worried or complained about your drinking in the past year?

(1)   **Eye-openers**—Do you sometimes take a drink in the morning when you first get up?

(1)   **Amnesia** (blackouts)—Has a friend or family member ever told you about things you said or did while you were drinking that you could not remember?

(1)   **K** (C) Cut Down—Do you sometimes feel the need to cut down on your drinking?

- To score the test, a 7-point scale is used.
- The Tolerance–hold question scores 2 points if the respondent is able to hold six or more drinks.
- The Tolerance–high question scores 2 points if three or more drinks are needed to feel high.

A total score of 2 or more indicates that patients are likely to be risk drinkers. A score of 3 or greater identifies harmful drinking or alcoholism.

Figure 17.3. The TWEAK questionnaire.

and validated for assessing alcohol misuse in pregnant women and may outperform the CAGE in women (103).

Women are more likely to develop alcohol dependence after a lesser duration of drinking, and suicide, trauma, and liver disease are more common in female than male alcoholics (104, 105). Alcoholism decreases a woman's average life expectancy by 15 years (105, 106). Complications of alcoholism in women are discussed in Chapter 5.

Women who initiate heroin use are more likely than men are to have been influenced by a partner who uses heroin (107, 108). Unlike men, who are more likely to use by injection, women tend to snort heroin (109). One study suggests that women who use heroin develop dependence more quickly than men do (110). There appears to be no gender differences in complications or mortality related to heroin addiction.

Compared to men, women use cocaine at an earlier age, develop a problem earlier, are more frequently living with an addicted partner, are of lower socioeconomic status, and are more likely to have comorbid depression (111). Women are more likely than men are to use by smoking and injection, rather than intranasally (112). Women may also trade sex for crack cocaine, putting themselves at high risk for sexually transmitted diseases.

There is little data on gender differences related to marijuana use. Cigarette smoking, however, appears to be particularly problematic for women, with a common belief that smoking can control weight and that cessation will contribute to unacceptable weight gain (113, 114). Women are also more likely than men are to identify smoking as a way to reduce stress (115). Adolescent females who smoke are more likely than nonsmokers are to also use amphetamines to control weight (116).

Treatment

There are some particular obstacles to addiction treatment for women. Historically, because of stigma, women have been more likely to be "hidden" users of drugs and alcohol. Once in treatment, women are more likely to need provision of child care, and alcoholic women tend to have less spousal support than alcoholic men do. Women have been found to respond well to brief intervention for alcoholism, especially if they are pregnant (117). Over the last 20 years many treatment programs have been developed specifically for women (118). However, even among these programs, most do not provide child care. Women attending self-help groups should seek other women to be their sponsors.

Pregnancy

Estimates of substance abuse during pregnancy range from 0.4% to 27% depending on inclusion of nicotine and population studied (119–121). In a national survey of pregnant women aged 15 to 17 years, the prevalence of substance abuse was 15.1%, which is slightly greater than the rate of 14.1 % for nonpregnant women of the same age (3). In a 2003 survey, 4.1% of pregnant women reported binge drinking and 4.3% reported using illicit drugs in the previous month (3). In the same survey, 18.0% of pregnant women aged 15 to 44 smoked cigarettes in the past month, compared to 30.7% of matched nonpregnant women. The most recent survey of women who gave birth in the United States found that 5.5% tested positive for use of illicit drugs (122).

Many reported ill effects of drugs of abuse on fetal development are based on animal studies (in which massive doses of drugs are administered) or case reports. For most substances of abuse, the major risk to the fetus appears to be possible growth retardation. A summary of reported effects of drugs of abuse on the fetus is found in Table 17.3. Of the drugs of abuse, alcohol is the most harmful to the fetus. Fetal alcohol syndrome (FAS), the most preventable cause of mental retardation (123), was first described as a well-defined syndrome in 1973 (124). FAS is defined by (1) maternal drinking during pregnancy, (2) characteristic pattern of facial anomalies (short palpebral fissures and abnormalities of the premaxillary area—flat upper lip, flattened philtrum, flat midface), (3) growth retardation and neurodevelopmental abnormalities, and (4) structural brain abnormalities. The amount of alcohol intake needed to cause FAS is unknown

Table 17.3. Reported abnormalities on the fetus/neonate by substances of abuse

Substance	Impact
Alcohol	Spontaneous abortion; microcephaly; intrauterine growth restriction; central nervous system dysfunction including mental retardation and behavioral abnormalities; craniofacial abnormalities
Sedatives: benzodiazepines	Mild reduction in head circumference at birth; hypotonia and decreased suckling at birth, mild impairment in gross motor development
Opioids	No anomalies; intrauterine growth restriction; depressed breathing movements; preterm rupture of the membranes; preterm labor; meconium-stained amniotic fluid
Marijuana	No anomalies; mild behavioral alterations
Stimulants: methamphetamines, cocaine, methylphenidate	Urinary tract defects; intrauterine growth restriction; hyperactivity in utero; placental abruption; neonatal necrotizing enterocolitis
Hallucinogens	No anomalies; increased spontaneous abortions; dysmorphic face; behavioral problems
Inhalants	Similar to alcohol; increases risk of childhood leukemia
Nicotine	No anomalies; spontaneous abortion; mild intrauterine growth restriction; preterm birth; placenta previa; placental abruption

and all pregnant women should be advised to be abstinent from alcohol.

Cocaine use during pregnancy has been associated with increased risk of placenta previa, placental abruption, and premature labor (125, 126). Much political clamor on the detrimental long-term developmental effects of prenatal cocaine exposure has made some states attempt to criminalize cocaine use during pregnancy. However, the concurrent abuse of other drugs, including alcohol and opiates, has confounded most studies of cocaine risk during pregnancy. Studies differ as to whether infants born to cocaine-using women have lower birth weight (127–129). Environmental factors appear to play a role in reports of neurobehavioral effects of prenatal exposure to cocaine (130, 131). A systematic review of the literature, which included 36 papers, failed to find evidence that prenatal cocaine exposure was associated with developmental toxic effects in children (132).

For opiates, the infant may be born opiate-dependent and require treatment for withdrawal at birth (133, 134). Signs of opiate withdrawal in a neonate include tremor, high-pitched cry, increased muscle tone, hyperactivity, poor feeding, diarrhea, and sweating. Prenatal marijuana exposure has been reported to cause placental abruption (135), low birth weight (136), increased risk of prematurity (137), and neurologic disturbances (138).

Treatment of addiction in pregnant women is mostly similar to that for other individuals. Some programs include specific considerations such as education related to pregnancy and parenting. Clinical trials of pharmacotherapy for addiction, including treatment of withdrawal, have generally excluded pregnant women. As a result, recommendations for treatment of addiction in pregnant women have been based on expert opinion, with avoidance of medications that clearly can put the fetus at risk for developing abnormalities. Additional consideration must be given after delivery, as most medications do pass into breast milk.

For treatment of alcohol withdrawal in pregnant women, the benzodiazepines should be prescribed (preferably diazepam) as described in Chapter 5. Both prospective and retrospective clinical trials have not found an association between diazepam use and birth defects (139, 140). Studies that have reported risk for benzodiazepines have been small and included women using other substances, including alcohol. The anticonvulsant drugs carbamazepine and valproic acid, sometimes prescribed for treatment of alcohol withdrawal, should not be used in pregnant women because of teratogenic risk (141, 142).

For prevention of relapse to drinking, disulfiram should be avoided in pregnant women. Drinking after taking disulfiram could lead to high levels of acetaldehyde that may be dangerous to the mother and fetus. Additionally, fetal abnormalities have been reported with first-trimester exposure to disulfiram (143, 144). There is no data to support the use or safety of naltrexone or acamprosate in treating alcohol dependence in pregnant women.

Opiate withdrawal in pregnant women has mostly been treated with methadone, followed by either a taper or maintenance. The advantage of maintenance is the obvious continued engagement of pregnant women in addiction treatment. There are no reports of birth defects associated with methadone; however, there are reports of lower birth weight and smaller head circumference (145). Babies born to women receiving methadone will be opiate-dependent and require treatment for withdrawal. There is no evidence that these babies will have long-term cognitive abnormalities (146). Clonidine, discussed in Chapter 7, is often used as an adjunct in the treatment of opiate withdrawal and is safe during pregnancy (147).

Buprenorphine, discussed in Chapter 7, has been used successfully in several clinical trials to treat opiate dependence in pregnant women (148, 149). Babies born to women receiving buprenorphine maintenance have less opiate withdrawal; some do not require treatment (150). Reports on the use of naltrexone for opiate dependence in pregnant women are limited to a study of seven women who received oral naltrexone (151) and a study of eight women who received subcutaneous pellet implants of naltrexone (152). Both study groups had no adverse outcomes.

All pregnant women should be encouraged to quit smoking. Nicotine replacement therapies in pregnant women result in serum nicotine levels similar to those obtained from cigarettes (153). Tapered use of nicotine replacement is preferable to maintenance, as nicotine may reduce uterine blood flow (154). The safety of the use of bupropion for smoking cessation during pregnancy is unclear, with the manufacturer's registry showing increased risk of congenital anomalies (155).

Intimate Partner Abuse

Intimate partner abuse (also referred to as domestic violence or victimization) can be defined as the debilitating experience of physical, psychological, or sexual abuse, often associated with increased isolation from the outside world and limited personal freedom and accessibility to resources. This occurs in all demographic and socioeconomic strata (156). It is especially prevalent in women whose partners abuse alcohol or other drugs and in women who themselves abuse substances (157, 158). It is estimated that 75% of wives of alcoholics have been threatened and 45% have been assaulted by their alcoholic partners (159). A study of 842 female college students found a direct relationship between amount of weekly drinking and the risk of sexual victimization (160). Similarly, female high school students who drink alcohol are more likely to be victims of date violence (161). In a survey of women in a residential drug treatment center, 73% of women had been raped at least once during their lifetime (162), and in a similar study of women in a methadone treatment program, 60% reported physical or sexual abuse by an intimate partner (163).

Nearly 5.3 million intimate partner victimizations occur each year among U.S. women ages 18 and older, and this violence results in nearly 2 million injuries and nearly 1300 deaths (164). Most of these women never seek help from health care providers for the consequences of domestic violence. Brief screening for domestic violence should be incorporated into the medical interview of all women. Because some women may not initially recognize themselves as victims of domestic violence, questioning should be specific (Figure 17.4). The issue should be dealt with sensitively,

Integrating domestic violence inquiry into interview as part of social history:

"Because abuse and violence have unfortunately become a common part of a woman's life, I ask all my patients about it routinely."

> We all occasionally fight at home. What happens when you and your partner disagree?
>
> Have you ever been treated badly or threatened by your partner?
>
> Has your partner ever prevented you from leaving the house, seeing friends, getting a job, or continuing your education?
>
> Does your partner ever force you to have sex or force you to engage in sex that is uncomfortable to you?

(if appropriate) You mentioned your partner drinks (uses drugs). How does he (or she) act when he (or she) is drinking (using drugs)?

Figure 17.4.   Screening patients for domestic violence.

validating the difficulty most women have in discussing the issue. There may be reluctance to disclose information because of shame, humiliation, low self-esteem, or fear of retaliation by the perpetrator. Some women may also believe that they deserve the abuse and do not deserve help or that they need to protect their partner, who is often their only source of affection and support. There may also be a belief on the part of the victim that the medical provider will not understand the problem or believe her.

In addition to screening, certain patient problems should alert the practitioner to the possibility of domestic violence (Table 17.4). Women with a history of intimate partner abuse report 60% higher rates of all health problems than do women with no history of abuse (165). Problems may range from direct evidence of physical trauma (contusions, abrasions, broken bones) to nonspecific complaints of fatigue and difficulty concentrating. The screening information and medical history related to domestic violence must be well documented in the medical record, because they provide evidence that may be used in a legal case. The record should include detailed descriptions of any injuries and, if possible, photographs of injuries sustained.

Once evidence of abuse is obtained, one must validate the seriousness of the situation to the patient. This must occur even if the patient is not yet ready to leave the abusive spouse. In addition, the immediate safety of the woman should be assessed. Unfortunately, the level of severity of past violence may not be a predictor of the severity of future violence. If safety is in question, the woman (and her children) should be advised to stay with family or friends or at a shelter that specializes in caring for abused women and their families. Medical attention may also be needed for abused children in the household. When women resist taking action, the provider should continue to show concern and work to motivate the patient toward taking action. The National

Table 17.4.   Clinical signs and symptoms suggestive of domestic violence

Alcohol or drug abuse
Anxiety
Atypical chest pain
Change in appetite
Chronic headaches
Chronic pain of unclear etiology
Depressed mood
Difficulty concentrating
Dizziness
Fatigue
Frequent minor trauma
Frequent requests for pain medications or tranquilizers
Frequent vague somatic complaints
Gastrointestinal upset, diarrhea, or dyspepsia
Insomnia
Palpitations
Panic attacks
Paresthesias
Pelvic pain
Suicide attempts or gestures

Domestic Violence Hotline (1-800-799-7233) is a 24-hour service that helps women with crisis intervention. Unfortunately, women with recent substance abuse are sometimes denied shelter by organizations that assist victims of intimate partner violence. As an alternative, women's recovery houses that are sensitive and able to meet the needs of women in crisis should be sought. For women with addiction and victimization, recovery from addiction is closely tied to recovery from victimization (166).

FAMILIES AND CODEPENDENCE

Codependence is maladaptive or dysfunctional behavior that is associated with living with, working with, treating, or being close to a person with addiction (167). Codependence affects families, friends, professionals, and communities. Signs and symptoms of codependence include behaviors aimed at protecting the individual with addiction (enabling), psychological symptoms (anxiety, depression, insomnia, aggressiveness, eating disorder, or suicidal gestures), psychosomatic illness, family violence, and drug addiction (168). Health professionals may fail to diagnose addiction and incorrectly treat symptoms with sedatives, antidepressants, or narcotics. Society often chooses not to confront relatives, friends, and colleagues who are obviously impaired by addiction.

When a patient has unexplained somatic or psychological symptoms, it is helpful to ask whether the patient is concerned about the drinking or drug use of "someone" close to him or her. For an affirmative response, the patient should be asked to describe the problem. One can also ask the patient with possible codependence to answer CAGE questions or the questions on the MAST as though they were addressed to, and answered honestly by, the "someone." A positive score on one of these is a strong indication of codependence.

Initially, the psychological and behavioral expressions of the individual with codependence are normal responses to an abnormal situation. However, these adaptive responses eventually become dysfunctional. Codependence is chronic and progressive, characterized by denial, ill health, and/or maladaptive behavior and by a lack of knowledge about addiction.

The major strategies in treating a patient with codependence are similar to those for treating an individual with addiction—gaining acceptance of the diagnosis of codependence, motivating the patient to get help, and referring the patient to Al-Anon or Nar-Anon; as with AA or NA referrals, a good understanding of the Al-Anon or Nar-Anon process (see Table 17.5) on the part of the referring physician is critical to successful referral. Additionally,

Table 17.5. The Al-Anon process

Al-Anon began in the 1940s as an Alcoholics Anonymous (AA) auxiliary and was initially called AA Family Groups. In 1952, the wives of the founders of AA established Al-Anon.

Al-Anon is a fellowship of family members of alcoholics who meet together to share their experiences, strengths, and hopes so that they can achieve health and serenity. The organization is modeled after AA and uses the 12 Steps of AA as its principles. Its focus is not on the alcoholic but on the family members, freeing families from their "dependence" on the alcoholic. In some areas, Al-Anon members have begun groups for adult children of alcoholics. These groups offer help to adults who may no longer live with an alcoholic family member but whose lives continue to be adversely affected by the legacy of growing up in an alcoholic home.

Al-Anon meetings are all open to the public and often meet at the same time and location as AA meetings. The Web site www. al-anon.org has a directory of meetings.

Al-Anon meetings generally last 1 hour and follow the format of AA meetings, but they are usually smaller.

Al-Anon is also the sponsor of Ala-Teen and Ala-Tots, which are organizations for teenage and young children of alcoholics, respectively. These groups follow the Al-Anon discussion format and in general are not open to the non-alcoholic public, but helping professionals are usually welcome if they request to attend ahead of time.

Al-Anon publishes a number of pamphlets that are available at meetings for families. *Al-Anon Faces Alcoholism,* Al-Anon's "Big Book," describes the family's plight with alcoholism through a variety of stories that graphically describe how families become sick in response to the alcoholic. More information can be obtained from www.al-anon.org.

the provider may refer the patient or the family for additional therapy, especially group therapy. If appropriate, assistance in getting the individual with addiction into treatment can be provided.

Codependence includes actions of health care providers that enable individuals with addiction to remain enmeshed in their disease. Enabling behavior often coexists with otherwise excellent clinical skills (169). The Professional Enablers Screening Test (Figure 17.5) is useful for identifying the ways in which

	Yes	No
1. Do you sometimes avoid raising sensitive issues related to drinking because it might offend your patient or make him or her angry or feel bad?	(2)	
2. Do you generally treat the heavy-drinking person's problems without focusing most of the treatment on the drinking behavior?	(5)	
3. Do you avoid confronting your heavy-drinking patient when there is good evidence that he or she has misinformed you about his or her drinking?	(2)	
4. Do you generally suggest to your alcoholic patients that they cut down on their drinking?	(3)	
5. Do you believe what your heavy-drinking patient tells you about his or her drinking without using other sources such as a spouse, employer, screening test, blood alcohol test, or other laboratory test?	(5)	
6. Do you generally prescribe a sedative or minor tranquilizer for the nervous conditions or sleep problems of your alcoholic patients?	(5)	
7. Do you refer most of your alcoholic patients to attend Alcoholics Anonymous meetings regularly?		(5)
8. Do you refer many of your alcoholic patients to an alcoholism therapy group?		(5)
9. Do you prescribe disulfiram (Antabuse) to many of your alcoholic patients?		(3)
10. When your alcoholic patient has a minor crisis requiring hospitalization, do you routinely hospitalize him or her in a community hospital general ward?	(5)	
11. Do you refer most of the spouses of family members of your alcoholic patients to attend Al-Anon meetings regularly?		(5)
12. Do you subscribe to the theory that most alcoholics have an underlying psychological disorder that is the major cause of the alcoholism?	(5)	
13. Do you believe that most alcoholics will not respond positively to treatment for their alcoholism?	(5)	

Note: Numbers in parentheses are the scores recommended for the corresponding responses. A score of 0 to 3 points indicates a probable non-enabler, 4 to 6 points may indicate a possible enabler, and 7 points or more indicates a probable enabler.

Figure 17.5.   Professional Enablers Screening Test.

enabling may occur in the context of medical care. Societal norms, one's own beliefs related to the use of alcohol or other drugs, and a lack of awareness of approaches to diagnosis, motivation, and treatment of the alcoholic are the major reasons for codependence in health care providers. To overcome enabling behavior, health care providers should update their knowledge of addiction, attend some AA, NA, and Al-Anon meetings, and try using the interviewing skills described in Chapter 3. Increased comfort in treating codependence occurs as the provider helps increasing numbers of patients and their families through the recovery process.

REFERENCES

1. Kessler, R. C., P. Berglund, O. Demler, et al. 2005. Lifetime prevalence and age-of-onset distributions of DSM-IV disorders in the National Comorbidity Survey Replication. *Arch. Gen. Psychiatry* 62:59–602.

2. *The Monitoring the Future National Results on Adolescent Drug Use: Overview of Key Findings 2001.* Department of Health and Human Services, Bethesda, MD. Available at http://www.drugabuse.gov

3. Substance Abuse and Mental Health Services Administration. 2004. *Results from the 2003 National Survey on Drug Use and Health: National Findings* (Office of Applied Studies, NSDUH Series H-25, DHHS Publication No. SMA 04-3964). Rockville, MD.

4. Banken, A. 2004. Drug abuse trends among youth in the United States. *Ann. N.Y. Acad. Sci.* 1025:465–471.

5. Substance Abuse and Mental Health Services Administration. *The NSDUH Report—Inhalant use and delinquent behaviors among young adolescents.* Available at http://www.oas.samhsa.org

6. McCabe, S. E., C. J. Teter, C. J. Boyd, et al. 2005. Non-medical use of prescription opioids among U.S. college students: Prevalence and correlates from a national survey. *Addict. Behav.* 30:789–805.

7. McCabe, S. E., C. J. Boyd, and C. J. Teter. 2005. Illicit use of opioid analgesics by high school seniors. *J. Subst. Abuse Treat.* 28:225–230.

8. Elster, A., and N. Kuznets. 1994. *AMA Guidelines for Adolescent Preventive Services (GAPS).* Baltimore, MD: Williams & Wilkins.

9. American Academy of Pediatrics. 1998. Tobacco, alcohol, and other drugs: The role of the pediatrician in prevention and management of substance abuse. *Pediatrics* 101:125–128.

10. American Academy of Pediatrics. 1997. *Periodic Survey of Fellows #31: Practices and attitudes toward adolescent drug screening.* Elk Grove Village, IL: American Academy of Pediatrics, Division of Child Health Research.

11. Knight, J. R., L. A. Shrier, T. D. Bravender, et al. 1999. A new brief screen for adolescent substance abuse. *Arch. Pediatr. Adolesc. Med.* 153:591–596.

12. Knight, J. R., L. Sherritt, L. A. Shrier, et al. 2002. Validity of the CRAFFT substance abuse screening test among general adolescent clinic patients. *Arch. Pediatr. Adolesc. Med.* 156:607–614. *This study of 538 patients ages 14–18 (68.4% were female and*

75.8% were from racial / ethnic minorities) had diagnostic classifications for substance use during the past 12 months as no use (49.6%), occasional use (23.6%), problem use (10.6%), abuse (9.5%), and dependence (6.7%). A CRAFFT score of 2 or higher was optimal for identifying any problem (sensitivity, 76%; specificity, 94%; positive predictive value, 83%; and negative predictive value, 91%) and dependence (sensitivity, 92%; specificity, 80%; positive predictive value, 25%; and negative predictive value 99%). Validity was not significantly affected by age, sex, or race.

13. Levy, S., L. Sherritt, S. K. Harris, et al. 2004. Test-retest reliability of adolescents' self-report of substance use. *Alcohol Clin. Exp. Res.* 28:1236–1241.

14. Wilson, C. R., L. Sherritt, E. Gates, and J. R. Knight. 2004. Are clinical impressions of adolescent substance use accurate? *Pediatrics* 114:536–540. *Secondary analysis of data from a validation study of the CRAFFT substance abuse screening test in 14- to 18-year-old medical clinic patients (n = 533) and their corresponding medical care providers (n = 109). Of 100 patients with problem substance use, providers correctly identified 18; of 50 patients with a diagnosis of alcohol or drug abuse, providers identified 10; and of 36 patients with a diagnosis of alcohol or drug dependence, providers identified none.*

15. Cornelius, J. R., S. A. Maisto, N. K. Pollock, et al. 1995. Withdrawal and dependency symptoms among adolescent alcohol and drug abusers. *Addiction* 90:627–635.

16. Federal Bureau of Investigation. 2004, October. *Crime in the United States, 2003.*

17. National Institute of Justice. 2002. *Preliminary data on drug use & related matters among adult arrestees & juvenile detainees.* Available at http://www.whitehousedrugpolicy.gov

18. Grunbaum, J. A., L. Kann, S. A. Kinchen, et al. 2002. Youth risk behavior surveillance—United States, 2001. *MMWR* 51:1–62.

19. Substance Abuse and Mental Health Services Administration. *Emergency Department Trends from the Drug Abuse Warning Network, Final Estimates 1995–2002.* Available at http://www.dawninfo.samhsa.gov

20. Biederman, J., T. Wilens, E. Mick, et al. 1997. Is ADHD a risk factor for psychoactive substance use disorders? Findings from a four-year prospective follow-up study. *J. Am. Acad. Child Adolesc. Psych.* 36:21–29.

21. Deykin, E. Y., J. C. Levy, and V. Wells. 1987. Adolescent depression, alcohol and drug abuse. *Am. J. Pub. Health* 77:178–182.

22. Molina, B. S., and W. E. Pelham. 2003. Childhood predictors of adolescent substance use in a longitudinal study of children with ADHD. *J. Abnormal Psych.* 112:497–507.

23. Esposito-Smythers, C., and A. Spirito. 2004. Adolescent substance use and suicidal behavior: A review with implications for treatment research. *Alcohol Clin. Exp. Res.* 28:77S–88S.

24. Shaffer, D., M. S. Gould, P. Fisher, et al. 1996. Psychiatric diagnosis in child and adolescent suicide. *Arch. Gen. Psych.* 53:339–348.

25. Clark, D. B., K. G. Lynch, J. D. Donovan, et al. 2001. Health problems in adolescents with alcohol use disorders: Self-report, liver injury and physical examination findings. *Alcohol Clin. Exper. Res.* 25:1350–1359.

26. Levy, S., B. L. Vaughan, and J. R. Knight. 2002. Office-based intervention for adolescent substance abuse. *Pediatr. Clin. North Am.* 49:329–343.

27. Weddle, M., and P. Kokotailo. 2002. Adolescent substance abuse. Confidentiality and consent. *Pediatr. Clin. North Am.* 49:301–315.

28. Brown, S. A., S. F. Tapert, S. R. Tate, and A. M. Abrantes. 2000. The role of alcohol in adolescent relapse and outcome. *J. Psychoactive Drugs* 32:107–115.

29. Liddle, H. A., G. A. Dakof, K. Parker, et al. 2001. Multidimensional family therapy for adolescent drug abuse: Results of a randomized clinical trial. *Am. J. Drug Alcohol Abuse* 27:651–688.

30. Belenko, S., and T. K. Logan. 2003. Delivering more effective treatment to adolescents: Improving the juvenile drug court model. *J. Subst. Abuse Treat.* 25:189–211.

31. Sells, S. B., and D. D. Simpson. 1980. The case for drug abuse treatment effectiveness, based on the DARP research program. *Br. J. Addict.* 75:117–131.

32. Federal Bureau of Prisons. 2005, March. *Federal Bureau of Prisons Quick Facts,* U.S. Department of Justice. Available at http://www.bop.gov

33. National Institute of Justice. 2003. *Drug and alcohol use and related matters among arrestees.* Available at http://www.ojp.usdoj.gov/nij

34. Lo, C. C., and R. C. Stephens. 2000. Drugs and prisoners: Treatment needs on entering prison. *Am. J. Drug Alcohol Abuse* 26:229–245.

35. Welsh, W. N., and G. Zajac. 2004. A census of prison-based drug treatment programs: Implications for programming, policy and evaluation. *Crime Delinquency* 50:108–133.

36. *Substance abuse and treatment-state and federal prisoners.* 2000. Bureau of Justice Statistics. Available at http://www.ojp.usdoj.gov/bjs

37. Substance Abuse and Mental Health Services Administration. 2000. *Substance abuse treatment in adult and juvenile correctional facilities.* Available at http://www.oas.samhsa.gov

38. Rossiter, L. F. 1983. Prescribed medicines: Findings from the national medical care expenditure survey. *Am. J. Public Health* 73:1312–1315.

39. Bristow, M. F., and A. W. Clare. 1992. Prevalence and characteristics of at-risk drinkers among elderly acute medical inpatients. *Br. J. Addict.* 87:291–294.

40. McKim, W. A., and L. T. Quinlan. 1991. Changes in alcohol consumption with age. *Can. J. Pub. Health* 82:231–234.

41. Molgaard, C. A., C. M. Nakamura, E. P. Stanford, et al. 1990. Prevalence of alcohol consumption among older persons. *J. Commun. Health* 15:239–251.

42. Eaton, W. W., M. Kromer, J. C. Anthony, et al. 1989. The incidence of specific DIS/DSM-III mental disorders: Data from the NIMH Epidemiologic Catchment Area program. *Acta Psychiatr. Scand.* 79:163–178.

43. Molgaard, C. A., C. M. Nakamura, E. P. Stanford, et al. 1990. Prevalence of alcohol consumption among older persons. *J.*

Commun. Health 15:239–251. *The Epidemiologic Catchment Area (ECA) study interviewed 805 men and 1305 women over the age of 65 in five different geographic areas—Baltimore, New Haven, Durham, St. Louis, and Los Angeles. Prevalence of alcohol abuse ranged from 1.5% in Durham to 3.7% in Baltimore. The prevalence among men was greater than it was among women and declined with age.*

44. Adams, W. L., P. J. Garry, R. Rhyre, et al. 1990. Alcohol intake in the healthy elderly: Changes with age in a cross-sectional and longitudinal study. *J. Am. Geriatr. Soc.* 38:211–216.

45. Moore, A. A., R. D. Hays, G. A. Greendale, et al. 1999. Drinking habits among older persons: Findings from the NHANES I Epidemiologic follow-up study (1982–84). *J. Am. Geriatr. Soc.* 47:412–416.

46. Adams, W. L., K. Mageder-Habib, S. Trued, and H. L. Bromme. 1992. Alcohol abuse in elderly emergency department patients. *J. Am. Geriatr. Soc.* 40:1236–1240.

47. Adams, W. L., Z. Yuan, J. J. Barboriak, and A. A. Rimm. 1993. Alcohol-related hospitalizations of elderly people: Prevalence and geographic variation in the United States. *JAMA* 270:1222–1225.

48. Curtis, J. R., L. Geller, E. J. Stokes, et al. 1989. Characteristics, diagnosis and treatment of alcoholism in elderly patients. *J. Am. Geriatr. Soc.* 97:310–316.

49. Mangion, D. M., J. S. Platt, and V. Syam. 1992. Alcohol and acute medical admission of elderly people. *Age Ageing* 21:362–367.

50. Stinson, F. S., M. C. Dufour, and D. Bertolucci. 1989. Alcohol-related morbidity in the aging population. *Alcohol Health Res.* 13:80–87.

51. Graham, K. 1986. Identifying and measuring alcohol abuse among the elderly: Serious problems with existing instrumentation. *J. Stud. Alcohol.* 47:322–326.

52. Buchsbaum, D. G., R. G. Buchanan, J. Welsh, et al. 1992. Screening for drinking disorders in the elderly using the CAGE questionnaire. *J. Am. Geriatr. Soc.* 40:662–665.

53. Jones, T. V., B. A. Lindsey, P. Yount, et al. 1993. Alcoholism screening questionnaires: Are they valid in elderly medical outpatients? *J. Gen. Intern. Med.* 8:674–678.

54. Bercsi, S. J., P. W. Brickner, and D. C. Saha. 1993. Alcohol use and abuse in the frail, homebound elderly: A clinical analysis of 103 persons. *Drug Alcohol Depend.* 33:139–149.

55. Adams, W. L., K. L. Barry, and M. F. Fleming. 1996. Screening for problem drinking in older primary care patients. *JAMA* 276:1964–1967. *Five thousand sixty-five consecutive patients older than 60 years were administered questions about the quantity and frequency of regular drinking in the last 3 months, the number of episodes of binge drinking (≥6 drinks/occasion), and the CAGE questionnaire. Fifteen percent of men and 12% of women drank in excess of recommended limits (>7 drinks/week for women and >14 drinks/week for men), while 9% of men and 3% of women screened positive on the CAGE (≥2 positive answers) for alcohol abuse within 3 months. The authors concluded that asking about the quantity and frequency of drinking in addition to the CAGE increases the number of problem drinkers detected.*

56. Blow, F. C., K. J. Brower, J. E. Schulenberg, et al. 1992. The Michigan Alcoholism Screening Test-Geriatric version (MAST-G): A new elderly-specific screening instrument. *Alcoholism: Clin. Exp. Res.* 16:372.

57. Joseph, C. L., L. Ganzin, and R. M. Atkinson. 1995. Screening for alcohol use disorders in the nursing home. *J. Am. Geriatr. Soc.* 43:368–373.

58. MacNeil, P. D., J. W. Campbell, and L. Vernon. 1994. Screening for alcoholism in the elderly. *J. Am. Geriatr. Soc.* 42:SA7.

59. Adams, S. L., and S. A. Waskel. 1991. Late onset of alcoholism among older midwestern men in treatment. *Psychol. Rep.* 68:432–434.

60. Atkinson, R. M., R. L. Tolson, and J. A. Turner. 1990. Late versus early onset drinking in older men. *Alcoholism: Clin. Exp. Res.* 14:574–579.

61. Brennan, P. L., and R. H. Moos. 1991. Functioning, life context and help-seeking among late-onset problem drinkers: Comparison with non-problem and early onset heavy drinkers on skidrow. *Br. J. Addict.* 86:1139–1150.

62. Hurt, R. D., R. E. Finlayson, R. M. Morse, and L. J. Davis. 1988. Alcoholism in elderly persons: Medical aspects and prognosis of 216 inpatients. *Mayo Clin. Proc.* 63:753–760.

63. Pozzato, G., M. Moretti, F. Franzin, et al. 1995. Ethanol metabolism and aging: The role of first pass metabolism and gastric alcohol dehydrogenase activity. *J. Gerontol.* 50:135–141.

64. Vestal, R. E., E. A. McGuire, J. D. Tobin, et al. 1977. Aging and ethanol metabolism. *Clin. Pharmacol. Ther.* 21:343–354.

65. Seitz, H. K., U. A. Simanowski, R. Waldherr, et al. 1993. Human gastric alcohol dehydrogenase activity: Effect of age, sex and alcoholism. *Gut* 34:1433–1437.

66. Scott, R. B. 1989. Alcohol effects on the elderly. *Compr. Ther.* 15:8–12.

67. Grant, B. F., M. C. Dufour, and T. C. Hartford. 1988. Epidemiology of alcoholic liver disease. *Sem. Liver Dis.* 812–825.

68. Potter, J. F., and O. F. James. 1987. Clinical features and prognosis of alcoholic liver disease in respect to advancing age. *Gerontology* 33:380–387.

69. Atkinson, J. H., and M. A. Schuckit. 1983. Geriatric alcohol and drug misuse and abuse. *Adv. Sub. Abuse* 3:195–237.

70. Brower, K. J., S. Mudd, F. C. Blow, et al. 1994. Severity and treatment of alcohol withdrawal in elderly versus younger patients. *Alcoholism: Clin. Exp. Res.* 18:196–201.

71. National Institute on Alcohol Abuse and Alcoholism. 2000. *Alcohol and health.* Tenth Special Report to the U.S. Congress from the Secretary of Health and Human Services.

72. Janik, S. W., and R. G. Dunham. 1983. A nationwide examination of the need for specific alcoholism treatment programs for the elderly. *J. Stud. Alcohol.* 44:307–317.

73. Amadeo, M. 1990. Treating the late life alcoholic. Guidelines for working through denial integrating individual, family and group approaches. *J. Geriatr. Psych.* 23:91–105.

74. Kofoed, L. L., R. L. Tolson, R. M. Atkinson, et al. 1987. Treatment compliance of older alcoholics: An elder-specific approach is superior to mainstreaming. *J. Stud. Alcohol.* 48:47–51.

75. Schonfeld, L., and L. W. Dupree. 1995. Treatment approaches for older problem drinkers. *Int. J. Addiction* 30:1819–1842.
76. Atkinson, R. M., R. L. Tolson, and J. A. Turner. 1993. Factors affecting outpatient treatment compliance of older male problem drinkers. *J. Stud. Alcohol.* 54:102–106.
77. Capel, W. L., and L. G. Peppers. 1978. The aging narcotic addict: A longitudinal study of known abusers. *Addictive Diseases* 3:389–403.
78. Ancill, R. J., G. D. Emburg, G. W. Mac Ewan, and J. S. Kennedy. 1988. The use and misuse of psychotropic prescribing for elderly psychiatric patients. *Can. J. Psychiatry* 33:585–589.
79. Finlayson, R. E., and L. J. Davis. 1994. Prescription drug dependence in the elderly population: Demographic and clinical features of 100 inpatients. *Mayo Clin. Proc.* 69:1137–1145.
80. Szwabo, P. A. 1993. Substance abuse in older women. *Clin. Geriatr. Med.* 9:197–208.
81. Moore, R. D., L. Mead, and T. A. Pearson. 1990. Youthful precursors of alcohol abuse in physicians. *Am. J. Med.* 88:332–336.
82. Hughes, P. H., N. Brandeburg, and C. L. Baldwin. 1992. Prevalence of substance use among U.S. physicians. *JAMA* 267:2333–2339. *National survey of 9600 physicians (response rate 59%) found they were less likely to have used illicit substances in the past year than their age and gender counterparts in the National Household Survey on Drug Abuse but were more likely to have used alcohol, minor opiates, and benzodiazepines. Prescription substances were used primarily for self-treatment, whereas illicit substances and alcohol were used primarily for recreation. Current daily use of illicit or controlled substances was rare.*
83. Hughes, P. H., C. L. Storr, N. A. Brandenburg, et al. 1999. Physician substance use by medical specialty. *Addict. Dis.* 18:23–37.
84. Paris, R. T., and D. I. Canavan. 1999. Physician substance abuse impairment: Anesthesiologists vs. other specialties. *J. Addict. Dis.* 18:1–7.
85. Booth, J. V., D. Grossman, J. Moore, et al. 2002. Substance abuse among physicians: A survey of academic anesthesiology programs. *Anesth. Analg.* 95:1024–1030.
86. Knight, J. R., L. T. Sanchez, L. Sherritt, et al. 2002. Monitoring physician drug problems: Attitudes of participants. *J. Addict. Dis.* 21:27–36. *Study of 87 physicians in a treatment program—identified sources of referral were self (32.2%), a friend/colleague (31%), the state medical board (14.9%), a hospital chief (11.5%), or a family member (3.4%).*
87. Brooke, D., G. Edwards, and C. Taylor. 1991. Addiction as an occupational hazard: 144 doctors with drug and alcohol problems. *Br. J. Addict.* 86:1011–1016. *A retrospective descriptive study of 144 doctors (mean age 43.1) who received treatment for drug and alcohol abuse; mean duration prior to entering treatment was 6.4 years for drug users and 6.7 years for alcohol users. Alcohol was the current problem for 41.6% and drugs for 26.4%; 31.3% were using both alcohol and drugs.*
88. Smith, P. C., and J. D. Smith. 1991. Treatment outcomes of impaired physicians in Oklahoma. *J. Okla. State Med. Assoc.* 84:599–603.
89. Carlson, H. B., S. L. Dilts, and S. Radcliff. 1994. Physicians with substance abuse problems and their recovery environment: A survey. *J. Subst. Abuse Treat.* 11:113–119.

90. Galanter, M., D. Talbott, K. Gallegos, and E. Rubenstone. 1990. Combined Alcoholics Anonymous and professional care for addicted physicians. *Am. J. Psychiatry* 147:64–68.

91. Domin, K. B., T. F. Hornbein, N. L. Polissar, et al. 2005. Risk factors for relapse in health care professionals with substance use disorders. *JAMA* 293:1453–1460. *Retrospective cohort study of 292 health care professionals; 74 (25%) of 292 had at least one relapse. The risk of relapse increased for family history of a substance use disorder (hazard ratio [HR]: 2.29); use of an opioid increased the risk of relapse significantly in the presence of a coexisting psychiatric disorder (HR: 5.79) but not in the absence of a coexisting psychiatric disorder (HR: 0.85). The presence of all three factors (opioid use, psychiatric illness, and family history) markedly increased the risk of relapse (HR: 13.25). The risk of subsequent relapses increased after the first relapse (HR: 1.69).*

92. Gualtieri, A. C., J. P. Consentino, and J. S. Becker. 1983. The California experience with a diversion program for impaired physicians. *JAMA* 249:226–229.

93. Shore, J. H. 1987. The Oregon experience with impaired physicians on probation. *JAMA* 257:2931–2934.

94. Reading, E. G. 1992. Nine years experience with chemically dependent physicians: The New Jersey experience. *Md. Med. J.* 41:325–329.

95. Gallegos, K. V., B. H. Lubin, C. Bowers, et al. 1992. Relapse and recovery: Five to ten year follow-up study of chemically dependent physicians—the Georgia experience. *Md. Med. J.* 41:315–319.

96. Substance Abuse and Mental Health Services Administration. *Emergency Department Trends from the Drug Abuse Warning Network, Final Estimates 1995–2002.*

97. Centers for Disease Control and Prevention. *Deaths: Final Data for 2001.* Available at http://www.cdc.gov

98. Substance Abuse and Mental Health Services Administration. *Treatment Episode Data (TEDS) Highlights—2002.* Available at http://www.samhsa.gov

99. Wilsnack, R., S. Wilsnack, and A. Klassen. 1984. Women's drinking and drinking problems: Patterns from a 1981 national survey. *Am. J. Public Health* 74:1231–1238.

100. Redgrave, G. W., K. L. Swartz, and A. J. Romanoski. 2003. Alcohol misuse by women. *Int. Rev. Psychiatry* 15:256–268.

101. Bradley, K. A., J. Boyd-Wickizer, S. H. Powell, and M. L. Burman. 1998. Alcohol screening questionnaires in women: A critical review. *JAMA* 280:166–171.

102. Cherpital, C. J. 1999. Screening for alcohol problems in the U.S. general population: A comparison of the CAGE and TWEAK by gender, ethnicity, and services utilization. *J. Stud. Alcohol.* 60:705–711.

103. Russell, M., S. S. Martier, R. J. Sokol, et al. 1994. Screening for pregnancy risk-drinking. *Alcohol Clin. Exp. Res.* 18:1156–1161.

104. Wilsnack, S. C., and R. W. Wilsnack. 1991. Epidemiology of women's drinking. *J. Subst. Abuse Treat.* 3:133–157.

105. Roman, P. M. 1988. Biological features of women's alcohol use: A review. *Public Health Rep.* 103:628–637.

106. Smith, E. M., C. R. Cloninger, and S. Bradford. 1983. Predictors of mortality in alcoholic women: A prospective follow-up study. *Alcohol Clin. Exp. Res.* 7:237–243.

107. Hser, Y., M. Anglin, and W. McGlothin. 1987. Sex differences in addict careers, I: Initiation of use. *Am. J. Drug Alcohol Abuse* 13:33–57.

108. Gossop, M., P. Griffiths, and J. Strang. 1994. Sex differences in patterns of drug taking behaviour. A study at a London community drug team. *Br. J. Psychiatry* 164:101–104.

109. Powis, B., P. Griffiths, M. Gossop, and M. Strang. 1996. The differences between male and female drug users: Community samples of heroin and cocaine users compared. *Subst. Use Misuse* 31:529–543.

110. Ellinwood, E., W. Smith, and G. Vaillant. 1966. Narcotic addictions in males and females: A comparison. *Int. J. Addict.* 1:33–45.

111. Griffin, M. L., R. D. Weiss, S. M. Mirin, and U. Lange. 1989. A comparison of male and female cocaine abusers. *Arch. Gen. Psychiatry* 46:122–126.

112. McCance-Katz, E., K. Carroll, and B. Rounsaville. 1999. Gender differences in treatment-seeking cocaine abusers—implications for treatment and prognosis *Am. J. Addict.* 8:300–311.

113. Charlton, A. 1984. Smoking and weight control in teenagers. *Public Health* 98:277–281.

114. Rigotti, N. 1989. Cigarette smoking and body weight. *N. Engl. J. Med.* 320:931–933.

115. Gritz, E., I. Nielsen, and L. Brooks. 1996. Smoking cessation and gender: The influence of physiological, psychological, and behavioral factors. *J. Am. Med. Women's Assoc.* 51:35–42.

116. Gritz, E., and L. Crane. 1991. Use of diet pills and amphetamines to lose weight among smoking and non-smoking high school seniors. *Health Psychol.* 10:330–335.

117. Manwell, L. B., M. F. Fleming, M. P. Mundt, et al. 2000. Treatment of problem alcohol use in women of childbearing age: Results of a brief intervention trial. *Alcohol Clin. Exper. Res.* 24:1517–1524. *Two hundred five female patients ages 18–40 were randomized to brief intervention (two 15-minute physician-delivered counseling visits) or control group and were followed for 48 months. The intervention significantly reduced both 7-day alcohol use (p = 0.0039) and binge-drinking episodes (p = 0.0021).*

118. Grella, C. E., and L. Greenwell. 2004. Substance abuse treatment for women: Changes in the settings where women received treatment and types of services provided, 1987–1998. *J. Behav. Health Serv. Res.* 31:367–383.

119. Bachi, K., M. Varner, and R. Chase. 1993. The prevalence of substance abuse among pregnant women in Utah. *Am. J. Obstet. Gynecol.* 81:239–242.

120. Chasnoff, I. J., H. Landress, and M. Barrett. 1990. The prevalence of illicit drug and alcohol use during pregnancy and discrepancies in mandatory reporting in Pinellas County, Florida. *N. Engl. J. Med.* 322:1202–1206.

121. Hollinshead, W. H., J. F. Brin, H. D. Scot, and M. E. Burke. 1990. Current statewide prevalence of illicit drug use by pregnant women: Rhode Island. *MMWR* 39:225–227.

122. National Pregnancy and Health Survey. 1996. *Drug use among women delivering live births* (Publication no. BKD192). Rockville, MD: National Clearinghouse for Alcohol and Drug Information.

123. Warren, K., and L. Foudin. 2001. Alcohol-related birth defects, the past, present and future. *Alcohol Res. Health* 25:153–158.

124. Jones, K., D. Smith, C. Ulleland, and P. Streissguth. 1973. Pattern of malformation in offspring of chronic alcoholic mothers. *Lancet* 301:1267–1271.

125. Macones, G., H. Sehdev, S. Parry, et al. 1997. The association between maternal cocaine use and placenta previa. *Am. J. Obstet. Gynecol.* 177:1097–1100.

126. Acker, D., B. P. Sachs, K. J. Tracey, and W. E. Wise. 1983. Abruptio placentae associated with cocaine use. *Am. J. Obstet. Gynecol.* 146:220–221.

127. Miller, J., M. Boudreaux, and F. Regan. 1995. A case-control study of cocaine use in pregnancy. *Am. J. Obstet. Gynecol.* 172:180–185.

128. Hulse, G., D. English, E. Milne, et al. 1997. Maternal cocaine use and low birth weight newborns: A meta-analysis. *Addiction* 92:1561–1570. *A meta-analysis of five studies presenting data for "any" prenatal cocaine exposure, adjusted for tobacco smoking but not for gestational age, produced a pooled relative risk estimate of 2.15. Other lifestyle factors not controlled for may account for the observed effects.*

129. Sprauve, M., M. Lindsay, S. Herbert, and W. Graves. 1997. Adverse perinatal outcome in parturients who use crack cocaine. *Obstet. Gynecol.* 89:674–678.

130. Chasnoff, I., A. Anson, R. Hatcher, et al. 1998. Prenatal exposure to cocaine and other drugs. Outcome at four to six years. *Ann. NY Acad. Sci.* 846:314–328. *Ninety-five children born to mothers who used cocaine and other drugs during pregnancy were compared with 75 matched, nonexposed children born to mothers who had no evidence of alcohol or illicit substance use during pregnancy. Prenatal exposure to cocaine and other drugs had no direct effect on the child's cognitive outcome (measured as IQ), but there was an effect mediated through the home environment.*

131. Koren, G., I. Nulman, J. Rovet, et al. 1998. Long-term neurodevelopmental risks in children exposed in utero to cocaine. The Toronto Adoption Study. *Ann. NY Acad. Sci.* 846:306–313.

132. Frank, D. A., M. Augustyn, W. G. Knight, et al. 2001. Growth, development, and behavior in early childhood following prenatal cocaine exposure: A systematic review. *JAMA* 285:1613–1625.

133. Werler, M. M., B. R. Pober, and L. B. Holmes. 1985. Smoking and pregnancy. *Teratology* 32:473–481.

134. Himmelberger, D., B. Brown, and E. Cohen. 1978. Cigarette smoking during pregnancy and the occurrence of spontaneous abortion and congenital abnormality. *Am. J. Epidemiol.* 108:470–479.

135. Williams, M. A., E. Lieberman, R. Mittendorf, et al. 1991. Risk factors for abruptio placentae. *Am. J. Epidemiol.* 134:965–972.

136. Zuckerman, B., D. A. Frank, R. Hingson, et al. 1989. Effects of maternal marijuana and cocaine use on fetal growth. *N. Engl. J. Med.* 320:762–768.

137. Gibson, G. T., P. A. Baghurst, and D. P. Colley. 1983. Maternal alcohol, tobacco and cannabis consumption and the outcome of pregnancy. *Aust. N. Z. J. Obstet. Gynaecol.* 23:15–19.

138. Fried, P. A. 1982. Marihuana use by pregnant women and effects on offspring: An update. *Neurobehav. Toxicol. Teratol.* 4:451–454.

139. Rosenberg, L., A. A. Mitchell, J. L. Parsells, et al. 1983. Lack of relation of oral clefts to diazepam use during pregnancy. *N. Engl. J. Med.* 309:1282–1285.

140. Ornoy, A., J. Arnon, S. Shechtman, et al. 1998. Is benzodiazepine use during pregnancy really teratogenic? *Reprod. Toxicol.* 12:511–515. *In 460 pregnancies in which women reported using benzodiazepines, the incidence of congenital anomalies (3.1%) was not significantly different from that in 424 control pregnancies (2.6%).*

141. Matalon, S., S. Schechtman, G. Goldzweig, and A. Ornoy. 2002. The teratogenic effect of carbamazepine: A meta-analysis of 1255 exposures. *Reprod. Toxicol.* 16:9–17.

142. Wide, K., B. Winbladh, T. Tomson, et al. 2000. Psychomotor development and minor anomalies in children exposed to antiepileptic drugs in utero: A prospective population-based study. *Dev. Med. Child Neurol.* 42:87–92.

143. Helmbrecht, G. D., and I. A. Hoskins. 1993. First trimester disulfiram exposure: Report of two cases. *Am. J. Perinatal.* 10:5–7.

144. Reitnauer, J., N. P. Callanan, R. A. Farber, and A. S. Aylsworth. 1997. Prenatal exposure to disulfiram implicated in the cause of malformations in discordant monozygotic twins. *Teratology* 56:358–362.

145. Blinick, G. E., E. Jerez, and R. C. Wallach. 1973. Methadone maintenance, pregnancy and progeny. *JAMA* 225:477–479.

146. Kaltenbach, K. A., and L. P. Finnegan. 1989. Prenatal narcotic exposure: Perinatal and developmental effects. *Neurotoxicology* 10:597–604.

147. Dashe, J. S., G. L. Jackson, D. A. Olscher, et al. 1998. Opioid detoxification in pregnancy. *Obstet. Gynecol.* 92:854–858.

148. Fischer, G., R. E. Johnson, H. Eder, et al. 2000. Treatment of opioid-dependent pregnant women with buprenorphine. *Addiction* 95:239–244. *Case series of 15 opioid-dependent pregnant women who received sublingual buprenorphine for opioid withdrawal. Buprenorphine was well tolerated during induction and 91% of women remained opioid negative. All maternal, fetal, and neonatal safety laboratory measures were within normal limits or not of clinical significance. Opioid withdrawal was absent, mild (without treatment), and moderate (with treatment) in eight, four, and three neonates, respectively. The mean duration of withdrawal was 1.1 days.*

149. Johnson, R. E., H. E. Jones, and G. Fischer. 2003. Use of buprenorphine in pregnancy: Patient management and effects on the neonate. *Drug Alcohol Depend.* 70:S87–S101.

150. Johnson, R. E., H. E. Jones, and G. Fischer. 2003. Use of buprenorphine in pregnancy: Patient management and effects on the neonate. *Drug Alcohol Depend.* 70(2 Suppl.):S87–S101. *Review of 15 cohorts of infants exposed to buprenorphine in utero. Of approximately 309 infants exposed, neonatal abstinence syndrome (NAS) occurred in 62% of the infants with 48% requiring treatment; 40% of these cases were confounded by illicit drug use.*

151. Hulse, G. K., G. O'Neill, C. Pereira, and C. Brewer. 2001. Obstetric and neonatal outcomes associated with maternal naltrexone exposure. *Aust. N. Z. J. Obstet. Gynaecol.* 41:424–428.

152. Hulse, G., and G. O'Neil. 2002. Using naltrexone implants in the management of the pregnant heroin user. *Aust. N. Z. J. Obstet. Gynaecol.* 42:569–573.

153. Ogburn, P., R. Hurt, J. Croghan, et al. 1999. Nicotine patch use in pregnancy: Nicotine and cotinine levels and fetal effects. *Am. J. Obstet. Gynecol.* 181:736–743.

154. Clark, K. E., and G. L. Irion. 1992. Fetal hemodynamic response to maternal intravenous nicotine administration. *Am. J. Obstet. Gynecol.* 167:1624–1631.

155. Glaxo Wellcome Bupropion Pregnancy Registry. 2003. September 1, 1997 to February 28, 2003, Glaxo Wellcome, p. 22. Research Triangle Park, NC.

156. Heise, L., and C. Garcia-Moreno. 2002. Violence by intimate partners. *World Report on Violence and Health.* Geneva: World Health Organization.

157. Weinsheimer, R. L., C. R. Schermer, L. H. Malcoe, et al. 2005. Severe intimate partner violence and alcohol use among female trauma patients. *J. Trauma* 58:22–29. *Survey of 95 consecutive adult female trauma patients; 46.3% reported a lifetime history of severe intimate partner violence (IPV), and 26% experienced severe IPV in the past year. Past-year IPV was identified more often in women screening positive for drinking problems (59.1% vs. 12.7%) and when the partner was a problem drinker (55.2% vs. 8.3%). On multivariate analysis, female problem drinking (OR = 5.8) and partner problem drinking (OR = 8.9) were independent predictors of past-year severe IPV.*

158. Miller, B. A., S. C. Wilsnack, and C. B. Cunradi. 2000. Family violence and victimization: Treatment issues for women with alcohol problems. *Alcohol Clin. Exp. Res.* 24:1287–1297.

159. Eisenstat, S. A., and L. Bancroft. 1999. Primary care: Domestic violence. *N. Engl. J. Med.* 341:886–892.

160. Gross, W., and R. Billingham. 1998. Alcohol consumption and sexual victimization among college women. *Psychol. Rep.* 82:80–82.

161. Malik, S., S. Sorenson, and C. Aneshensel. 1997. Community and dating violence among adolescents: Perpetration and victimization. *J. Adolesc. Health* 21:291–302.

162. Teets, J. M. 1997. The incidence and experience of rape among chemically dependent women. *J. Psychoactive Drugs* 29:331–336.

163. Gilbert, L., N. el-Bassel, R. F. Schilling, and E. Friedman. 1997. Childhood abuse as a risk for partner abuse among women in

methadone maintenance. *Am. J. Drug Alcohol Abuse* 23:581–595.

164. Centers for Disease Control and Prevention. *Intimate partner violence in the United States.* Available at http://www.cdc.gov/ncipc/pub-res/ipv

165. Campbell, J., A. S. Jones, J. Dienemann, et al. 2002. Intimate partner violence and physical health consequences. *Arch. Intern. Med.* 162:1157–1163.

166. Liebschutz, J. M., K. P. Mulvey, and J. H. Samet. 1997. Victimization among substance-abusing women. Worse health outcomes. *Arch. Intern. Med.* 157:1093–1097.

167. Young, E. 1987. Co-alcoholism as a disease: Implications for psychotherapy. *J. Psychoactive Drugs* 19:257–268.

168. Hurcom, C., A. Copello, and J. Orford. 2000. The family and alcohol: Effects of excessive drinking and conceptualizations of spouses over recent decades. *Subst. Use Misuse* 35:473–502.

169. Williams, E., L. Bissell, and E. Sullivan. 1991. The effects of codependence on physicians and nurses. *Br. J. Addict.* 86:37–42.

Appendix A. DSM-IV Criteria for Substance Dependence

Substance dependence is a syndrome characterized by a maladaptive pattern of substance use, leading to clinically significant impairment or distress, as manifested by three (or more) of the following, occurring at any time in the same 12-month period:

(1) Tolerance, as defined by either of the following:
   (a) a need for markedly increased amounts of the substance to achieve intoxication or desired effect, or
   (b) markedly diminished effect with continued use of the same amount of the substance.
(2) Withdrawal, as manifested by either of the following:
   (a) the characteristic withdrawal syndrome for the substance, or
   (b) the same (or a closely related) substance is taken to relieve or avoid withdrawal symptoms.
(3) The substance is often taken in larger amounts or over longer period than was intended.
(4) There is a persistent desire or unsuccessful efforts to cut down or control substance use.
(5) A great deal of time is spent in activities necessary to obtain the substance (e.g., visiting multiple doctors or driving long distances), use the substance (e.g., chain-smoking), or recover from its effects.
(6) Important social, occupational, or recreational activities are given up or reduced because of substance use.
(7) The substance use is continued despite knowledge of having a persistent or recurrent physical or psychological problem that is likely to have been caused or exacerbated by the substance (e.g., current cocaine use despite recognition of cocaine-induced depression, or continued drinking despite recognition that an ulcer was made worse by alcohol consumption).

Source: American Psychiatric Association. 2000. *Diagnostic and statistical manual of mental disorders.* 4th ed. (text revision). Used with permission.

B

Appendix B. DSM-IV Criteria for Substance Abuse

A. A maladaptive pattern of substance use leading to clinically significant impairment or distress, as manifested by one (or more) of the following, occurring within a 12-month period:

    (a) Recurrent substance use resulting in a failure to fulfill major role obligations at work, school, or home (e.g., repeated absences or poor work performance related to substance use; substance-related absences, suspensions, or expulsions from school; neglect of children or household)

    (b) Recurrent substance use in situations in which it is physically hazardous (e.g., driving an automobile or operating a machine when impaired by substance use)

    (c) Recurrent substance-related legal problems (e.g., arrests for substance-related disorderly conduct)

    (d) Continued substance use despite having persistent or recurrent social or interpersonal problem caused or exacerbated by the effects of the substance (e.g., arguments with spouse about consequences of intoxication, physical fights)

B. The symptoms have never met the criteria for substance dependence for this class of substance.

Source: American Psychiatric Association. 2000. *Diagnostic and statistical manual of mental disorders* 4th ed. (text revision). Used with permission.

Index